What the Experts Are Saying About *The Whole Pregnancy Handbook*:

"This is by far the most comprehensive book available on becoming pregnant and carrying through to a healthy childbirth. Dr. Evans has left no topic uncovered, and his breadth and depth of knowledge is matched only by his unique ability to integrate high-tech medicine and natural-health approaches. Whether you are easily pregnant or struggling with fertility issues, this book will guide you gently and wisely through the whole process."
Martin L. Rossman, MD, Department of Medicine, University of California, San Francisco, author of *Preparing for Childbirth* and *Guided Imagery for Self-Healing*

"*The Whole Pregnancy Handbook* is one of the best prenatal guides available. It presents pregnancy as a fulfilling, natural life process instead of a medical problem. This is integrative health care at its best."
Larry Dossey, MD, author of *Healing Beyond the Body*, *Reinventing Medicine*, and *Healing Words*

"Every OB/GYN and pregnant woman should use this book as their reference for all aspects of pregnancy. It is a comprehensive, well-researched, and easy-to-read book on everything one needs to know in order to have a healthy pregnancy. It is the ideal book for obstetricians to give to their pregnant patients as a reference guide . . . it is an amazing body of work!"
Judith Balk, MD, MPH, assistant professor, University of Pittsburgh, Magee-Womens Hospital

"A tour de force! Everything the pregnant woman needs to know to optimize her health and the health of her baby. I especially like the stories of real patient experiences. Dr. Evan's effective integration of conventional and natural medicine provides comprehensive, authoritative guidance."
Joe Pizzorno, MD, president emeritus, Bastyr University; coauthor of the *Encyclopedia of Natural Medicine*

"We have needed *The Whole Pregnancy Handbook* for several years. The information surrounding how to optimize the outcome of pregnancy for the baby and mother has been exponentially growing the past decade. The problem has been making this information easily accessible. Dr. Evans, who is both board certified in obstetrics and gynecology as well as an expert in integrative medicine, has captured the latest information on how to improve the outcome of pregnancy and delivers this message in a manner that is readily applicable. On behalf of the many doctors and their patients who will find value in this book, I applaud Dr. Evans' efforts."
Jeffrey Bland, PhD, chairman, Institute for Functional Medicine

"I learned so much while skimming and skimming again through *The Whole Pregnancy Handbook* that I'll recommend it to pregnant women and health professionals as well."
Michel Odent, MD, author of *Birth Reborn* and *The Caesarean*

"*The Whole Pregnancy Handbook* is a wonderful gift for women. Dr. Evans has created a gold mine of information—practical and comprehensive."
Leo Galland, MD, author of *Superimmunity for Kids*

The
Whole Pregnancy
HANDBOOK

An Obstetrician's Guide
to Integrating Conventional
and Alternative Medicine
Before, During,
and After Pregnancy

JOEL M. EVANS, MD, Ob/Gyn,

with ROBIN ARONSON

GOTHAM BOOKS

This book is dedicated to my sons, Jarad and Spencer,
who continually help me to understand,
on a deeply personal level, the true miracle of birth.
My love and connection to them cannot be described.
I thank you both for constantly reminding me
that our future is in good hands.

—J. E.

GOTHAM BOOKS
Published by Penguin Group (USA) Inc.
375 Hudson Street, New York, New York 10014, U.S.A.

Penguin Group (Canada), 10 Alcorn Avenue, Toronto, Ontario, Canada M4V 3B2 (a division of Pearson Penguin Canada Inc.); Penguin Books Ltd, 80 Strand, London WC2R 0RL, England; Penguin Ireland, 25 St Stephen's Green, Dublin 2, Ireland (a division of Penguin Books Ltd); Penguin Group (Australia), 250 Camberwell Road, Camberwell, Victoria 3124, Australia (a division of Pearson Australia Group Pty Ltd); Penguin Books India Pvt Ltd, 11 Community Centre, Panchsheel Park, New Delhi - 110 017, India; Penguin Group (NZ), Cnr Airborne and Rosedale Roads, Albany, Auckland, New Zealand (a division of Pearson New Zealand Ltd); Penguin Books (South Africa) (Pty) Ltd, 24 Sturdee Avenue, Rosebank, Johannesburg 2196, South Africa

Penguin Books Ltd, Registered Offices: 80 Strand, London WC2R 0RL, England

Published by Gotham Books, a division of Penguin Group (USA) Inc.

First printing, March 2005
10 9 8 7

Human karyotype photo (page 289) copyright © SIU BioMed/Custom Medical Stock Photo

Copyright © 2005 by Joel M. Evans, MD, and Robin Aronson
All rights reserved

Gotham Books and the skyscraper logo are trademarks of Penguin Group (USA) Inc.

Library of Congress Cataloging-in-Publication Data

Evans, Joel M.
   The whole pregnancy handbook : an obstetrician's guide to integrating conventional and alternative medicine before, during, and after pregnancy / Joel M. Evans and Robin Aronson.
      p. cm.
   ISBN 1-592-40111-2 (alk. paper)
   1. Pregnancy—Popular works. 2. Childbirth—Popular works. 3. Holistic medicine. I. Aronson, Robin. II. Title.
   RG525.E823 2005
   618.2—dc22

2005041268

Printed in the United States of America
Set in Garamond 3, New Caledonia, and Univers
Designed by Victoria Hartman

Contents

Foreword

Whenever I have a question about pregnancy or childbirth, fertility or women's health, Dr. Joel Evans is the first one I call. Now I have a book—this book—I can refer to and one that I can recommend to patients, friends, and colleagues.

I've worked closely with Joel for almost ten years. I liked him the first time I met him, when he came as a young obstetrician/gynecologist to the Center for Mind-Body Medicine's (CMBM) weeklong training in MindBodySpirit medicine. He is very bright, inquisitive, open-minded, and openhearted.

In the years since then, I've come to know him well as a member of the CMBM faculty in the U.S. and abroad, and as a close colleague and friend. I've come to deeply respect his professional judgment, to appreciate his mastery of the science of medicine, and to enjoy his warmth and kindness. It is these qualities—professional expertise, calm, thoughtful judgment, and generous heart—that make Joel Evans such a wonderful guide to the experience of pregnancy and childbirth, and that make *The Whole Pregnancy Handbook* so valuable.

One of the abiding problems of childbirth in the United States is the sense so many mothers have that birth is a medical enterprise that is both incomprehensible and frightening. *The Whole Pregnancy Handbook* provides another, far more encouraging perspective. Joel Evans demystifies the biochemistry and physiology of menstruation, ovulation, and fertilization. He carefully explains the changes in the three trimesters of pregnancy, and the stages of labor and delivery. His message is clear, useful, and hopeful: This is your body. Understand and enjoy it. A safe, healthy, and happy birth is *your* birthright.

He answers the questions that pregnant women, and women hoping to become pregnant, most often ask. He encourages you to engage in an ongoing dialogue with your obstetricians and midwives. He offers new ways to think about fertility and to promote it, and tells you what you need to know about genetic testing. He explains the variety of symptoms you may encounter during pregnancy, and offers ways to ease them—and to understand what they do, and don't, signify.

Joel Evans's expertise, however, extends far beyond a thorough understanding of the conventional approaches to obstetrics and women's health. He has devoted a major portion of his time to the study and integration of a variety of complementary approaches to health and healing. A majority of women may be using these approaches, and almost everyone wants to know more about them. What you need is a guide who can help you differentiate what is safe from what is suspect and give you the tools to participate in the process. Dr. Evans does this in *The Whole Pregnancy Handbook*.

Dr. Evans's greatest expertise in integrative approaches is probably in the use of food, vitamins, minerals, and herbs in promoting fertility and facilitating a healthy pregnancy. He presents detailed, scientifically based, easy to understand and follow nutrition recommendations. He is also skilled in integrating mind-body approaches (including relaxation, meditation, and biofeedback) into the care and lives of pregnant women and their partners. He recommends and guides women in the use of Chinese medicine, massage, exercise, homeopathy, and such hands-on "energy" healing methods as therapeutic touch and Reiki, and provides powerful group support for women who are, or want to become, pregnant.

"Here is what I've seen and experienced," Joel Evans says on every page of this book, "and what the research literature shows us. Take a look for yourself. Share this information with your partner and your obstetrician or midwife. Make your own judgments."

Perhaps most importantly, this book is informed by Joel Evans's kindness and compassion for his patients and for the children they will bring into the world. On every page, you will feel the presence of a scientist who celebrates the wondrous biology of conception, pregnancy, and childbirth; of a physician who is as caring as he is knowledgeable; and of a man who genuinely respects and loves the women and their partners to whom he's offering guidance.

James S. Gordon, MD
Founder and Director of the Center for Mind-Body Medicine;
Former Chair, the White House Commission on
Complementary and Alternative Medicine Policy

Introduction

Pregnancy is a magical and mysterious time of life. As it progresses and you move toward parenthood, you're aware of all the profound ways life is about to change—it will be filled with joy and responsibility, challenges and love. It can all be exhilarating and overwhelming. The purpose of this book is to help you make the best choices for yourself and your child from before you conceive all the way to the first weeks after birth. It's my hope that *The Whole Pregnancy Handbook* will help you experience your pregnancy as a fulfilling and transforming first phase in your life as a parent.

Embracing a Holistic Philosophy

Over the years, it's been my privilege to participate in the physical and emotional journey of pregnancy both as a doctor and a father. In that time, my approach to my entire medical practice has changed. I started out as a classically trained, conventional ob-gyn, but through a series of lessons taught to me by patients, I gradually began to practice integrative medicine, embracing a holistic philosophy that focuses on self-care and the principle that true wellness reflects the coming together of emotional, spiritual, *and* physical well-being.

My orientation shifted to a holistic approach about five years into my medical practice. Over the course of a couple of months, two colleagues, nurses whom I had worked closely with, came to me after being diagnosed with cancer. Both were told by their oncologists that there was "nothing" they could do but show up for their chemotherapy treatments. They were told to relax and let the chemotherapy fight their cancer, but they didn't feel comfortable with that. Both wanted to be more proactive in their care. So, after each asked me questions that I couldn't answer about what she could do to help heal her cancer, we began a journey together, discovering how mind-body medicine combined with alternative modalities like acupuncture and herbal medicine could improve not only their responses to treatment, but also the quality of their day-to-day lives.

The lessons I learned with these women about the importance of self-motivation and participation resonated with what I'd learned practicing prenatal care. As a young obstetrician just out of residency, I quickly realized that my approach was too dogmatic. I'd often say to a pregnant woman, "This is the way it is—just do what I say." In that situation, the woman might do what I asked, but she didn't believe in my recommendation. This problem hit home after a birth where a woman had experienced complications in labor and required a C-section. Afterward, she developed a wound infection, a not-unusual postoperative event that meant she had to come into the office two or three times a week. As she was leaving one of these visits, she said under her breath, "This never would have happened if I hadn't had the C-section." I was surprised that she felt that way because she was basically okay and her baby was healthy. So I asked her to stay to talk about the Cesarean. I learned that she didn't trust my decision to perform the Cesarean because she hadn't felt she'd been a part of it. I realized that this lack of trust and her sense that she was an observer instead of a participant in her birth experience couldn't have begun in the labor room. Instead, I believe it reflected the fact that over the course of the nine months of her pregnancy, we hadn't developed a real partnership.

That single, under-the-breath comment was the "aha" that helped me to see that I needed to change, to become a source of support, information, and comfort to pregnant women, someone they could turn to for guidance, but not someone who would impose proscriptive or dogmatic opinions. I changed my entire approach to prenatal care. I learned how to be open and listen to my patients in a new way, to follow their lead as we work together with the shared goals of a healthful, vital pregnancy, a childbirth anticipated with excitement instead of fear and anxiety, and a newborn brought into the world in a room filled with love, all the while realizing the mystery and sacredness that surrounds the experience.

REAL VOICES
For me in childbirth it was important to have a provider that I trusted, who would include me in the decision-making along the way and treat me as a partner—because you just can't anticipate every little thing that's going to happen.

Martha*, mom of two

Over the last ten years, as I explored a holistic approach with all of my patients, I began to practice mindful meditation on my own. I studied nutritional, herbal, and mind-body medicine and collaborated with experts in traditional Chinese medicine/acupuncture, craniosacral therapy, reflexology, and Reiki. Through this work, I've been able to create an integrative medical practice, one that combines the best of conventional and complementary medicine.

I'm now a senior faculty member of the Center for Mind-Body Medicine in Washington, D.C., through which I've participated in and/or planned mind-body workshops in the Middle East, Macedonia, and in New York, working with firefighters after 9/11. I became the first and only (as of this writing) physician in Connecticut to be board certified in both obstetrics/gynecology and holistic medicine. As an assistant clinical professor at both the Albert Einstein College of Medicine and the College of Physicians and Surgeons of Columbia University, I teach medical students and doctors-in-training about holistic care.

My own journey has been both intellectually fascinating and personally rewarding—and I truly believe that my patients are better served as a result of my embrace of a holistic philosophy of care.

Holistic Obstetrics

What does it mean for an obstetrician to practice holistic medicine? It means that I look to the women I work with, my patients, to be active participants in their care. It means that instead of focusing on individual symptoms, I try also to understand a woman's emotions and how the situations she faces in her daily life may be affecting her health. It means I always try to use gentle, noninvasive treatments that promote overall wellness and build on the body's ability to heal.

---

*Some names have been changed in "Real Voices" throughout.

This approach is especially important when a woman is pregnant or trying to conceive. I firmly believe that conception, pregnancy, and childbirth are extraordinary biological events that the body has the wisdom to guide. I see my role as that of a helper who stays in touch with a woman's physical and emotional experiences, someone who tries to uncover and allay any fears that being pregnant may generate. I never expect complications or difficulties, and I never think of pregnancy as a series of medical disasters waiting to happen. But if something starts to go wrong during a pregnancy, I can apply my medical training to the situation.

At the same time, over the course of most pregnancies, I can offer the tools of complementary and alternative medical treatments to relieve typical pregnancy aches and pains, help prepare a woman for a positive childbirth, and support her overall physical and emotional health.

The Whole Pregnancy Philosophy

This book is designed to help you make choices that are right for you, your child, and your family. As in my practice, I don't try to dictate what you should do. For example, I don't believe there's a "right" way or a "wrong" way to approach pain management in labor. For some women, an epidural is a good choice; for others, a medication-free approach to childbirth is best. And while I *do* recommend using mind-body exercises to start to prepare for labor as early as the start of the second trimester, these are only suggestions. You can, and should, pick and choose what feels right for you on every front.

The goal of this book is simply to give you the information you need to make your own decisions. To show how an integrative approach to preconception, prenatal, and postpartum care can bring together the very best of conventional medicine with the best of complementary and alternative medicine. I try to answer questions you may have and help you experience the joy, confront the fears, and meet the challenges that pregnancy can bring. I hope that by presenting you with a range of approaches not only to your prenatal care but also to your own unique experience as a pregnant woman, this special time can become one of empowerment and self-discovery.

How to Use This Book

You can read this book straight through, but it's designed to be a resource you can turn to at any point, from before conception through postpartum. You can plunge in wherever you like and find the material you need. Whether you're thinking about getting pregnant, actively trying to conceive, currently pregnant, or have just given birth, there's something here for you.

The Whole Pregnancy Handbook is loosely chronological. The first chapters cover preconception, fertility, and the first trimester. Then comes a chapter that provides an overview of all nine months. It includes a discussion of the physical and emotional milestones of pregnancy; a description of fetal development and prenatal care; and mind-body techniques you can use to connect with your child emotionally, energetically, and physically, and to prepare for childbirth. Later chapters are on common physical symptoms of pregnancy; nutrition; exercise; prenatal tests; complications; and miscarriage, so you can easily find what you need when and if *you* need it. The final chapters of the book go through preparing for childbirth; the contours of labor and childbirth; and life postpartum.

Throughout, you'll find the voices of women describing their own experiences, as well as interviews with experts—complementary practitioners, midwives, doulas, and others—who have important insights to contribute to understanding pregnancy.

Contributors

Cynthia Chazotte, MD, perinatologist: Cynthia is professor of clinical obstetrics and gynecology and women's health and director of obstetrics and perinatology at the Weiler Hospital of the Albert Einstein College of Medicine/Montefiore Medical Center.

Monique Class, MS, CS, APRN: Monique is a certified family nurse practitioner, childbirth educator, and nutrition counselor at the Center for Women's Health. She's also certified in imagery and visualization by the Psychosynthesis Institute in New York City. A senior faculty member of the Center for Mind-Body Medicine in Washington, D.C., Monique is also assistant professor of nursing in the holistic masters program at the College of New Rochelle School of Nursing.

Bobby Clennell, illustrator: A professional animator, Bobby Clennell was certified by B. K. S. Iyengar as a yoga instructor in 1977 and continues to study at the Iyengar Institute in India. Bobby now teaches yoga full-time and is a core faculty member of the New York Iyengar Institute. She is the author of *A Woman's Yoga Practice: Poses for the Menstrual Cycle* (Rodmell Press, 2005).

Libby Cohen, CNM: Libby, mother of three boys, is a certified nurse midwife who's been in solo practice for nearly twenty years.

Jacques Depardieu, MSOM, L/Ac, acupuncture, traditional Chinese medicine: Jacques specializes in women's health using acupuncture, acupressure, Chinese herbs, diet, and qi gong. In addition to his private practice, he's the director of integrative Chinese medicine at the Center for Women's Health.

Robin D. Evans, MD, dermatology: Robin, Joel's wife, is a dermatologist and the founder and director of the Southern Connecticut Dermatology Skin and Laser Center in Stamford, Connecticut. She is also a clinical instructor at the Albert Einstein College of Medicine.

Janet Hall, CD (DONA), CCE, doula: Janet was the first doula in Connecticut and only the seventeenth in the U.S. to be certified through Doulas of North America (DONA). The founder of Birth Partners, a doula agency, she's a certified childbirth educator and a member of the Community Advisory Board for the Birthplace at St. Mary's Hospital. Janet serves on the board of directors for the Nurture by Nature Network and was the recipient of the 2000 Community Achievement Award from the National Association of Childbearing Centers.

Tullia Forlani Kidde, MSC, NCACII, NBCCH: Tullia is a holistic psychotherapist, interfaith minister, and clinical hypnotherapist. She is affiliated with the Center for Women's Health and has a private practice in Stamford, Connecticut.

Alma Largey, prenatal yoga: Alma came to yoga through a career as a modern dancer and choreographer. She teaches prenatal yoga, *vinyasa*-style yoga, and kids' yoga both privately and in yoga studios throughout New York City. Ms. Largey is also a contributor to *American Baby* magazine.

Richard Mandelbaum, AHG, herbalist: Richard has been a practicing clinical herbalist with a background in Chinese and Western herbs since 1997. He lectures on a wide range of topics related to herbal medicine and holistic health, and teaches at the herbalist training program at the Lehigh Valley Healing Arts Academy in Emmaus, Pennsylvania. An avid student of the plant world for more than eighteen years, Richard leads workshops on wild edible plants, including mushrooms. He has a private practice in New York City and Sullivan County, New York, and is a professional member of the American Herbalists Guild (AHG). Contact: (845) 796-1883; e-mail: *richardmandelbaum@hotmail.com.*

Kimberli McEwen, MPH, lactation consultant: Kimberli has studied lactation for eight years, and has worked with hundreds of breastfeeding mothers as a breastfeeding counselor. She provides breastfeeding education to both professionals and families.

Elizabeth Parr, CNM, MSN: Elizabeth is the coauthor of *Choosing a Nurse-Midwife* (John Wiley & Sons, 1994) and a faculty member of Philadelphia University's certificate program in nurse midwifery.

Jeffrey Perry, DO, osteopathy: Jeffrey is a specialist in the field of pain management with expertise in the treatment of spinal disorders. He's an attending physician at New York City's Hospital for Joint Diseases Spine Center and serves as the medical adviser to the Occupational and Industrial Orthopaedic Center, also in New York City.

Lauren Pueraro, MD, anesthesia: Lauren is an attending anesthesiologist at the Stamford Hospital, Stamford, Connecticut.

Suzanne Roth, BA, LMT, craniosacral therapy: Suzanne is a Reiki master/teacher, certified reflexologist, and craniosacral practitioner. She has practiced the healing arts in both the U.S. and Europe since 1989.

Penny Simkin, PT, birth doula: Penny has been a doula and childbirth educator for over thirty-five years. One of the founders of DONA (Doulas of North America, *www.dona.org*), she's the author of many books, including *The Birth Partner* (Harvard Common Press, 2001) and, most recently, *When Survivors Give Birth* (Classic Day Publishing, 2004).

Joan White, prenatal yoga: Joan has been practicing yoga since 1968 and teaching since 1971, and has studied with B. K. S. Iyengar, author of *Light on Yoga*, since 1973. She also studies with Geeta Iyengar, author of *Yoga: A Gem for Women*. She holds an Advanced Iyengar Teacher Certificate and is chairperson of the U.S. Iyengar Yoga teacher certification program. She has her own school of Iyengar Yoga in Philadelphia, where she both teaches and trains teachers. She gives workshops throughout the U.S.

Publisher's Note

Neither the publisher nor the author is engaged in rendering professional advice or services to the individual reader. The ideas, procedures, and suggestions contained in this book are not intended as a substitute for consulting with your physician. All matters regarding your health require medical supervision. Neither the author nor the publisher shall be liable or responsible for any loss or damage allegedly arising from any information or suggestion in this book.

Part One

Part One

1

Holistic Medicine

Holistic medicine; alternative, complementary, and integrative medicine—these terms are sometimes used interchangeably, but they're not exactly interchangeable. To clarify what I mean when I use them, here are basic definitions of terms I use throughout this book, along with a discussion of how to find practitioners who are right for you.

◆ ◆ ◆

In this chapter you'll find:

- Defining Holistic Medicine
- Finding a Complementary or Alternative Medicine Practitioner
  - Quality matters
  - Figure out your needs
  - Collect names
  - Set up a consultation

Defining Holistic Medicine

• *Holistic medicine* is based on the fundamental principle that good health comes from physical, emotional, and spiritual well-being. Holistic practitioners believe that each of these elements—body, mind, and spirit—needs to be accounted for in any medical treatment. In other words, no one symptom—for example, chronic headaches or gastrointestinal problems—is understood or treated as an isolated event. Holistic medicine embraces prevention and self-care, using noninvasive treatments that support a person's natural abilities to heal.

• *Alternative medicine* generally refers to diagnostic and treatment methods (also known as "modalities") that are independent of those taught and practiced in most American medical schools and hospitals. Because they often encompass entire systems of medical theory that developed separately from what we in the West know as conventional medicine, they are typically considered "alternative" only in the U.S. Ayurveda, Tibetan medicine, traditional Chinese medicine, and herbal medicine are all examples of alternative medicine. In theory, alternative medicine is used independently of conventional medicine—and some alternative treatments must be used alone. In practice, alternative treatments are often used alongside conventional care. Medical schools in the U.S. are now beginning to teach some modalities of alternative medicine (primarily herbal medicine and nutritional therapies). However, knowledge of alternative medicine is not required for a medical license in any state.

• *Complementary medicine* combines alternative and conventional medical treatment. For example, using regular massage therapy sessions to reduce stress and lower high blood pressure or having acupuncture to supplement fertility treatment.

• *CAM* is an abbreviation for "complementary and alternative medicine." CAM is most often confused with complementary medicine, but CAM is the umbrella term for both complementary and alternative medicine.

• *Conventional* or *allopathic medicine* is the mainstream medicine taught in U.S. medical schools and delivered in U.S. hospitals by licensed professionals, such as a medical doctor, physician's assistant, or certified nurse-midwife.

• *Integrative medicine* shares holistic medicine's philosophy; it emphasizes prevention and self-care, and uses conventional medicines and surgery only when necessary. An integrative medical doctor understands how alternative and complementary treatments can be used alongside or instead of conventional medical care.

• *Functional medicine* also shares the principles of disease prevention, self-healing, and noninvasive treatment with holistic medicine. It fine-tunes that approach by focusing on improving the function of the body's digestive, immune, and hormonal systems, primarily through nutrition, dietary supplements, and lifestyle changes.

There are hundreds of types of complementary and alternative medicine modalities. In this book I focus on those that are widely available and generally recognized as effective and safe during pregnancy. These are: mind-body medicine; acupuncture and Chinese herbs; nutrition and dietary supplements; herbal medicine; and manual therapies like chiropractic, massage, craniosacral therapy, and reflexology. I also discuss the therapeutic role exercise and yoga can play during pregnancy. (For a description of these complementary and alternative modalities, see the Glossary of CAM Terms, page 525.)

Note: Homeopathy is a well-known form of alternative medicine that uses individualized remedies to treat specific physical complaints and illnesses. Generally speaking, during pregnancy, homeopathic remedies may be used to treat various nonthreatening but uncomfortable side effects, as well as everyday viruses and bugs, as long as your primary medical practitioner knows you're using them. Homeopathic remedies sold in health food stores have such small amounts of the active ingredients that they shouldn't pose a problem. (*Avoid* any preparation—homeopathic or otherwise—containing blue cohosh, which is used to stimulate uterine contractions.)

Classic homeopathic remedies are tailored to the individual, and require a long, in-depth patient-practitioner interview before they can be prepared. In the United States, homeopathy lacks standard accreditation or licensing in any state. Therefore, its safety and effectiveness depend heavily on the skills of the practitioner. For these reasons I don't use it regularly in my own obstetric practice, and, for the most part, it won't be included in this book.

Q: Do you always recommend the same complementary or alternative treatments for particular problems?

Dr. Evans: No. In some cases I may recommend a particular therapeutic approach, but for the most part, I don't. For example, for pregnancy-related back pain in the second and third trimesters, acupuncture, massage, and chiropractic are all treatments that can help. If a patient wants to work with an alternative practitioner for typical, pregnancy-related back-pain relief, I will ask about her preferences—does she like to be touched, is she afraid of needles—and explain what each treatment is like. Then, I leave it up to the patient to decide which

Complementary and Alternative Medicine:
Do You Need a Study to Know It Is Safe?

✦ As consumers, we're bombarded with information every day about the latest study on this or that new drug or supplement. We're taught to think that the medicine we're given by doctors has been stringently studied before we take it. But that's not always the case. In fact, not every conventional medical treatment has substantial data behind it, *especially* when we're talking about medication in pregnancy. Even over-the-counter medicines have not always been subject to in-depth clinical studies on humans. (The ethical issues are enormously complicated.) Doctors often decide on or guide a patient toward a course of action based primarily on their patient's individual needs and wishes combined with their clinical experience, meaning their experience practicing medicine day-to-day and the knowledge they've gained from teachers and peers.

Studies of alternative and complementary therapies that are constructed according to the standards of Western science are in an early stage in the U.S. and Europe. The information we have from these clinical trials about CAM therapies—as opposed to the knowledge about CAM that's been disseminated by practitioners over time, sometimes centuries—is scanty. Clinical studies are hard to design because many CAM therapies, and the philosophies behind them, require that treatment be tailored to the individual. To complicate things even more, it's difficult to run an ethical clinical trial of any medication—conventional or herbal—to assess safety in pregnancy. Finally, even with conventional allopathic medicine, scientific studies aren't always available to give us answers for every clinical situation.

Is it best to avoid even "safe" medications and herbs during pregnancy? Yes. Is that always realistic? No. The odds are that at some point during a pregnancy, you'll get a cold or have indigestion or back pain, which a conventional or alternative treatment can help. Will the treatment work? Probably (there's no 100 percent guarantee for *any* treatment). Is the treatment or medication safe? If an experienced, well-trained doctor or midwife recommends you take something—be it medicine or herb—if you trust her as a prenatal care provider, you can trust that she wouldn't suggest a treatment if she didn't believe it to be safe for you and your baby. That said, you can choose whether or not to take something, and you can do your own research on drug safety and ask your provider any questions you may have.

Likewise if you're working with a Chinese or Western herbalist or homeopath who's experienced working with pregnant women, ask what his philosophy is. Is he cautious in giving herbs to pregnant women? Where does he get his information about herb safety? (For example, Commission E, the German FDA, is a recognized authority on botanical medicine.) How long has he been using this herb with pregnant women and where does he get his herbs? If you're not familiar with any of his answers, feel free to take notes and do follow-up research. In general, you probably can trust that established, experienced practitioners would err on the side of caution when working with herbs during the preconception, pregnancy, and postpartum periods. But just as with your medical provider, it's important to ask the questions. And you should check with your doctor or midwife before taking anything.

Ultimately, when it comes to safety in all health-related matters, but especially in pregnancy, there are no absolutes, only our best knowledge at any given moment in time.

approach is right for her. Sometimes, since I work with a group of alternative practitioners regularly, I'll recommend massage therapy over acupuncture simply because I sense the patient will get along especially well with the massage therapist. And if a patient asks for a specific recommendation, I always give one that takes into account the personality of patient and practitioner, and the nature of the treatment.

That said, there are times when I recommend one treatment over others because my clinical experience has shown it to be especially effective. For example, I always recommend acupuncture combined with herbal treatment for women with elevated levels of follicle-stimulating hormone (FSH) or other symptoms of early menopause (known as perimenopause) because in my practice, we've had consistently good results with that approach. (For more on elevated FSH, see page 38.)

Finding a Complementary
or Alternative Medicine Practitioner

Just as when you're looking for a new doctor or nurse-practitioner, when you set out to find an alternative practitioner you want to find someone who's not only well qualified, but who's also a good match for your personality and needs. Finding an experienced practitioner whose approach you agree with and personality you click with may not be easy, but it's worth the effort. It can make a world of difference in your treatment, its result, and your emotional experience along the way.

Quality matters

Complementary and alternative health care providers most often go through extensive training in their individual fields. But because alternative medicine is relatively new in this country, national and state standards for licensing and accreditation have yet to be uniformly established. Unfortunately, that means "buyer beware"; it may be worth your while to do a little research to find out not only what qualifications a practitioner has, but also what qualifications she should have to be considered in good standing professionally. The Web can be a great resource; a quick online search of sites devoted to specific treatments should tell you what the accreditation/licensing standards are. When checking credentials, bear in mind:

- *Licensing* is administered by state governments, and requirements change from state to state. Keep in mind that standards can vary according to prior professional training. For example, with acupuncture, medical doctors may have fewer requirements for licensure than nonmedical professionals.
- *Accreditation* and *certification* are generally administered by voluntary, nonprofit organizations or trade associations.

Once you have some names, feel free to ask questions: If there's a state licensing board where you live, you can check with it to make sure that a practitioner is registered. If there isn't a state board, you can check with the specialty's major professional organizations to learn more about accreditation and find out if the practitioner is in good standing. Finally, don't be shy about asking a practitioner if he's accredited or licensed, and what that means in terms of his training.

Finding a qualified practitioner isn't always easy, but it's important to learn how caregivers are licensed so you can choose from a well-qualified group of practitioners.

Figure out your needs

No matter what kind of practitioner you're looking for—massage therapist, chiropractor, herbalist, acupuncturist—when you set out to find a complementary or alternative practitioner, first take some time to figure out what's important to you.

• *Office setting:* Some people work out of their homes; some will come to your house; still others work out of professional spaces. If you have a strong preference for one environment over another, pay attention to it and look for someone who works in a space where you'll be comfortable.

• *Travel time:* If you're lucky, you'll only get the names of people who work near your home or office. But your friend may know a great acupuncturist or massage therapist who lives forty-five minutes away. Decide in advance how important a convenient location is to you. Keep in mind that complementary and alternative therapies often involve regular sessions, so you may be making this trip as often as once a week.

FIRST QUESTIONS

Before the consultation, prepare a list of questions. You can ask about anything that you're wondering about. For example:

• What kind of training do you have?
• How long have you been practicing?
• What's your experience with women's health issues in general and pregnancy in particular?
• How can *you* help *me*?
• Is there scientific literature supporting your approach? (It's okay if there aren't many conventional, controlled studies of the modality, but you should know what's out there—and the practitioner should be able to tell you.)

• *Cost:* How often you see a practitioner may depend not only on travel time, but also on price. Since a new baby means new costs, set a reasonable budget for what you need. When you talk with a practitioner, ask if her fee structure changes based on the frequency of your visits. If she's out of your price range, see if she can recommend someone whose fees are more affordable. Also, check with your insurance company to see if the treatment is covered. Many insurance companies now cover a range of complementary and alternative treatment options, but they often require a referral from your primary care physician.

• *Expertise:* Most important, since you're either pregnant or trying to be, look for someone who specializes in women's health and pregnancy care. If you're already pregnant, check with your doctor or midwife before you try a new treatment.

Collect names

Once you have a general sense of what kind of practitioner you're looking for, begin to assemble a list of names.

Is This Practitioner Good for Me?

✦ Jacques Depardieu, MSOM, L/Ac, treats patients with acupuncture, Chinese herbs, diet, and qi gong. He works with me at the Center for Women's Health. Specializing in women's health, Jacques speaks widely on acupuncture, Chinese medicine, and herbal medicine.

Q: How do you know if a practitioner is good?

Jacques Depardieu: First, the match of experience to condition has to be right. Some acupuncturists are phenomenal at back pain, and some practitioners are incredible for gastrointestinal problems, but not everyone is great for everything. And you should get results relatively quickly. Not for everything—an internal issue like a fibroid can take months. But for pain, you should start feeling better after a couple of treatments. If you've had more than, say, four treatments and you're not feeling better, I would strongly suggest that the practitioner may not be good for your specific problem.

Another key thing is to find a connection with a practitioner and to cultivate that connection. In the U.S., you get so many different types of practitioners and styles of acupuncture, as well as other modalities of complementary medicine. You as the patient need to feel a practitioner is there for you and listening to you. Really, feeling connected to a practitioner can be more important than the modality itself.

Finally, I believe that a practitioner should empower a patient. As a patient, you should understand that it's your body's intelligence receiving the treatment, making sense of it, and then integrating it. The practitioner isn't some big "Healer"; your body is doing the work. So when you see someone, be open to being critical and engaged. Question them. Why? Why are you giving me those herbs? What can I do for myself? Can I change my diet? Do you suggest I do yoga or qi gong? Do you think I should take naps? The point is that the practitioner should be able to help you engage in your own healing process.

REAL VOICES

I'd moved to a new city, and I wanted to find a craniosacral therapist because I'd recently miscarried and I thought it would help me feel more centered and energetic. I called one woman whose name I found online. She seemed to have a lot of experience, but when we talked, I felt like I had to keep repeating myself for her to get what I was saying. I thought, this can't be right. I never went to her, but after asking around I did find a great massage therapist who really helped me.

Rebecca, pregnant

1. Ask your doctor, midwife, or nurse-practitioner. As complementary and alternative treatments become more popular, more medical professionals are developing a network of practitioners they work with regularly.
2. Ask friends, coworkers, and family members for recommendations.
3. Check with your health insurance company, which may have a list of recommended or in-network practitioners.
4. Look for ads for practitioners in alternative newspapers, magazines, and health food stores.
5. Search online: Even though these listings may be incomplete or out-of-date, an online search can be a good way to get started.
6. Get a list of licensed practitioners in your state—for example, licensed massage therapists.
7. Get a list of practitioners in your area who are accredited by the national organization for that discipline—for example, herbalists who are members of the American Herbalists Guild.

Set up a consultation

Once you have a couple of names, start calling. See if you can set up a pretreatment interview and, if you have time, a tour of the workspace. If a practitioner isn't willing to have a consultation or let you tour his workspace, look for someone else. Ask about special consultation fees—the visit may be free or a practitioner may have a lower consultation-only fee. Let the practitioner know whether you're pregnant or trying to conceive and what you're specifically interested in working on. You may find the perfect match right away, or it may take talking to several practitioners. Odds are, when you find someone you can work with, you will know.

Before the interview, take a few breaths to help focus. Throughout your talk, pay attention to how you are feeling. Does the practitioner inspire confidence? Do you like her voice? Does he understand what you're there for? Do her explanations make sense to you? If you're touring the workspace, take a few minutes in the parking lot

WHAT TO WATCH FOR

- *Locking you into multiple sessions:* A practitioner might recommend that you come in regularly, and he may even offer a discount if you purchase a number of visits in advance, but you should not *have* to pay for multiple sessions up front.
- *Dirty space or disheveled appearance:* A workspace may have unusual decor, but it needs to be clean. Likewise, a practitioner needs to look professional and put together.
- *No questions asked:* A practitioner should have a lot of questions about your current health, your health history, and your treatment goals. If a practitioner doesn't ask thorough questions, you need to find someone else.

before you go in to check in with how you feel. When you walk in, notice your sensations. Does the space feel comfortable to you? Do you like the smell? All these signals contribute to your gut feeling about the practitioner, and if something feels off, look for someone else.

2

First Steps: Preconception Health

When you decide you're ready to become pregnant, you start a process that will bring excitement, new physical experiences, emotional challenges, and life changes. As you start trying to conceive, one wonderful thing you can do for yourself is take a step back to check in with where you are right now physically and emotionally; make an appointment with your doctor or nurse practitioner; and evaluate your lifestyle and emotional habits.

In holistic medicine, we often talk about "optimal health." The process of preparing for pregnancy that I'm recommending isn't about making a complicated series of changes in order to optimize your health before pregnancy. If anything, evaluating your emotional and physical world is about simplifying your life. It's about understanding how the choices you make each day can help you improve your overall sense of well-being and how you can feel stronger physically and emotionally as you set out to have a child. *That's* what optimal preconception health is all about.

◆ ◆ ◆

In this chapter you'll find:

- A Preconception Visit: The Medical Intake
  - Medical history
  - Genetic screening

- The Emotional Side of Preconception Health
  - Building your own emotional intake

Now's a Good Time!

✦ If you're already pregnant, don't worry—it's never too late to take good care of yourself! In early pregnancy, your body will tell you what it needs; all you really have to do is listen. You may find you want to rest, take walks, eat (or not), stare out the window—these quiet moments in the first trimester present wonderful opportunities to help your body physically by simply resting and help your emotional world adjust to the idea of pregnancy, giving yourself time to reflect on everything that's happening right now. (For more on first trimester health, nutrition, and emotions, see chapter 9.)

A Preconception Visit: The Medical Intake

Ideally, before you become pregnant, you'll have a chance to talk with your gynecological provider, either at a special appointment—what's often called a *preconception visit*—or during your annual well-care visit/Pap smear. When a woman has a preconception visit with me, our discussion typically goes through three stages. First, we thoroughly review her medical history, then we talk about how she feels about getting pregnant, and finally, we talk about steps she can take to improve her health before she conceives.

Q: Do I need to have a preconception visit?

Dr. Evans: I always recommend a preconception visit because it gives both caregiver and patient the chance to have a real conversation about optimal health and early prenatal care before pregnancy begins. Often women will bring up their pregnancy plans during an annual appointment instead of scheduling a separate preconception visit, and for the most part that's fine. But if you've had a difficult pregnancy or a pregnancy loss, or if you have a chronic, preexisting condition, such as high blood pressure, epilepsy, or diabetes, it's important to schedule a special visit for a preconception discussion with your caregiver.

Note: If you were born in 1974 or before, I always ask if your mother took diethylstilbestrol (DES) while she was pregnant with you. The drug was given to women from 1947 through the early 1970s to treat pregnancy bleeding and to help prevent miscarriage, but it has caused health problems in the children of women who took it. In women, these problems include abnormalities in the genital tract, which can lead to cancers, pregnancy-related complications, and/or difficulty conceiving.

♦ ♦ ♦

Here is how a typical preconception visit unfolds.

Medical history

Understanding your medical history is the first step toward providing sound medical care throughout your pregnancy.

• *Family history:* Any medical history will include questions not only about your own health but also about the health of your family members—for example, if there's a family history of heart disease, diabetes, or, with pregnancy, neural tube defects. A medical history will also include questions about your ethnic background as well as the potential father's, which helps a provider determine if genetic testing is appropriate. (For more on genetic testing, see pages 16–18.)

• *Immunity:* Your provider will ask about immunity to German measles (also known as rubella) and prior exposure to chicken pox (also known as varicella). You can be immune to chicken pox if you were around someone who had it, even though you never got it yourself. If you're not sure if you've ever had chicken pox, a simple blood test can determine immunity. Likewise, even though most women were immunized against German measles as children, the vaccine can become weaker over time. A blood test at a preconception or first prenatal visit can determine if you're still immune—important information because German measles, while rare, is extremely dangerous to a developing fetus. If the test is done at a preconception visit and it turns out you are not immune to German measles, you may be vaccinated as long as you're not pregnant; after receiving the vaccination, you should wait three months before trying to conceive.

If you work with small children or spend a lot of time around small children, you're at risk for contracting fifth disease (parvovirus) and your immunity should be tested.

Note: If you're already pregnant, you'll be tested for immunity to German measles and chicken pox at your first prenatal visit, and if you're at risk, your immunity to fifth disease will be tested as well. If you're not immune, particularly to chicken pox, you can take simple precautions like asking friends with small children if their kids have recently been exposed to chicken pox and staying away if they have, as well as washing your hands before and after being around small children.

- *Menstrual/reproductive history:* Learning about a woman's menstrual and reproductive history is the final component of a standard medical intake exam.
  - For the *menstrual* history, I ask questions like "When did you have your first period? Are your periods regular? What happens physically and emotionally before and during menstruation?"
  - Taking a *reproductive* history simply means finding out what happened in past pregnancies, basically so I know if there's something special to watch or plan for. For example, if you had a relatively straightforward vaginal delivery, odds are good that you won't have complications with your next childbirth. If you had a C-section or induced labor, we would explore a different set of questions when we start planning for your next birth. (For more on labor and birth, see chapters 19–22.)
  - *Previous pregnancies:* Similarly, I need to know if a woman has had a miscarriage, no matter how early in the pregnancy it occurred, and if any testing was done afterward. (For more about miscarriage prevention and treatment, see chapter 18). Finally, the reproductive history is not complete unless I know if a woman has had an abortion, no matter how long ago. From a medical perspective this is important for a couple of reasons. First, it's actually useful to know that someone has conceived in the past; and second, a provider needs to know if there were any complications, such as an infection, that *might* affect a patient's fertility. However, a prior abortion, free from complications, shouldn't affect either your fertility or your ability to carry a pregnancy to term.

Genetic screening

Certain families and ethnic and racial groups have a higher incidence of specific genetic disorders that are passed to a fetus by either a recessive or dominant gene. When a *recessive* gene carries a condition, both parents have to carry the gene for the fetus to be at an increased risk. When a *dominant* gene carries a condition, the disease can be passed on if only one parent (and it could be *either* parent) carried the gene. In general, the diseases for which you'll be tested are all carried by recessive genes;

therefore, the baby's father would only have to be tested for a gene if you were to test positive.

Note: Genetic conditions like those described below are different from *chromosomal* abnormalities such as Down syndrome. Chromosomal abnormalities occur spontaneously, and their likelihood usually can't be predicted by anything identifiable in the parents' genes, although a family history of a chromosomal abnormality does increase the risk of one occurring in a pregnancy.

If you're a member of one of the groups described below, you'll probably be asked to have a blood test either at a preconception or first prenatal visit to determine if you carry the genes associated with the specific diseases in question. If you learn that you have one of the genes, it *does not* mean that you have the disease or that your child will. It does mean that the father should be tested. If his test results are also positive, you will probably meet with a genetic counselor. Once again, even if both parents carry the gene for the disease, it simply means the risks are greater. Even if only the male in a couple is a member of one of these groups, I still strongly urge a woman to be tested—while it's extremely unlikely that both individuals are carriers of one of these conditions, you just never know; the stakes are high and the test is relatively simple.

If you're adopted or if you're unsure of your ethnic or racial history, you can discuss what tests make sense for you with your doctor or midwife.

If you'll be trying to conceive with donated sperm or a donated egg, in addition to the genetic testing that's appropriate for your situation, be sure to get all the genetic information that you need from the donor, whether known or anonymous. If you're working with an anonymous donor, reputable clinics should supply this information.

Ethnic Group and Genetic Screening Tests

• *Eastern European Jewish (Ashkenazi) descent:* You'll be screened by a blood test for Tay-Sachs, a rare and fatal condition that affects a child's nervous system; it's passed by a recessive gene; therefore both parents must be carriers for the child to be at risk. Ashkenazi Jews are often screened for several other diseases, all of which are carried by recessive genes and occur with more frequency in this population. They include: Canavan disease, cystic fibrosis, Gaucher's disease, Bloom's syndrome, Niemann-Pick disease, and familial dysautonomia.

Certain *French Canadian* and *Cajun* population groups should also be screened for Tay-Sachs.

• *North African, Middle Eastern, and Sephardic Jewish (Mediterranean, North African, and Middle Eastern) descent:* You'll be tested for cystic fibrosis and Fanconi's anemia. Both are passed by a recessive gene; therefore both parents must be carriers for a child to be at risk.

• *African, African-American, or Latino descent:* You'll be screened for sickle-cell anemia. This blood disorder is passed by a recessive gene; therefore both parents must be carriers for a child to be at risk.

• *Mediterranean or Southeast Asian descent:* You'll be screened for sickle-cell anemia, as well as for an anemia called thalassemia. Parents with roots in the Mediterranean region are more likely to be carriers of beta-thalassemia, also called Cooley's anemia or Mediterranean anemia. People with roots in Southeast Asia, including India, Pakistan, and Sri Lanka, are more likely to be carriers of alpha-thalassemia. Both alpha- and beta-thalassemia, like sickle-cell anemia, are carried by recessive genes.

• *All couples* are advised to have cystic fibrosis (CF) screening—ideally at a preconception visit and certainly at a first prenatal care exam. White couples especially should be tested, because CF occurs much more often among Caucasians.

To conclude your preconception visit, your caregiver will probably prescribe prenatal vitamins (see page 25), discuss how long it can take to conceive (on average six to eight months, see page 40), and how you know when you're most fertile (see pages 42–44).

The Emotional Side of Preconception Health

As a holistic physician, I believe it's important for every woman who's trying to become pregnant to start thinking about the emotional questions that the idea of having a child raise for her—because our minds, our emotional lives, and our general outlook on life all have indelible effects on our bodies and our physical experiences. For example, think of how external stresses can trigger headaches or disrupt the menstrual cycle.

Before and during pregnancy, confusion, stress, fear, ambivalence, or anxiety may have obvious *or* subtle physical impacts. Trying to conceive means inviting huge changes into our lives. While most of those changes are exciting and wonderful, it's human to feel some trepidation, even if it isn't often talked about. Even though it's difficult, I don't believe that keeping the complexity of our emotional lives quiet will make them easier to manage. The only way to move through "negative" emotions, emotions we wish we didn't feel because they cause us pain or because we think we shouldn't have them, is to feel them. Once we can feel and acknowledge these emotions, they often don't seem so overwhelming or stressful—they just seem like feelings, and their effect on our physical well-being will lessen. The process of transforming "negative" emotions by acknowledging them can happen naturally over time, after using mind-body techniques, or by working with a therapist. But you can't transform emotions that aren't acknowledged and experienced.

Opening yourself up to *all* the feelings that a pregnancy inspires may be an ongoing process. Since I hope to support a woman as she engages her mind, body, and spirit in her pregnancy, I feel that a preconception visit offers a good opportunity for me to ask about some of the more complicated emotional issues that can accompany pregnancy and begin a dialogue that will continue throughout our relationship.

I call this part of a preconception visit the "emotional intake." To start off, I try to feel out where a woman is and what she feels comfortable sharing. I only engage in these discussions when a woman seems open to it; I never push anyone to discuss anything.

• *Work and Parenthood:* We might begin by talking about work: Does she like it? Is she concerned about the effects a pregnancy and child might have on her career? If a woman's job is very stressful and she works long hours, we might strategize about how she can better manage and maybe reduce some of the stress she lives with now. I might teach her some relaxation techniques, which in turn will help her body function a little more easily by soothing the nervous system. (For a description of some of these exercises, see page 62.)

• *Getting pregnant:* After talking about work, we might move on to a discussion of how a woman feels about getting pregnant. Is this something she wants for herself, or does she feel pressure from other people in her life—her partner, parents, even friends? Is she excited about becoming a mother? Does she feel good about how she was parented? How was/is her relationship with her mom? Finally, we may talk about any other experiences she has had with pregnancy.

• *Past pregnancies:* If a woman miscarried in a previous pregnancy, I might ask if she feels she's had enough time to mourn, if she feels any responsibility for what happened, if she feels emotionally and physically ready to try again. (For more on trying after miscarriage, see page 377.)

If a woman has had an abortion, and if she's open to talking about it, I might ask how she feels about it—for example, conflicted, comfortable, or guilty.

• *Being pregnant:* Finally, I'll ask a woman how she feels about actually, physically being pregnant. Does she know someone who had a very good experience, and are her expectations very high? Or maybe someone she's close to had a very bad experience, and she's nervous, even afraid. Is she very concerned about labor? Does she feel excited by the idea of it?

Questions like these help both of us learn about where a woman is emotionally. Our discussion may introduce issues or concerns that need to be worked through, either with me or a trained therapist, so the woman I'm working with can have as exciting and rewarding an experience as possible, from conception forward. I understand that the questions I ask could tap into very big, very personal issues, but this conversation isn't about finding answers, it's about opening up a sincere, serious self-exploration.

REAL VOICES

At the time we started to try, I had a lot of anxiety about my body in pregnancy. Would I be very sick? My older sister was violently ill in both of her pregnancies. But I just knew that my body was different from hers and that I had no idea how I was really going to feel. So even though I was very nervous about nausea and vomiting, part of me said, "I can't give in to this." We really wanted to start a family, we'd been married four years, I felt ready to start a family, and I knew if I waited for my anxiety to go away, it never would. I just didn't want to hold myself back.

Mary, mom of two

When we started to try, we'd been married seven years, and we were finally both in a place where we wanted to have children. So we were pretty excited about it—there were no reservations.

Rochelle, mom of three

Building your own emotional intake

If you won't have the chance to have an "emotional intake" with your caregiver, you can explore some of these questions either on your own or with a mental health professional. If you're going to work on your own, set aside a time and space where you won't be disturbed. Ask and answer questions either by writing in a journal or talking into a tape recorder. Reread or play back your answers. How did they make you feel? Are you surprised by your responses? There are many questions you can ask yourself, on a wide range of topics—work, your relationship, any past experiences with pregnancy, or even a friend's pregnancy. Here are some sample questions to help you get started:

1. What five words pop into your head when you think about having a baby? Talk a little about what each word means to you, and why you think it came to you.
2. What do you think about when you put together "work" and "baby"? Do you see yourself as a "working" mom? How do you imagine yourself in both "jobs"?
3. Is anything particularly exciting to you about being pregnant? Is any one aspect of pregnancy particularly frightening to you?
4. You're six months pregnant. How do you feel? What do you look like? Are you doing anything in particular?
5. You're pregnant and with your partner. Where are you? What are you doing? What are you feeling?
6. Can you imagine telling your mom or dad you're pregnant? What does that scene look like?
7. You're with your baby and your partner. How does that feel?

These questions may seem very abstract just now, when you're not yet or you're newly pregnant and don't already have a child. But they're simply meant to help you identify some of the issues around pregnancy and having children that are most important to you *right now*. Sometimes the answers to questions like these come very easily; sometimes they build excitement about having a baby; sometimes they trigger confusing feelings. While you might be surprised if you feel somewhat ambivalent about the idea of pregnancy, my experience is clear: You are not alone.

Don't label or judge your emotions as "right" or "wrong." Just acknowledge and experience whatever you feel, regardless of whether you think it's "good" or "bad." If you find that you have a very strong response to certain questions, or if you simply want to think about some of these issues with the help of a professional, consider talking with your doctor or midwife; she may be able to help you or suggest a professional counselor.

Moving Toward Optimal Preconception Health

3

Because pregnancy is physically demanding, it's useful to think about reasonable changes to diet and lifestyle that you might make in order to improve your general health and well-being and prepare the way for pregnancy. You may want to discuss this with your caregiver during a preconception visit, or you may want to think about what changes you can make on your own.

◆ ◆ ◆

In this chapter you'll find:

- Preconception Diet and Weight
- Prenatal Vitamins and Supplements
- Preconception Lifestyle: Simple Adjustments for Optimal Health
- When You Stop Birth Control: Common Questions

Preconception Diet and Weight

Diet

When it comes to what you eat before you conceive, healthy choices make sense for two reasons:

1. *Reducing your chemical load:* When you eat foods that have a lot of additives and preservatives, you consume chemicals that are more difficult for the body to break down. Generally speaking, the body cleans these out efficiently, but if you want to begin your pregnancy with your body functioning as well as it can, it's better to eat foods with fewer chemicals. Overall, that means eating whole grains and five to seven daily servings of (preferably organic) fruits and vegetables, and avoiding foods with artificial sweeteners as well as packaged foods (like snack foods) with a long shelf life.

2. *Preparing for pregnancy:* Once you become pregnant, you need more vitamins and minerals like calcium, iron, zinc, and folic acid; you don't need that many more calories daily. (The latest research shows that the number of calories you need depends on two factors: (1) your pre-pregnancy weight, and (2) what trimester you're in; see page 241). Since changing eating habits is most successful when you do it slowly, it may be helpful to start tweaking your diet now—picking an apple over a cookie, or a lowfat yogurt over a bowl of ice cream. (Of course, every so often the only smart thing to do is hunker down with a cookie *and* a bowl of ice cream.) If you gradually replace less healthy choices with better ones, it'll be easier to maintain good eating habits once you're pregnant and beyond. (For food and nutrition during pregnancy, see chapter 13.)

REAL VOICES

Before starting to try with my first pregnancy, I made sure to drink a lot of wine and eat a lot of sushi, since I knew I wouldn't be able to enjoy those things for a long time!

Kate, mom of one, pregnant

Weight

Does pre-pregnancy weight matter? Most often pre-pregnancy weight doesn't affect a woman's ability to conceive or her pregnancy, although if a woman's weight is in the "normal" range before pregnancy, it'll be easier for her to return to her typical body weight after she has her baby. Because weight is such a loaded issue in our culture, I try to focus my patients on how they feel, instead of how much they weigh. If they feel good in their bodies before conceiving, that's what's most important.

Pre-pregnancy weight can have an impact, however, if a woman is either significantly under- or overweight. Both very underweight and very overweight women

Organic Foods: What's in a Label?

+ I recommend choosing organic foods whenever possible (that is, when they're available and affordable). But what does "organic" really mean? The USDA has established labeling standards for foods that have organic ingredients. Under the new rules, organic means:

• Chemical fertilizers or sewage sludge is not used for growing crops.
• Crop rotation and plant and animal fertilizer are used to maintain the soil.
• Pests are controlled by nonchemical methods.
• Weeds are controlled by mulching, mowing, hand weeding, or mechanical cultivation instead of herbicide.
• Products are not genetically engineered or irradiated.

Organic Food Labels

There are several different types of labels used on organic food packages. Here's what they mean:

• *100% organic:* A product contains only organically produced ingredients (other than water and salt).
• *Organic:* A product contains at least 95 percent organic ingredients.
• *Made with organic ingredients:* A product contains at least 70 percent organic ingredients.

Products with less than 70 percent organic ingredients may designate organic ingredients on the ingredients panel.

may have irregular periods because of their body mass level. Likewise, both groups are at a higher risk for various complications. For example, underweight women are at risk for low-birth-weight babies, and a low birth weight means the child has a greater risk of health complications. Similarly, very overweight women are at risk for both preterm labor and very large babies, which can mean a difficult delivery (421).

If pre-pregnancy weight is a concern, talk it over with your doctor or midwife.

What's the "Right" Weight for Me?

✦ If you're wondering exactly where in the weight spectrum you fall, use the chart in appendix 4 to find out your body mass index (BMI), the measurement many doctors and nutritionists now use to establish that someone's at a healthy weight for her height.

It's always a bad idea to try to lose weight during pregnancy. (For more information about pregnancy weight gain see page 243.)

Prenatal Vitamins and Supplements

• *Do I need to take them?* That's the question many women have. There's no doubt that a pregnant woman needs more folic acid, iron, zinc, and calcium than she's likely to eat in a normal diet. If you eat a well-rounded diet, with five to seven servings of organic fruits and vegetables daily as well as whole grains, adequate sources of iron, zinc, calcium, folic acid, and protein, then you probably don't need to take any supplements. But in my experience, that ideal diet is hard to maintain day-to-day. For this reason, I recommend taking prenatal vitamins and omega-3 fatty acid supplements because they insure that no matter what a woman eats on any given day, she gets the basic nutrients she needs.

• *What if I hate them?* Unfortunately, many women don't like taking prenatal vitamins. They're big and can be difficult to swallow. Plus, they have extra iron, which later in pregnancy helps the blood carry more oxygen to the growing baby, but makes some women nauseous or constipated, particularly early in pregnancy.

If prenatal vitamins make you queasy, particularly if you're already experiencing morning sickness, or if you just hate taking them, here are some alternatives:

— Take folic acid supplements (at least 400 mcg a day) and a children's chewable vitamin.

— Take a prenatal vitamin every other day, or at night before bed. That way, you'll sleep through any side effects.

— Take a prenatal vitamin with food. Having something in your stomach in addition to the vitamin may relieve some of the nausea.

— Ask your caregiver about prescription liquid prenatal vitamins or liquid folic acid supplements. They're often easier for some women to tolerate.

Q: What if it takes me a long time to conceive? Should I take prenatal vitamins the whole time?

Dr. Evans: Yes. Prenatal vitamins are simply vitamins, and even though they're designed for pregnancy, they're safe to take and good for you, even when you're not pregnant.

Q: Why do I need extra folic acid before I'm even pregnant?

Dr. Evans: Folic acid, also known as folate, is a nutrient in the B-complex vitamin group (there are eight B vitamins altogether). It's been shown to reduce the rate of fetal abnormalities, particularly defects to the brain and spinal cord such as spina bifida (an opening in the spine), by 50 to 70 percent. It also reduces the *recurrence* rate of these defects in subsequent children by as much as 80 percent. In addition, animal studies have shown that prenatal folic acid reduces the incidence of childhood cancers. Folic acid also offers important health benefits to adults, lowering the risk of heart disease, certain cancers, depression, and abnormal Pap smears.

Four hundred micrograms (or 0.4 mg) is the minimum amount of folic acid recommended for women trying to conceive, and most over-the-counter prenatal vitamins contain either 400 or 800 mcg of folic acid; prescription prenatal vitamins contain 1,000 micrograms (or 1 mg) of folic acid. I recommend a minimum of 800 mcg a day.

Because the spinal column and brain begin to develop almost immediately after conception, it's ideal to have been taking folic acid while trying to conceive—no matter how long it takes. However, if you haven't been taking prenatal vitamins while trying to conceive, increasing your folic acid right after you learn you're pregnant is still a good idea for you and your developing child.

If you have a family history of brain or spinal cord defects, let your doctor know; you should probably take around 4 milligrams of folic acid daily before you conceive and throughout your pregnancy.

• *Calcium supplements:* In addition to the calcium in a prenatal vitamin (typically about 250 mg), I recommend a supplement to bring your total calcium intake to 1,000 mg a day while you're trying to conceive. (I recommend this to all women of childbearing age.) Once you become pregnant, I recommend increasing your calcium to 1,500 mg a day. You can get calcium through food, supplements, or some combination thereof. (For a discussion of the calcium content of various foods, see pages 218–220.) The government recommended daily allowance of calcium for pregnant and nursing women is 1,250 mg a day—but calcium is such an important nutrient, not only for bone strength, but also for smooth muscle function and circulation, that a little extra always comes in handy when your body works as hard as it will during pregnancy. There are two main types of calcium supplements: calcium carbonate and calcium citrate. I suggest calcium citrate because it's more easily absorbed and, unlike calcium carbonate, you don't have to take it with food. However, calcium carbonate tends to be less expensive and is fundamentally just as good. (For food sources of calcium, see the charts on pages 220–222.)

• *Omega-3 essential fatty acid (EFA) supplements:* I always recommend omega-3 essential fatty acid supplements to my preconception and pregnant patients, for two reasons. First, recent studies have shown that EPA (eicosapentaenoic acid) and DHA (docosahexaenoic acid), both omega-3 EFAs, promote fetal brain development—especially DHA. Because brain and spinal cord development take place in the earliest days of a pregnancy, it's good to be prepared before you conceive or soon after you find out you're pregnant.

Second, omega-3 EFAs are anti-inflammatory agents, EPA in particular. They can help calm an overstimulated immune system, symptoms of which include headaches, joint pain, eczema, rashes, or a constantly runny nose—and, in some cases, delayed conception. Therefore, when a woman I'm working with wants to increase her chances of conceiving quickly, I recommend these supplements, even if she doesn't have any of these symptoms.

Omega-3 essential fatty acid supplements are available over-the-counter. Take at least 400 mg each of DHA and EPA daily. *Only buy an omega-3 EFA supplement that guarantees it's free of PCBs and heavy metals.* (See page 522 for resources.)

Preconception Lifestyle: Simple Adjustments for Optimal Health

In my view, moderation is the key to every aspect of long-term good health. Here are the dietary and lifestyle items that cause the most confusion to women trying to conceive.

• *Caffeine:* Is too much caffeine a problem before and during pregnancy? Yes. More than 300 mg of caffeine a day—the equivalent of two eight-ounce cups of

Detoxification

✦ With the growing popularity of natural remedies, the idea of "detoxifying" has become more prevalent, too. "Detoxifying" is commonly taken to mean fasting or following a supervised regimen of acupuncture or homeopathy, possibly having a colonic, in order to cleanse your system of excess toxins. Some adherents of detoxification go on juice fasts for extended periods of time—a practice I don't recommend if you're trying to conceive, because it's extremely taxing, draining energy you'll need should you become pregnant. If you wish to detoxify before trying to conceive, I recommend working with a professional practitioner who has experience working with women wishing to "detoxify" in preparation for pregnancy.

Keep in mind that, for the most part, the body efficiently rids itself of toxins. The liver does the bulk of this work in a two-phase process. Phase I prepares the toxins for elimination, after which the toxins are still quite potent. Phase II turns them into water-soluble substances that can be eliminated through urine and stool. If Phase II isn't as efficient as Phase I, the half-processed toxins themselves can cause significant problems in the body.

There are medical tests that can evaluate whether or not each phase is working efficiently. These tests fall under the heading of "functional medicine" (see page 56), and not all conventional doctors administer them. I usually recommend them when a woman has symptoms such as chronic fatigue, chronic headaches, eczema, and fibromyalgia. (Inefficient detoxification has also been linked to cancer, autism, attention deficit disorder, and Parkinson's disease.)

I also recommend detoxification testing to women who've been trying to conceive and feel that there might be a problem but don't necessarily want to move on to conventional fertility testing, as well as to women diagnosed with unexplained infertility. Sometimes a relatively minor adjustment to a woman's diet can make an enormous difference in her detoxification and hormonal balance, boosting her ability to conceive.

A Basic, Clean (Detoxifying) Diet

Whether or not you decide to have detoxification testing with a doctor or go through a "detoxification" process with an alternative practitioner, you can support your body's ability to detoxify by modifying your eating habits and following a basic, clean diet, something I suggest to all couples trying to get pregnant.

• Drink spring or filtered water.
• Eat brown rice and whole grain pastas and breads instead of white rice and products made with bleached or processed flour.
• Avoid processed foods, foods with chemical additives, and canned vegetables, which are usually very salty.
• Choose organic fruits and vegetables when possible. If they are not available or are overpriced, clean all vegetables very thoroughly (opt for fresh vegetables first, then frozen). (To wash your produce, put it in the bowl of a salad spinner, add *one drop* of dishwashing soap, and fill the bowl with water. Let the produce soak for fifteen minutes, and then rinse it *thoroughly*. This should get rid of most, if not all, pesticide residue.)
• Eat brightly colored fruits and vegetables like carrots, apricots, squash, tomatoes, peppers, mangoes, berries, grapes, and pomegranates.
• Eat cruciferous vegetables like cauliflower, cabbage, watercress, and bok choy, as well as citrus fruits like tangerines and oranges.
• Season food with garlic, onion, cumin, and turmeric.
• Reduce red meat consumption and get protein from sources like tofu, fish, and organic, free-range chicken.
• Increase consumption of omega-3 essential fatty acids. They're found in cold-water fish like salmon, mackerel, and halibut, as well as in flaxseeds, flaxseed oil, canola oil, soybeans, soybean oil, pumpkin seeds, pumpkin seed oil, purslane, perilla seed oil, walnuts, and walnut oil. Omega-3 essential fatty acid supplements are also available over-the-counter. *Only buy a supplement that guarantees it's free of PCBs and heavy metals.* (See page 522 for resources.)

Note: If you plan to breastfeed, it's a very good idea to eat a clean, detoxifying diet before, during, and after pregnancy. From a health perspective, breast milk is the most nutritious and beneficial food you can give your baby. Breast-fed babies have lower rates of asthma, diabetes, and some childhood cancers. They have lower risks of ear infections, diarrhea, and pneumonia. For mothers, breastfeeding reduces the risk of breast cancer and ovarian cancer.

But because we live in a world that's full of environmental toxins, breast milk has been shown to contain certain persistent organic pollutants (POPs)—specifically DDT, dioxin, PCBs (polychlorinated biphenyls), and the fire-retardant PBDEs (polybrominated diphenyl ethers), which are used in products like foam cushions, computers, and televisions. In fact, because of how swiftly blood and breast-milk concentrations of PBDEs have risen, they are now banned in Sweden and the European Union (California signed a ban in 2003, effective 2008), and there's a movement to ban them in the U.S. How heavy and what kind of toxic load a woman carries depends on many factors, such as where she lives (women in industrialized areas tend to have more PCBs; those in rural areas have higher levels of residue from DDT, which is now a banned substance) and whether a pollutant was manufactured near her home.

This is an extraordinarily complex topic, and my goal here is simply to raise awareness; *in no way* do I want to discourage breastfeeding. The bottom line is that even with the pollutants in breast milk, it is *still* the best food for your child, for however long you choose to nurse—be it one day or a year. But I *don't* believe parents should make uninformed choices about what to feed their children. Hiding information never helps anyone. Knowing that environmental toxins cycle through our bodies and land in breast milk can motivate us to make healthier choices in our diets and lifestyle—avoiding preservatives and pesticides as much as we can, eating cleaner foods, and exercising regularly.

Further, I believe environmental toxins are a political issue. The overall level of environmental toxins has gone down in Europe and the U.S. over the last thirty years because of political awareness and activism. But uninformed parents are silent parents. Regardless of your feelings about environmental politics and activism, we all have the right to all the information that's currently available about matters that affect our health and that of our children.

brewed coffee—could interfere with your fertility, and some studies have shown that high levels of caffeine can cause calcium loss. But one to two eight-ounce cups a day is just fine—and if you think your morning coffee is as essential as breathing, there's absolutely no reason to cut it out. Keep in mind, however, that it's not always easy to get an eight-ounce cup of coffee. For example, at Dunkin' Donuts, a "serving size" of coffee is ten ounces, while at Starbucks, a "tall" coffee is twelve ounces, a grande is sixteen ounces, and a venti is a whopping twenty ounces. (Note: Starbucks doesn't give estimates of the caffeine content of its drinks.) Ask the barista at your local café the size of each drink they serve.

• *Alcohol:* Because no one knows how little alcohol will harm a fetus, many physicians recommend abstaining from alcohol altogether while trying to conceive.

However, *moderate* alcohol consumption while trying to conceive (by "moderate" I mean a glass of wine with dinner one or two nights a week) should neither diminish fertility nor harm the developing fetus *before a pregnancy is confirmed* (after all, I would guess more than a few of us were conceived after a couple of drinks). But, again, no one can say for sure. While trying to conceive, some women choose not to drink any alcohol after they know they've ovulated. If you decide to drink *moderately* while trying to conceive, your own comfort level can be a gauge for when it's time to stop drinking before you have had a pregnancy test. Once you know you are pregnant, it's definitely time to stop drinking entirely for the first trimester. (For more on alcohol during pregnancy, see page 98.)

REAL VOICES

Oh yeah, like any good girl who reads the books, when we started trying I got on folic acid, started taking a multivitamin. I don't know that I stopped drinking all the time—we tried for two years—but I was conscious every single month of trying to live a healthy life.

Katherine, mom of twins

• *Smoking:* It's extremely difficult to quit smoking, but now there are more reasons for you to do it. Smoking can decrease both a woman's ability to conceive and a man's sperm count. During pregnancy, it creates multiple risks to the baby, including miscarriage and preterm labor. In addition to the medical implications for pregnancy, from a holistic perspective, smoking introduces a host of chemicals that your body has to work overtime to process, limiting its effectiveness in keeping everything from the common cold to cancer at bay. If you're not yet pregnant, now is the best time to quit.

Since secondhand smoke is just as dangerous to you and your baby, if your partner smokes, he or she must quit or smoke outside the house. (For more on smoking and quitting during pregnancy, see page 100.)

• *Exercise:* If you exercise regularly, you can continue your workout regime while you're trying to conceive. In fact, you'll most likely be able to keep working out, with some adjustments, all the way through your pregnancy. Regular exercise while you're trying to conceive will not only help you stay fit, but also help you manage any stress that may develop when you're hoping to become pregnant. Working out before conception is only a problem if you exercise so much that you skip periods.

If you don't exercise on a regular basis, now is a good time to add a short, accessible workout to your daily life. Excellent pre-pregnancy exercise includes walking, swimming, weight lifting, and yoga—all of which you can continue during your pregnancy. (For more on exercise during pregnancy, see chapter 14.)

Q: How long should we wait between pregnancies?

Dr. Evans: There's no one answer to this question. Deciding when to have another child means understanding your physical and emotional readiness and evaluating your financial situation. Still, there's some scientific data to guide you. One recent study showed that if you get pregnant within six months of giving birth, your risk of delivering the next baby prematurely doubles (regardless of the mother's age and class). On the flip side, there's new evidence that waiting at least three years between children lowers the risks of premature birth and low birth weight. But what do those data mean for you? If you live a healthy lifestyle and especially if you're concerned about your age, you and your partner can decide on the timing that works best for you.

Q: I've had persistent back pain in the past and it finally went away. Will I be able to handle pregnancy without it coming back?

Dr. Evans: According to my colleague Dr. Jeffrey Perry, an osteopath who works with many women before, during, and after pregnancy, this is a common concern. As with all persistent pain, persistent back pain requires a thorough medical evaluation. Once serious problems are ruled out, most concerns about back pain are unwarranted, and there is no reason to assume that your back pain will return during your pregnancy. Plus, if you've taken steps to improve your back by doing regular strengthening exercises, you are probably in a better position to alleviate pregnancy-related back pain or avoid it altogether. It is also likely that you are tuned in to your posture, which is important because most pregnancy-related back pain is connected to poor posture.

When You Stop Birth Control: Common Questions

One of the first steps every woman must take in order to get pregnant is to stop using birth control. Unfortunately, that step isn't always straightforward. Here are some common questions about going off the Pill, removing an IUD before and after a confirmed pregnancy, and reversing tubal ligations and vasectomies. (For a complete discussion of how to pinpoint ovulation and conceive, see chapter 4.)

Q: I've been on the Pill for a long time—ten years—does that mean it will take longer to conceive when I stop taking it?

Dr. Evans: No. There are two basic types of birth control pills: (1) fixed-dose pills, also known as monophasic, which deliver a steady amount of either estrogen or progestin (a synthetic form of progesterone) throughout the cycle, and (2) sequential pills, also known as triphasics, which deliver varying amounts of estrogen and/or progesterone in a manner that mimics a typical menstrual cycle. (For a description of the menstrual cycle, see page 38.) Both work because they introduce additional hormones, which suppress ovulation. No egg, no baby. Birth control pills also thicken the mucus produced by cervical glands, making it more difficult for the sperm to travel or even live in the reproductive tract. These days, all birth control pills are low-dose, containing only 50 *micro*grams of estrogen or less, which results in fewer side effects like weight gain, acne, loss of libido, etc. (When the Pill was first introduced in 1960, hormones were delivered in doses of 5 *milli*grams—one thousand times as much as now.)

When you decide you'd like to get pregnant, you shouldn't have any problems conceiving because you've been taking the birth control pill—even if you've been taking it for years. After you go off the Pill, it might take a couple of months for your periods to become regular again. If your periods were regular before you went on the Pill, your cycle should regulate itself fairly quickly. If your menstrual cycles were somewhat irregular before you started the Pill, it may take up to four months for your periods to return. If you're waiting for your menstrual cycle to begin and it's taking a couple of months, take a daily calcium supplement to ensure calcium intake of 1,000 mg/day. (For a chart of the calcium content of many foods, see page 220.) Estrogen is produced during the menstrual cycle; among other functions, it limits the loss of calcium. When you aren't menstruating, estrogen production goes down, so making sure you get enough calcium is a proactive step you can take to protect your bones. If you don't get your period after three or four months and you know you're not pregnant, call your doctor or midwife.

Q: How long after going off the Pill can I start to try to conceive?

Dr. Evans: It's safe to start trying at any point, though it's not a bad idea to wait until your periods are regular, because due dates are calculated based on your last menstrual period and waiting will help you date your pregnancy once you conceive. In addition, by going through at least two cycles, your uterine lining will be optimally prepared. If you conceive the month after you stop taking the birth control pill—that is, if you go off the Pill and don't have a period the next month because you're pregnant, don't worry. The hormones from the Pill taken in the previous cycle won't harm the fetus in any way, since they don't stay in your body from cycle to cycle.

In the unlikely event that you find out you're pregnant when you're still on the Pill (it has about a 1 percent failure rate), stop taking the Pill immediately and call your doctor or nurse practitioner.

Q: I have an IUD, and I want to get pregnant. Do I just have it removed?

Dr. Evans: The intrauterine device (IUD), which is quite small, is placed in the uterus to prevent a pregnancy. In the great majority of cases, simply removing the IUD means you can become pregnant immediately and carry a healthy pregnancy to term. Sometimes, however, IUDs can cause infections, which can cause scarring that can interfere with your ability to conceive.

Q: I got pregnant with an IUD. I'd really like to have the baby. Will it be okay?

Dr. Evans: IUDs fail to prevent pregnancy at a rate of 0.1 percent, which is one in a thousand. If you're pregnant with an IUD, call your doctor or midwife immediately. You'll go to the office to check that the pregnancy has actually implanted in the uterus and not in the fallopian tube. (This is known as an ectopic pregnancy, see page 125.)

If the pregnancy is healthy, then your doctor will evaluate whether or not it can continue without removing the device. Depending on its location in the uterus, your doctor may feel that the IUD must be removed because it could break through the wall of the uterus. Don't be overly concerned, because it's often possible for a healthy pregnancy to continue after an IUD is taken out. But sometimes, removing an IUD does cause a miscarriage.

If the IUD can be safely left in, it'll be pushed up against the wall of the uterus as the baby grows. The IUD won't cause the membranes to rupture (or "water to break"), and the device is usually delivered with the placenta.

Overall, the risk of miscarriage in the first trimester when an IUD is in place is about 25 percent. (The miscarriage rate in the general population is 15 to 20 percent.)

Q: I had my tubes tied, and now I want to get pregnant. What are the chances a surgical reversal will work?

Dr. Evans: A tubal ligation, also known as having your "tubes tied," causes sterility by blocking off the fallopian tubes, the pathway between the ovary and the uterus where fertilization typically happens. It's almost impossible to give a percentage success rate for reversing a tubal ligation, because the outcome depends on several factors, including your age, how long ago the procedure was performed, and the technique the doctor used.

If you had the procedure less than fifteen years ago, statistically your chances for a successful reversal are improved. More important than when, though, is what technique was used to block the tubes. If the doctor cauterized, or burned, the tubes, it's unlikely a reversal would work, because cauterization typically causes too much damage to the tubes' lining to repair. If the tubes were either tied in a knot or clips were used to block off a small portion of each tube, the ligation is relatively easy to reverse—assuming there's enough healthy tube left. A doctor would surgically remove the clips or the tied portion of the tube and rejoin what remained to reestablish an open, healthy tube. To find out what kind of procedure you had, contact the doctor who performed it, or if the doctor is unavailable, have your medical records sent to your new doctor.

Before you do anything, however, the potential father should have his semen analyzed, and you should make sure that you're ovulating regularly. Regular ovulation, healthy sperm, and open fallopian tubes are the basic requirements for conception, so before you undergo a surgical procedure, it's important to make sure that your situation isn't more complicated than it seems. Keep in mind, also, that reversing a tubal ligation may require an overnight stay in the hospital and may not be covered by insurance.

If you don't want to attempt a reversal, you can still become pregnant with in vitro fertilization (IVF). In fact, blockage or scarring of the fallopian tubes is one of the original reasons IVF was developed to help women become pregnant. Not surprisingly, your age is an important factor in deciding whether or not to attempt a reversal. If you're much closer to forty than to thirty-five, you may want to try IVF and skip the reversal, because after forty-one, egg quality goes down along with the success rate of IVF. (For more on IVF and other assisted reproductive technologies, see chapter 5.)

If you think you want to try IVF without a reversal, check with your insurance carrier to find out what procedures and medications are covered when you're undertaking IVF after a tubal ligation.

Q: My husband had a vasectomy. What are the chances a reversal will work? What are our options if it doesn't?

Dr. Evans: As with reversing a tubal ligation, the type of procedure used for the vasectomy combined with when it was performed will determine the reversal's potential for success. A vasectomy blocks the ducts that carry sperm out of the testicles, where they're formed. A vasectomy is done either by cauterizing (burning) or knotting the duct. If the damaged area is small, and if the procedure was performed within the last fifteen years, the chances for a successful reversal are better. It's important to discuss a reversal with either the doctor who performed the surgery or a urologist specializing in male fertility who has your medical records readily available. Also, before undergoing a surgical reversal, you should be sure the potential mother is ovulating and her fallopian tubes are open. A reversal is usually an outpatient procedure, but, like reversing a tubal ligation, generally it's not covered by insurance.

If you decide that it's not worth attempting a reversal, you may still be able to retrieve sperm by a technique called testicular aspiration, during which a doctor extracts sperm from the testicles through a short needle.

4

Getting Pregnant

W hat you need to do to become pregnant is fairly straightforward, but it doesn't always happen right away. You may get pregnant within the first couple of months of trying, or it may take longer, but the odds are extremely good that you'll conceive within six to eight months or a year.

◆ ◆ ◆

In this chapter you'll find:

- The Menstrual Cycle: The Mind and Body Dance
  - The follicular phase
  - The luteal phase
- Peak Fertility: How to Improve Your Chances of Conceiving
  - How to get pregnant
- Pinpointing Ovulation
  - Ovulation predictor kits
  - Tracking mucus
  - Tracking basal body temperature

The Menstrual Cycle: The Mind and Body Dance

The menstrual cycle is the result of an amazing dance between a woman's brain and her reproductive organs. It happens in two phases: The first, known as the follicular (or estrogenic or proliferative) phase, leads up to and includes ovulation; the second, known as the luteal (or progestational or secretory) phase, extends from ovulation to menstruation.

The follicular phase

This first phase begins on day 1 of a menstrual cycle, which is the first day of steady bleeding in a period. During this phase, an egg matures within and is released from one of the approximately four hundred thousand follicles a woman has had since she first menstruated. The process can take anywhere from eight to thirty days, with any number of factors (diet, stress, exercise habits, etc.) contributing to its length. A stressful event in the middle of your cycle, or ongoing stress, can disrupt and lengthen the follicular phase, because the stress hormones the brain produces can interfere with the hormone signals the follicle and egg need for maturation and release.

Here's how a menstrual cycle typically unfolds. (Technically, the hormonal activity leading to ovulation begins before the period, but for simplicity's sake, I'll start with menstruation.) On the first day of your period (day 1 of the menstrual cycle), the hypothalamus, a gland in the brain, sends a hormonal message to the pituitary, a second gland, located just below the hypothalamus. When the pituitary receives the hypothalamus's message, it produces two more hormones—luteinizing hormone (LH) and follicle-stimulating hormone (FSH)—which trigger the ovaries to produce estrogen. As estrogen levels go up and ovulation approaches, a series of events occurs:

1. The pituitary produces lower levels of LH and FSH.
2. Between fifteen and twenty follicles begin to develop. Only one or—rarely—two, will become "dominant" and mature fully.
3. The lining of the uterus (the endometrium) begins to build up.
4. About five days before ovulation (for example, day 9 of a twenty-eight-day cycle), the glands that line the cervix, the canal between the uterus and vagina, begin to secrete mucus that's considered "fertile" because sperm can live in it for up to five days. (See "Tracking mucus," page 43.)

As the follicular phase continues, estrogen production increases until it reaches a peak and then drops off suddenly. The rapid drop-off tells the pituitary to increase LH production to six to ten times what it had been (this is the "LH surge" that's detected by ovulation predictor kits). Twelve to sixteen hours later, ovulation occurs. When it does, the egg pushes its way out of the follicle, and then tiny fingerlike projections called fimbria coax it into a fallopian tube. (Some women experience cramping when they ovulate, a phenomenon known as *mittelschmerz*. Some have a mucus "cascade," the sudden appearance of even more mucus.) On average, an egg survives between six and twelve hours in the fallopian tube—but it can survive as long as twenty-four hours.

You're most likely to conceive if sperm are already in the outer third of the fallopian tube (where fertilization typically takes place) when the egg is released. In fact, the three to five days preceding ovulation (the days when your cervical mucus production is highest) are considered very fertile. Couples should have intercourse frequently during this period, and women conceiving by artificial insemination may want to inseminate the day or two before as well as the day of ovulation.

Note: An egg released from one ovary won't necessarily travel down the fallopian tube on the same side. A chemical attraction between the egg and tube determines in which tube the egg will travel, meaning that an egg can be released from the left ovary but travel down the right fallopian tube. The practical implication of this is a woman only needs one open tube and one working ovary to get pregnant, and the ovary and tube don't have to be on the same side.

The luteal phase

After releasing a mature egg, the follicle turns into what's known as a *corpus luteum* (literally "yellow body," because it turns yellow), which immediately begins to produce a lot of progesterone and some estrogen. Progesterone is extremely important for a new pregnancy; among many functions, it triggers the final thickening of the uterine lining, creating a nutrient-rich environment to nurture an embryo. If a woman becomes pregnant, the corpus luteum will keep producing progesterone until the placenta matures and takes over—around week 11 or 12.

By one week after ovulation, the uterine lining will be thick enough to support an embryo. Assuming a twenty-eight-day cycle, an embryo conceived around day 14 will arrive in the uterus sometime after day 21. It will start to dig itself into the uterine lining (sometimes causing spotting) and by around day 25, the embryo will begin to release the pregnancy hormone HCG (human chorionic gonadotropin—this is what's measured in both urine and blood pregnancy tests). The HCG signals to the corpus luteum to stay alive and keep producing progesterone, which in turn insures that the uterus will stay thick and filled with nutrients the embryo needs to thrive.

If, however, a woman doesn't become pregnant, the corpus luteum will stop producing progesterone after twelve to sixteen days, and the uterine lining will slough off in menstrual bleeding.

In spite of the complexity of the menstrual cycle and the many natural variations that can occur, the overwhelming majority of women have cycles that are considered normal—with regularity, they produce an egg and then hormones necessary to support an embryo's growth into a healthy baby.

Peak Fertility: How to
Improve Your Chances of Conceiving

We all know what it takes to get pregnant; the only question is when to do what it takes. In its own way, your body lets you know when the time is right.

How to get pregnant

Every month, on average, a couple has between a 15 and 25 percent chance of conceiving. Even though the media is full of stories about how hard it is to get pregnant, most healthy couples—about 85 percent—will become pregnant within six to eight months of starting to have unprotected, mid-cycle sex. Many of the remaining 15 percent will get pregnant after another few months of trying. Given these statistics, when I first talk with a patient about pregnancy at a preconception visit (see page 14), I simply encourage her to have sex whenever she and her partner are in the mood—which is one of the body's signs that you're in a fertile period—and the majority of my patients do conceive that way. (There's actually new data to back up this approach. In a small study, sixty-eight women who still ovulated and had had either a tubal ligation or used an IUD were asked to keep track when, in one month, they had intercourse. They also had regular blood tests to monitor their hormone production and fertility. Researchers found that the women had intercourse spontaneously 24 percent more often during the six days when their fertility, based on their hormone levels, was at its peak.)

Having said that, one reason it can take six to eight months to conceive is that couples might not be having sex when a woman is most fertile. If after a few months of untimed, unprotected sex, a patient hasn't conceived, we'll discuss how she can identify ovulation so she and her partner can time intercourse appropriately.

REAL VOICES

For me, the biggest change (in my sex drive) was when I first went off the Pill and I was ovulating. I could almost pinpoint when I was ovulating based on my sex drive!

Kate, mom of one, pregnant

If your periods are regular, the *simplest* way to figure out *approximately* when you're likely to ovulate is to count back fourteen days from the day you expect to get your period. If your cycles are twenty-eight days, this would be day 14 (day 1 is the first day of your period). Keep in mind that though ovulation usually occurs fourteen days before menstruation, it can occur anywhere from twelve to sixteen days before, or days 10 to 16 of a twenty-eight-day cycle. If you use this method, you won't know the *exact* day you ovulate, but you'll have a good idea of the days during which you're most fertile. As I've noted, studies have shown that you're likely to conceive when you've had intercourse at least one day before ovulation. Therefore, if your cycles are regular, to be sure you're in your fertile range, begin to have intercourse once daily or every other day two or three days before you expect to ovulate and keep going through the day after you ovulate. For many this fertile range is between day 11 and day 17.

If you don't have regular cycles, have daily intercourse starting three days before the earliest possible ovulation day. For example, if your cycle varies between twenty-five and twenty-seven days, you might ovulate as early as day 11, so you'd start having sex daily on day 8 and continue through day 12. If you want to have more exact information about when you ovulate, or if your cycle varies by more than a few days, use an ovulation predictor kit or one of the other methods described here to help you pinpoint ovulation (see page 42).

REAL VOICES

The first time I got pregnant, it happened right away. The second time, it took longer—I think about six months. But I realized after about four months that my cycle had changed and I was off by five days—and those are five crucial days.

Martha, mom of two

Q: I've heard we should "conserve sperm" and only have sex every other day during the week I ovulate. I've also heard that we should abstain from any sex for five days before we start trying. Should we do both?

Dr. Evans: Sex every day won't diminish your partner's sperm count, unless he has a lowered count to begin with. (For more about sperm count, see page 51.) If it's fun and relaxing, have sex once every day from a few days before and continuing through the day after ovulation (for example days 11 to 17). But if daily sex feels like too much, regardless of sperm count, don't push it. Having sex every other day during your fertile week will still give you a very good chance of conceiving.

As for the "five-day rule," the latest studies show that the freshest sperm is most fertile. Abstaining makes sperm stale, so have sex whenever you feel like it before your fertile period begins and as often as is comfortable during the days leading up to and including ovulation.

Pinpointing Ovulation

If you want to figure out exactly when you ovulate, you can use any of the three methods described below, either alone or in combination. Each will give you a clear picture of your cycle, especially when used over the course of several months. There's no "right" method; the one that works best for you is the one you should use.

Ovulation predictor kits

Many women I work with find ovulation predictor kits to be an easy way to identify ovulation. Although they're expensive, they're extremely simple. To use the kit, simply urinate on the test stick provided. The instructions will recommend when to start testing based on the average length of your cycle.

About twelve to sixteen hours before you ovulate, your body releases a surge of LH (luteinizing hormone); the kits detect the extra LH in your urine. Once you surge, you're very fertile for the next twenty-four hours. But remember that your fertility increases starting a few days before you ovulate, so have intercourse frequently starting around the time you begin using the test sticks.

Once you've ovulated, keep track of the number of days between ovulation and menstruation (if you don't conceive). Subtract that number from the typical length of your cycle to predict when you are likely to ovulate next month.

Note: If you're using an ovulation predictor kit and you conceive, the kit may not ever pick up an LH surge. In other words, it may seem like you're having an "anovulatory cycle" (a cycle in which you do not produce an egg), when you're actually pregnant.

Using an Ovulation Predictor Kit in a 28-Day Cycle

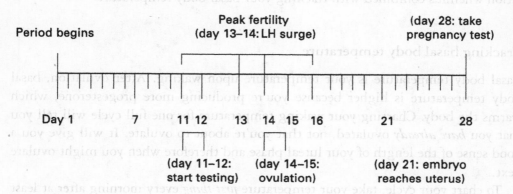

Period begins

Peak fertility
(day 13–14: LH surge)

(day 28: take pregnancy test)

Day 1   7   11 12   13   14 15   16   21   28

(day 11–12: start testing)

(day 14–15: ovulation)

(day 21: embryo reaches uterus)

Tracking mucus

In the first part of your cycle, rising estrogen levels tell the cervical glands to begin producing fertile mucus to prepare for ovulation and the presence of sperm. What makes mucus fertile? It's highly alkaline, just like semen, which means it allows sperm to live while they're in the vaginal tract. When you're not about to ovulate, the vagina is more acidic, which protects it from infections but kills sperm. Also, if you were to look at fertile mucus under a microscope, you'd see what's called "ferning," or lines that are more or less vertical, which encourage sperm's forward momentum. Once you ovulate, estrogen levels drop and fertile mucus production stops. (Cervical mucus that isn't fertile, which is secreted early in a cycle and after ovulation, is acidic and looks more honeycombed, so sperm can't thrive or travel easily in it.) Therefore, if you pay close attention to your mucus, you'll know when you've ovulated.

The week before ovulation, you may notice a slippery, wet sensation in your vagina (some women use panty liners during this time). This is steady lubrication from fertile mucus. It most often resembles egg whites, but it can also be yellow or pink/bloodstained from the normal light bleeding that can accompany ovulation.

Once mucus production slows considerably or stops, you know you've ovulated. Start counting the days until you menstruate. If you aren't pregnant, this will give you some idea of how long your luteal phase (the second half of a cycle) lasts. Subtract the length of your luteal phase, which is usually fourteen days, from the typical length of your cycle to predict approximately when you're likely to ovulate next month. (If you have a twenty-eight-day cycle and you ovulate on day 13, then your luteal phase is about 15 days.) Tracking mucus is more effective in pinpointing ovulation when it's combined with tracking your basal body temperature.

Tracking basal body temperature

Basal body temperature is your temperature upon waking. After ovulation, basal body temperature is higher because you're producing more progesterone, which warms the body. Charting your waking temperature for one full cycle will tell you that you *have already* ovulated, not that you're about to ovulate. It will give you a good sense of the length of your luteal phase and therefore when you might ovulate next.

To chart your cycle, take your temperature *first thing* every morning after at least three straight hours of rest (this should be at approximately the same time each day). Keep a thermometer by your bedside, and don't get up to go to the bathroom before taking your temperature. During the first half of your cycle, your waking temperature will vary from about 97.0 to 97.5 degrees Fahrenheit. A day or two after you've ovulated, your waking temperature will rise to about 97.6 to 98.6 degrees. Your temperature will be elevated until you get your period, then progesterone production will drop quickly, bringing your temperature back down to preovulation levels.

If you become pregnant (or if your period is late), your temperature will stay up because your progesterone levels will remain high.

(For more in-depth information about how to keep track of your ovulation, see the book *Taking Charge of Your Fertility: The Definitive Guide to Natural Birth Control, Pregnancy Achievement, and Reproduction Health*, by Toni Weschler, HarperCollins: 2002.)

> REAL VOICES
>
> I know a lot of women who didn't like charting their temperatures, but I really did. It gave me a sense of control. And when I did get pregnant, I knew right away—of course, I also knew even before my period each month when I didn't get pregnant.
>
> Karen, mom of 1

From My Office

✦ Recently, Emily*, a new patient, came to me to talk about getting pregnant. Immediately after I introduced myself, even before I could take a medical history, she began asking about the likelihood of conceiving at her age (she is forty-one) and pressing me about how quickly she could get on "fertility drugs." I felt overwhelmed by the pressure in her questions, and I wondered if she did, too. So instead of going into her medical options in depth, I asked if she could describe what she wanted from this consultation. Had she been trying to conceive for a while? Did she want to try "high tech" fertility treatments right away, or would she prefer to try some gentle, natural interventions first? She began to cry and said she felt enormous pressure from her husband to get pregnant, but she herself had real ambivalence about pursuing anything except natural interventions. Without me asking anything more, Emily got to the core of the issue: She felt that she couldn't talk to her husband about this because she was afraid he might leave her for a younger woman who could "give him children." At the end of our talk, she asked me what I thought she should do. I didn't answer directly, but instead asked her what she thought a good next step might be. She responded immediately: "Go to counseling to help me figure out what I really want." I agreed readily. Our talk gave Emily an opening to voice her *own* wishes and concerns, as well as an opportunity for *her* to come up with a "next step" that felt right. As her medical caregiver, it gave me much more insight into who she was as a person and how I could best help her with whatever medical care she wanted from me.

*All names of patients have been changed throughout.

Is this taking too long?

When is it time to investigate whether there's a reason you haven't become pregnant? The guidelines say that if a woman is forty or over, she and her partner should start testing after three months of regular mid-cycle sex; if she's between thirty-five and forty, she should go in after six months; and if she's under thirty-five, she and her partner should begin testing after a year of regular mid-cycle sex.

For the most part, I follow these guidelines in my practice. However, I always take my cues from the women I work with. If a thirty-three-year-old woman comes in and says she's been trying for four months but "something doesn't feel right," we will talk over what brought her in. Is she expressing a strong intuition? Does she know someone who has had difficulty getting pregnant and is she afraid she'll face the same situation? Is she feeling pressure from her partner, or does she just feel pressure because the news media say it's hard for a woman her age to get pregnant? Usually, by the end of our conversation, each of us will have a sense of what course of action best reflects her inner feelings. For some women, regardless of what the guidelines say, I am happy to order the initial medical tests to rule out a problem (see page 48). For others it will mean developing a daily meditation practice (see page 84); for still others it will mean a referral to an herbalist, acupuncturist/traditional Chinese medicine practitioner, or some other form of complementary therapy (see the CAM glossary in appendix 2). What's important in this conversation is for us to shift focus away from "What's wrong!?" and toward "What am I feeling right now?"

The bottom line is you have unique insight into your needs and your body. If you feel like something isn't right, but you haven't been trying for as long as the guidelines recommend, ask yourself what's driving those feelings. When you have a sense of what's behind your concerns, you can decide whether you want to get checked out by a doctor, nurse practitioner, or complementary practitioner such as an acupuncturist or herbalist. Often our own inner voices, as opposed to official medical guidelines, are our best guides.

5

When Pregnancy Is Delayed:
Fertility Tests, Treatments, and Technologies

If you decide it's time to investigate why you're not yet pregnant, you and your partner will have a series of tests to see if there's a problem. This chapter provides an overview of these tests, conditions that can impede fertility, and conventional interventions and treatments. I also discuss how complementary approaches to becoming pregnant, including functional testing, nutritional changes, acupuncture, and mind-body medicine, can play important roles in treatment and in helping you through what can be a very stressful experience.

❖ ❖ ❖

In this chapter you'll find:

- A Conventional Fertility Work-up
- Common Fertility Problems and Interventions
  - Endometriosis
  - Elevated FSH
  - Luteal phase defect (short luteal phase)
  - Polycystic ovarian syndrome (PCOS)
  - Unexplained infertility
- Assisted Reproductive Technologies

A Conventional Fertility Work-up

Conventional medicine investigates fertility problems by analyzing the basic requirements of conception: (1) Are you ovulating? (2) Are your hormones at appropriate levels, is your thyroid activity normal, and do you have any infections? (3) Are your fallopian tubes open, and is there any scarring in your uterus? (4) Is your partner's sperm healthy in terms of how much sperm is in the semen, its shape (morphology), and its movement (motility)?

For initial medical testing, you can work with an ob-gyn or a reproductive endocrinologist (RE). Some tests a midwife may order as well. REs are ob-gyns who've had several years of additional training during which they've developed an in-depth understanding of reproduction and reproductive medicine. If you decide to work with a specialist, ask your doctor or midwife for names and check with your insurance company to find out what's covered and if you need referrals from your general practitioner.

The tests described here are the starting point for a fertility work-up; based on their results and your treatment plan, other tests may be recommended.

• *Ovulation:* Ovulation is relatively easy to confirm. What I look for—above and beyond cycle length—is cycle regularity. Signs that a woman is ovulating include relatively regular periods, PMS symptoms, and mid-cycle cramping or spotting. To confirm ovulation, I recommend using an ovulation predictor kit to track cycle length (see page 42). If a woman has been charting her basal body temperature, I use that as added information, but for the purposes of an initial fertility work-up, I still ask that she use an ovulation predictor kit for at least one cycle. In addition to using an ovulation predictor kit, I'll ask a woman to have a blood test on day 3 of her cycle to measure her FSH. This provides a technically indirect but useful assessment of egg quality (for more information, see "Elevated FSH," page 53).

• *Hormones:* Blood tests given at different times in a cycle can confirm "normal" hormone production. These are the basic tests used:

- A blood test to measure *progesterone* seven days after ovulation (identified with an ovulation predictor kit) to confirm that you have ovulated and are producing enough progesterone to sustain a pregnancy (see "Luteal phase defect," page 54).

- A blood test to measure *prolactin*, the hormone that triggers breast milk production. Elevated prolactin levels can interfere with conception.

– A blood test to measure *thyroid function* (known as TSH). Proper thyroid functioning is very important not only for a healthy pregnancy, but also for fertility. If the thyroid is either over- or understimulated, it can be difficult for a woman to conceive.

• *Chlamydia and gonorrhea cultures:* Chlamydia and gonorrhea are two preventable causes of infertility. Chlamydia is one of the most commonly reported sexually transmitted diseases in the United States, and both infections can be present without any symptoms. A cervical culture taken with a simple swab (just like a like a Pap smear) can determine whether or not a woman is infected.

• *Ureaplasma/mycoplasma:* There's some disagreement over whether or not this infection interferes with fertility. It may cause inflammation of the uterine lining and the formation of sperm antibodies. The test sample for it is taken in a simple cervical swab, like a Pap smear, and if it's present, the infection may be treated with antibiotics.

• *Structural evaluation:* Once you know that ovulation and hormone production are normal, the basic conventional testing protocol calls for a hysterosalpingogram (HSG). In an HSG, dye is pushed through the fallopian tubes and uterus while an X-ray is taken. The test confirms that: (1) the fallopian tubes are open; (2) there's no scarring in the uterus that might interfere with implantation; and (3) the uterus is a normal pear shape. An HSG must be performed before ovulation, when you are absolutely positive you haven't conceived, and in many cases doctors have noted that their patients get pregnant the cycle they have the HSG or within the following three cycles.

Note: You may have heard of a "tipped" uterus. This refers to a uterus that lies back at an angle. As long as the uterus is mobile during a pelvic exam, a tipped uterus should not interfere with pregnancy at all. When a uterus seems more "fixed" in a position, it's potentially a sign of endometriosis (see page 51).

REAL VOICES

Before I had the HSG, my partner and I were wondering if we should even have it because we knew it increases your chances, so it seemed like a bigger emotional risk if we didn't get pregnant. But we still did it, and I didn't get pregnant and there were eggs there, and it was just hard. I was lucky, I got pregnant the next cycle, but people go through that for a long, long time, and I have the most empathy for them because I was a wreck after trying for what felt like a short time. It's just devastating when you feel like you're getting pregnant, you feel a little nauseous, and two weeks later you get your period.

Laura, mom of one, pregnant with twins

Fibroids and Fertility

◆ Fibroids are benign balls of connective and muscle tissue. They can be as small as a millimeter or as big as a honeydew melon. They can grow individually or in clusters within the uterine wall, toward the outside of it, or directly into the uterine cavity. Most fibroids will not interfere with becoming pregnant or carrying to term. If you have fibroids, however, talk over their size and placement with your doctor to be sure they won't cause any problems. If you work with a midwife, ask if you should have a consultation with the ob-gyn she works with because this issue may be beyond the scope of her practice.

We don't know what causes fibroids, but we do know they grow in response to estrogen. We also know a diet that is high in fiber and low in animal fat can help the body process and expel estrogen more efficiently, and thereby slow a fibroid's growth. Adding foods from the "basic clean" diet described on page 28 will also help the body get rid of excess estrogen.

The body turns the pesticide residue on conventionally grown fruits and vegetables into compounds that stimulate fibroid growth, so try to buy organic fruits and vegetables. However, if organic produce is not available or is too expensive, simply wash conventionally grown fruits and vegetables thoroughly, soaking them in soapy water and rinsing them completely, as described on page 29.

Once you're pregnant, any fibroid you have will grow because you'll be producing a lot of estrogen. Late in pregnancy, fibroids may cause some discomfort but are not likely to cause any complications. (For more on fibroids during pregnancy, see page 184.)

• *Sperm analysis:* In a sperm analysis a man provides a sample that's evaluated for count and quality as measured in sperm shape (morphology) and movement (motility). Over the last fifty years, sperm counts worldwide have been dropping annually (no one knows for sure why). Since male factors contribute to approximately 40 percent of all fertility problems, it's crucial that sperm count be tested.

Common Fertility Problems and Interventions

Here's a brief overview of common problems that can keep you from getting pregnant and treatments—both conventional and complementary—for them.

I don't address problems with male fertility since I don't handle them in my practice. That said, a man can prevent damaging sperm or lowering sperm count by doing the following:

1. Eat a basic, clean diet. (See page 28.)
2. Wear loose underwear to reduce the temperature around the scrotum. Likewise avoid hot baths and long bike rides.
3. Avoid recreational drugs, tobacco, and excess alcohol.

If your partner's sperm analysis comes back less than ideal, your doctor is likely to recommend seeing a reproductive endocrinologist or urologist who specializes in male fertility. Another option would be to see an experienced naturopath, nutritionist, or integrative doctor who has an interest in male fertility. Complementary and nutritional medicine can be very helpful and shouldn't interfere with conventional medical treatments, which are relatively limited for treating male fertility issues.

Endometriosis

• *What it is:* A condition in which uterine tissue grows outside of the uterus, endometriosis can be anywhere from quite mild to very severe. Twenty-five to 35 percent of women who have problems conceiving have some amount of endometriosis. In severe cases, it can produce cysts or scarring in the fallopian tubes or uterus, which can interfere with conception in the fallopian tube or an embryo's implantation in the uterus. Endometriosis can also cause inflammation on the site where the excess tissue is growing. Inflamed tissue may, in turn, overstimulate the immune system, which then *may* attack sperm or a fertilized egg.

No one knows why endometriosis develops, but, as with fibroids, we know excess estrogen can contribute to its growth. Symptoms of endometriosis include painful or heavy periods, pain during intercourse, and infertility. In fact, many women have no symptoms from their endometriosis other than not becoming pregnant. While endometriosis *can* cause severe pain, there's no direct relationship between the severity of the pain and the seriousness of the condition. Someone with terrible monthly menstrual pain may have very mild endometriosis, while someone with pain-free periods may have a very advanced case.

• *Diagnosis and conventional intervention:* While both a hysterosalpingogram (HSG) and a pelvic exam can suggest the presence of endometriosis, the only way to fully evaluate its severity is with a laparoscopy, an arthroscopic surgical procedure whereby a doctor can look directly into the uterus and tubes. If endometriosis is found, depending on how much there is, the doctor might choose to cut, burn, or laser away the excess tissue right then and there. A woman who wants to become pregnant is encouraged to try to become pregnant within six months of surgery, when her chances of conceiving are highest.

A laparoscopy is one of the two conventional treatments for endometriosis. The second uses medication, either the continuous use of birth control pills (with no inactive pills) or a course of treatment with Lupron, a drug that shuts down hormone production in the ovaries, to stop or slow the growth of the uterine tissue. Sometimes, the treatments are combined: Medication is prescribed for a brief period following surgery in order to prevent more endometrial tissue from forming. Once the growth is under control, a woman will stop the medication and start trying to conceive.

With severe endometriosis, even after surgery, in vitro fertilization (IVF, see page 59) may be necessary to get pregnant. Ironically, after pregnancy, a woman's endometriosis often improves substantially, and a clean, healthy diet (see page 28) can help keep it that way.

• *Nutritional medicine:* Diet can be very helpful in controlling endometriosis because certain foods can both reduce inflammation and lower the level of free estrogen, which, left unchecked, stimulates the growth of excess uterine tissue. Therefore, I often recommend a specific nutritional regimen in conjunction with surgery, based on a woman's individual needs.

To reduce inflammation, I begin with a round of functional testing. First, we take a blood sample to evaluate a woman's levels of different kinds of essential fatty acids. Certain fatty acids, like those found in salmon and flaxseed (EPA and DHA), reduce inflammation, while others, like those found in animal fat (arachidonic acid), promote it. Once we have the tests back, I'll work with a patient to adjust her diet in a way that balances out any problems the tests reveal. This usually involves reducing animal fats, shellfish, and cheese, eating more fatty fishes and natural sources of the omega-3 fatty acids (DHA, EPA, and DGLA), and taking supplements.

In addition to functional tests, I run a blood test for food sensitivities to determine if certain foods stimulate the immune system. Finally, we take a stool sample to test the intestinal tract for appropriate levels of "good bacteria." This test will also help determine how well the body is processing estrogen, since too many "bad" bacteria in the intestinal tract can increase estrogen levels, causing unwanted stimulation of the endometriosis. A situation like this is easily corrected through the use of supplements, including calcium D-glucarate, soluble fiber, and "good bacteria" like acidophilus.

• *Acupuncture and meditation:* Acupuncture can be extremely effective in relieving the chronic pain that may accompany endometriosis. Daily meditation has also been shown to aid pain management.

Elevated FSH

• *What it is:* Follicle-stimulating hormone, or FSH, is one of two key hormones the brain's pituitary gland produces during the menstrual cycle (see page 38). When it's measured on day 3 of the cycle (day 1 being the first day of heavy bleeding), it provides an indirect indication of egg quality. If FSH levels are below 10, they're considered normal, meaning the ovaries are still producing eggs that can be fertilized. An FSH level between 10 and 13, depending on a woman's age and the lab doing the analysis, is considered borderline. If the FSH level is 13 or above, it's unlikely that a woman is consistently producing healthy eggs.

• *Conventional intervention:* When a woman wants to become pregnant and her FSH is elevated, the typical conventional medical response is to try to stimulate a woman's ovaries so they produce a lot of eggs. This is done either before an intrauterine insemination (IUI) or as part of in vitro fertilization (IVF). Either way, the goal is to produce as many eggs as possible to improve the overall chances that a woman will produce a healthy egg, conceive, and carry to term.

• *Acupuncture and herbal medicine:* In my own practice, we've had repeated success treating women with elevated FSH levels with a combination of acupuncture, Chinese herbs, and Vitex, an herb that improves hormonal balance (the doses of Vitex and Chinese herbs depend entirely on the individual's situation). Supplementing this treatment with a program of mind-body relaxation techniques, a cleaner diet, and mindful exercise such as yoga helps women balance their energy, lower their stress levels, and feel better overall, which not only improves the chances of conceiving, but also improves the quality of their day-to-day lives. (For information on finding a complementary practitioner, see page 7.)

Luteal phase defect (short luteal phase)

• *What it is:* There's no consensus in the medical community about what's often called "luteal phase defect" or a short luteal phase. The diagnosis is used when the second half of the menstrual cycle—from ovulation to menstruation, or the "luteal phase"—lasts ten days or less. It's thought to be the result of a problem either with ovulation or with progesterone production. If some form of this condition is suspected, you'll be asked to have a blood test measuring progesterone on menstrual cycle day 21, and your doctor may recommend a procedure called an endometrial biopsy, which measures the thickness of the uterine lining. Because there can be variation between cycles, the classic diagnosis is reached after a short luteal phase has been observed in two consecutive menstrual cycles. In practice, depending on the woman, her age, and how aggressive she wants to be, I'll begin treatment after one such cycle.

• *Conventional intervention:* Because there's no real consensus about what causes a luteal phase defect, there's no real consensus about how to treat it. If it's understood as a problem with ovulation—the traditional approach—then the treatment is to stimulate the ovaries with clomiphene (Clomid); this may be combined with progesterone suppositories, which would make up for any progesterone deficiency.

Another somewhat less conventional approach is to try to extend the time from ovulation to menstruation to fourteen days by using natural micronized progesterone. This is the treatment I recommend, unless a patient prefers to take Clomid. Made from yams and soy extracts, the progesterone is called "natural" because the molecular structure is the same as that of the progesterone made by the body; "micronized" means it's been broken down into units that your body can process more easily. It comes in cream, lozenge, or pill form (Prometrium). The cream and lozenges can be bought without a prescription, but the doses are very low. I prefer using a prescription-strength form of natural progesterone.

Unless bloodwork shows a very marginal progesterone deficiency, in which case I would recommend a cream, I typically ask a patient to start with an oral form of progesterone and combine it with the herb Vitex, which helps balance the hormones. If a woman's cycle doesn't lengthen and she doesn't achieve normal progesterone levels after two months on this regimen, I increase the dosage. Since a woman with a short luteal phase has a higher risk of miscarrying (because her progesterone levels may be lower), until we've extended the luteal phase to fourteen days, I don't encourage her to actively try to conceive.

Even though there's a specific pharmacological intervention in this case, I recommend daily meditation to help manage stress throughout the treatment and in early pregnancy.

Polycystic ovarian syndrome (PCOS)

• *What it is:* This syndrome is marked by a hormonal imbalance that causes the ovaries to produce multiple follicles and cysts but not eggs. Symptoms vary, but besides irregular periods (often fewer than eight in a year), women with this condition may be overweight, and may have excess facial hair, mood swings, and elevated insulin levels (technically known as hyperinsulinemia).

• *Conventional intervention:* The standard medical intervention for PCOS is to use a drug that stimulates ovulation, such as clomiphene (Clomid), possibly combined with intrauterine insemination (IUI, see page 59).

• *Nutritional medicine:* With PCOS, it's very important that a woman's weight is within the "normal" BMI range (see chart in appendix 4). If a woman with PCOS is overweight, I work with her to slowly change her eating habits to a "low-glycemic-index" diet—essentially one that's low in carbohydrates such as white bread, white potatoes, most cold cereals, white rice, pasta, cake, and cookies, and is otherwise a generally clean, basic diet (see page 28).

Making dietary changes can be hard, so I recommend talking to your doctor, midwife, or a nutritionist to develop a reasonable plan that allows you to slowly and successfully change your eating habits. In addition, because exercise is crucial to maintaining weight loss and lowering insulin levels, for those who aren't already exercising regularly, it's important to find a form of exercise that you can do consistently.

Between the lifestyle changes and fertility interventions, treating and living with PCOS can be especially stressful, so I strongly recommend developing a daily meditation practice. Finally, there are support groups specifically for women coping with PCOS and many online resources as well.

Unexplained Infertility

• *What it is:* If you haven't conceived, you've been tested, and there are no abnormal results, you're likely to be diagnosed with "unexplained infertility." According to the Society of Reproductive Medicine, between 10 and 15 percent of couples undergoing fertility testing will receive this diagnosis.

• *Conventional treatment:* Assisted reproductive technologies such as intrauterine insemination (IUI) and in vitro fertilization (IVF) typically work well for couples in this situation. (For a description of both procedures, see page 59.)

• *Mind-body medicine:* Stress-relief through simple breathing exercises, meditation, and visualization techniques is extraordinarily important in dealing with all kinds of fertility problems, but especially unexplained infertility.

Functional Testing: Is It for You?

✦ Functional medicine is an approach taken by some medical doctors who have a holistic approach to patient care. Functional medicine, like holistic medicine, focuses on self-care and preventive medicine, but goes to another level through the use of laboratory analysis to investigate how well the interrelated systems of the body—hormonal, digestive, etc.—are working. In my own practice, I offer functional testing in addition to basic conventional fertility testing because it's my belief and experience that subtle imbalances of the hormones or even slightly inefficient detoxification can keep pregnancy from occurring. Once diagnosed, these imbalances are correctable by nutritional or herbal intervention. However, the tests can take more than a month to complete, the interventions can take a few months to take effect, and the tests aren't always covered by insurance. But for those interested in a "low-tech" approach to boosting fertility, these tests can be a good place to start.

Functional tests for fertility

• *A standard female profile:* Using a special kit at home, a woman will take eleven saliva samples throughout her cycle. Because the test uses samples from an entire cycle, it gives a more complete hormonal picture than bloodwork, which reflects the hormones only on the day the test was taken. For this reason, I recommend the functional test even if a woman's bloodwork is totally "normal." If there's even a slight imbalance, I recommend a combination of nutritional supplements and herbs tailored to the individual.

• *Detoxification evaluation:* The body has two interrelated systems that eliminate toxins and excess hormones, called the phase I and phase II detoxification systems. If either detoxification system is impaired, hormones and toxins may build up and disrupt the intricate conception process. To evaluate each phase of detoxification, a patient takes a substance like aspirin, and we then collect stool and saliva samples to see if it has been eliminated. When both detoxification phases are working well, the body will eliminate toxins and hormones efficiently. If, however, one of the detoxification systems isn't working well, the body's hormones may be out of balance. If this is the case, I'll work with a woman to create an individualized nutritional strategy that uses diet and supplements to promote balanced and efficient detoxification.

• *Detoxification genomic profile:* Our genes are responsible for everything that the body produces. There are specific genes that direct the production of detoxifying enzymes, and these genes can be tested for abnormalities. You wouldn't necessarily know if these genes were abnormal; your body would function fairly well. But if the enzymes were functioning less effectively because of a genetic abnormality (called a single nucleotide polymorphism, or SNP), the metabolism of hormones and many medications would be compromised. In this situation, I would work with a woman to develop a unique nutritional program to supplement and improve enzyme production, which in turn may subtly boost her fertility.

Note: These tests aren't widely used, and their results require individualized treatment plans. The lab I use, Great Smokies Diagnostic Laboratory/Genovations, will work with any doctor who requests their test kits. If your doctor or midwife does not regularly use these tests, he or she can administer them and you can work with a qualified nutritionist who has experience with these tests to develop a treatment plan based on the results. Or you can find a functional medicine practitioner who regularly uses them. To find a practitioner, contact Great Smokies Diagnostic (*www.gsdl.com*). The tests, which cost between $200 and $400, are sometimes covered by insurance.

Assisted Reproductive Technologies

Here's an overview of commonly used reproductive technologies:

• *Ovulation stimulation:* The theory behind ovulation stimulation goes that if you haven't conceived on your own, you need to produce eggs in order to increase your chance of conceiving in a given cycle. Clomiphene (Clomid) is often the first ovarian-stimulating drug prescribed; it promotes the development of more than one follicle, so it not only increases the likelihood of pregnancy, it also increases the chances of a multiple gestation (twins or triplets). (Identical twins, or twins that

Soy and Fertility

✦ Soy foods are rich in isoflavones, a class of phytoestrogens, which is a weak, non-steroidal type of estrogen with a wide range of health effects—most of them positive. For example, isoflavones from soy protein can lower LDL ("bad") cholesterol, act as antioxidants, and may help prevent cancers that are hormonally related, like breast and prostate cancer. Because of its estrogen content, some suspect that soy could contribute to both male-factor and female infertility. I *don't* agree, and I *don't* think eating moderate amounts of soy should be a concern to those trying to conceive. Moderation with soy is worthwhile, however, for two reasons. First, its hormonal component affects health when consumed in large quantities, and second, I think all foods are better for you when eaten in moderation. By moderate I mean no more than 75 to 100 mg of soy isoflavone per day (which, in fact, is probably more than most people eat). Bear in mind that various soy products have different levels of isoflavones (see chart).

When weighing whether or not a food is safe to eat or it interferes with fertility, I think it's helpful to consider its observed effects in countries where it's eaten consistently. In Asian countries where historical consumption of soy is high, women don't reduce the amount of soy they eat when trying to conceive. I believe that women who wish to become pregnant can safely consume *moderate* amounts of soy products; they are an easily digestible, healthy source of protein and other nutrients.

Product*	Average isoflavone content (mg) (amount may vary by brand)
Roasted soybeans (½ cup = 4 oz.)	167
Tempeh (uncooked ½ cup = 4 oz.)	61
Soy flour (¼ cup = 2 oz.)	44
Tofu (fresh, ½ cup = 4 oz.)	38
Soy milk (1 cup = 8 oz.)	20

*Mahan, L. Kathleen, and Escott-Stump, Sylvia. *Krause's Food, Nutrition, and Diet Therapy*, 10th ed. New York: Saunders Company, 2000.

result from the splitting of one fertilized egg, occur consistently in four of one thousand births worldwide. The frequency of fraternal twins, or twins from two fertilized eggs, varies widely by ethnic origin and culture.) Purified FSH, in medications such as Gonal-F or Perganol, will also stimulate ovulation. It's stronger than Clomid, and it's taken by injection. Both clomiphene and purified FSH injections may be used alone or in conjunction with intrauterine insemination (IUI).

• *Artificial insemination (AI)* and *intrauterine insemination (IUI):* These are relatively simple procedures. For AI, the sperm is pushed through a catheter and deposited just outside or inside of the cervix. In IUI, the catheter is threaded through the cervix and into the uterus itself and the sperm are pushed into the uterus. These procedures are timed to coincide with ovulation.

• *In vitro fertilization (IVF):* First developed for women with blocked or scarred fallopian tubes, this procedure is now used to treat many infertility problems, including unexplained infertility, male-factor infertility, and advanced maternal age. A woman's ovaries are stimulated to produce many eggs, which are then surgically collected and fertilized in a laboratory. The resulting embryos may be transferred— typically two, three, or five days after fertilization. In some cases of male-factor infertility, a procedure called intracytoplasmic sperm injection (ICSI) may be used. With ICSI, an embryologist inserts a sperm directly into an egg to achieve fertilization (although even with this technique, neither fertilization nor pregnancy is guaranteed).

• *Preimplantation genetic diagnosis (PGD):* This technique may be employed in conjunction with an IVF cycle. With it, one cell of a two-day-old embryo is removed and its chromosomes are analyzed for specific genetic abnormalities. This allows doctors to transfer only healthy embryos back into the uterus. A relatively new but fast-growing procedure, it's now performed more frequently at clinics nationwide. It's used primarily with older women (over forty), women who have miscarried two or more times, and couples with a high risk for a genetic illness or abnormality.

REAL VOICES
The month I got pregnant, I was in the middle of an IVF cycle, and they called it off the day of the retrieval because they said I had no eggs. But since my husband had this super sperm sample—he was so proud—they said, "Let's not waste it. Let's do an IUI, but it's not going to happen." That was the only time in two years that the doctors said forget about it. So that was the only day in two years I didn't go home, think about it, sit upside down— you know, all the stuff you do. Instead I went to the beach with my husband

and some friends and had a great time. I'd also just quit a stressful summer job, and I'd had a massage right before starting the IVF, thinking I would just do whatever I could to just be open to getting pregnant. They still tested me two weeks later because they had to, but I didn't think anything of it. We'd picked out this dog the day before the blood test, and we were going to go pick it up that weekend. It was a Sunday night and a nurse from the clinic calls me and starts chatting with me. Then the nurse said, "You're pregnant." I couldn't believe it. I was so stunned. After I got off the phone, I had to go to the drugstore to get a pregnancy test. I still have that stick, even though that grosses my husband out, because I'm still so proud I got that blue "positive" line—the only one I got in my life.

Katherine, mom of two

In this chapter you'll find

• Mind-Body Medicine

6

Mind-Body Medicine and Fertility

There's no question that trying to conceive can become stressful. Women often say that because they're "waiting" for something so big to happen, they have a hard time with decisions large and small—from planning a vacation to changing jobs to buying clothes ("Will this fit in three months?"). The way professionals talk about pregnancy can also be dispiriting: A woman "tries" to "achieve" a "successful" pregnancy, as if there were a way to try harder and be more successful.

To make matters worse, if you're trying to conceive, some well-meaning person (or two) will inevitably tell you to simply "relax." ("I have a friend who has a friend who tried for *years*. Finally, she gave up, went on vacation, and boom! Just *relax*.") But being told to relax just creates more stress! Could the stress from daily life keep you from conceiving? There's no definitive answer. But we do know that trying to conceive month after month creates stress, depression, and anxiety. And whether or not the stress and anxiety of trying to conceive can keep you from getting pregnant—studies show they may—they are painful and can make day-to-day life difficult. It's important to find relief from feeling overwhelmed and out of control if you're not getting pregnant, so you can improve the quality of your daily life—which ultimately may help you conceive. This is where mind-body medicine comes in.

◆ ◆ ◆

In this chapter you'll find:

- Mind-Body Exercises
  - Exercise one: belly breathing
  - Exercise two: visualization for emotional clarification
  - Exercise three: visualization before a procedure
  - Exercise four: daily meditation
- Mind-Body Medicine: The Power of Movement
- Mind-Body Medicine: Energy Work

Mind-Body Exercises

Mind-body exercises help you develop the tools to manage daily stress; develop insight into your emotions, wishes, and any life situations that feel out of control; and live more fully in the present moment, without regrets from the past or worries about the future. They can be used at any time, whether you're trying to conceive, in the midst of fertility treatments, or already pregnant. If you're having fertility testing or treatments done, these exercises can help you manage and even defuse the stress of the experience.

Here are four simple mind-body exercises to help you get started.

- *Exercise one:* "belly breathing" to help you move into a relaxed state wherever you are—at the office, in a parking lot, at home.
- *Exercise two:* A visualization exercise designed to help you clarify your feelings about pregnancy and parenthood, whether or not you're conscious of them.
- *Exercise three:* A visualization exercise to help you prepare for a procedure.
- *Exercise four:* A daily meditation to relieve stress and gain new perspectives on your day-to-day life.

Note: Just like any other kind of exercise, mind-body exercises can only be beneficial if they're practiced regularly. Even though at first they can feel funny or boring, or make you feel self-conscious, the way to benefit from them is to practice them on a consistent basis.

Exercise one: belly breathing

Belly breathing is so simple you can do it anywhere—at your desk, in a waiting room, anywhere. The technique stimulates the vagus nerve, which runs through the diaphragm and is part of the parasympathetic nervous system. The parasympathetic nervous system is one half of the autonomic (involuntary) nervous system; the sympathetic nervous system is the other half. The autonomic nervous system manages muscle response that you can't control directly, like your heart rate. The sympathetic nervous system speeds things up, for example when you're stressed, and the parasympathetic slows things down. When you purposefully stimulate a parasympathetic nerve like the vagus nerve, it responds by triggering what's come to be known as the relaxation response (technically known as a parasympathetic dominant state). As this happens, physical changes can be observed; for example, your heart rate slows, your blood pressure comes down, and people report feeling a sense of serenity.

The exercise goes like this: Sit or lie down in a comfortable position. Gently shut your eyes and let your hands rest on your thighs. Turn your attention away from any distractions and focus on your breath, breathing in through your nose, out through your mouth. Pay attention to the physical sensations you experience as you do this. Feel the air move up your nostrils, through your nose, and into your expanding lungs. Try to let the air flow all the way into the bottom of your belly, filling up your abdomen. Exhale slowly and completely through your mouth. With each slow, deep breath, focus on the air moving in and out of your body and on the movements of your abdomen. Try saying to yourself the word "soft" with each in breath and "belly" with each out breath. Continue breathing like this for one to five minutes. Slowly open your eyes and come back to your day. Pay attention to how you feel right now—maybe a little more relaxed?

Exercise two: visualization for emotional clarification

This visualization exercise is designed to help you begin to examine the complex and conflicted feelings that might accompany the idea of getting pregnant and becoming a parent. Don't read the instructions until you're ready to do the exercise; it will be less effective if you read the description ahead of time.

People don't often talk about the confusion or ambivalence that can spring up around the decision to have a child. They focus instead on the excitement and joy a baby brings. But becoming pregnant and then being a mother means making dramatic changes in your life, and anticipating those changes can stir up conflicting emotions. You may think you should only focus on the "positive," but when it comes to emotions, we have to acknowledge both the pleasant and the unpleasant in order to understand and move through them. Spending time with the full range of your emotions about pregnancy and parenthood—what makes you the most anxious or fearful, what feels best about it, what your secret wishes are—will give you the chance to better understand your motivations, conflicts, and priorities.

To begin, find a quiet place where you feel at ease. The temperature should be comfortable—not too hot, not too cold. Limit potential distractions: Turn off your cell phone and the ringer on your home phone, and let whoever is in the house know that for ten or fifteen minutes you don't want to be disturbed. Use any pillows or blankets you need to help you settle into a position in which you're comfortable and unlikely to fidget. You can sit or lie down, whichever feels best for you. The idea is to take away any physical distractions so you can become as calm and centered as possible. Ideally, any outside noise like roadwork or a neighbor's music would be minimal, but if it's there, try not to be aggravated by it. Instead, try to accept it as part of your surroundings—like the color of the walls.

Start by breathing deeply: in through your nose, out through your mouth. As you breathe, empty your mind of distractions—the work you have to do, what you're having for dinner—and just focus on your breath. You might want to start by using the belly breathing exercise described above to clear your mind and move into a relaxed state.

When you feel you're in a relaxed state, start to form a picture of yourself pregnant or holding a baby—whichever comes naturally to you. What do you see? How do you feel? Are there colors? What is the light like? Continue to slowly inhale and exhale. Focus on the image, paying close attention to its details and the emotions that come up while it is in your mind's eye. Are you happy? Sad? Excited? Ambivalent? Tired? Energized? When you have a strong sense of the image and feelings it inspires, stay with it for a couple of minutes, and then begin to emerge from your relaxed place. Let your breathing deepen and slowly open your eyes. When you're fully back, take some time to either draw or write down what you saw and felt. Try not to judge yourself or censor your feelings—there's no right or wrong answer here, no good or bad drawing—there's just what you saw and felt (maybe you were filled with excitement, worried about your body, nervous about money, loving toward your partner, scared of childbirth, or any combination of these feelings).

If you find you're feeling very centered and/or energized about the idea of pregnancy, you can explore the particulars of what excites and grounds you in your thinking about becoming a parent. If you find you're anxious, do your best to name what's worrying you. This exercise is not about trying to change anything; it's about identifying all of your emotions and gaining clarity about what's important to you at this point in your life.

There are many ways to explore what you learn through this exercise. Some people feel comfortable working with their feelings on their own—although if this exercise brought up very strong feelings, I would recommend working with a therapist. If you do choose to continue exploring on your own, try to meditate daily (see page 67), which can create more internal clarity, and check in with this visualization exercise every few days to a couple of weeks.

In my experience, women coping with fertility issues are helped enormously by exploring their feelings about pregnancy, whether it's through individual therapy or by joining either an infertility support group or a mind-body infertility group. You may find a therapist or support group through a friend, doctor, nurse practitioner/midwife, your clergyman or -woman, a community health center or local hospital, or a church or synagogue. Or contact Resolve, a national organization dedicated to helping women and couples manage fertility-related issues (you can find them online).

Recent studies have shown that women and couples coping with infertility who participated in support groups had a higher pregnancy rate than those in control groups who did not. Those who participated in prayer groups or prayed regularly were also shown to have higher pregnancy rates. Many insurance plans now offer some coverage for mental health services.

REAL VOICES

In the beginning it was exciting, moving, and exhilarating to try to conceive. Later it was stressful and a bit sad as I realized I might have a problem. Finally, I started taking private yoga lessons, and eventually went to an amazing therapist who specializes in fertility/adoption issues. I also found the Web site for Resolve, the infertility support group, incredibly helpful.

Laura, mom of two

Exercise three: visualization before a procedure

This visualization exercise is designed to prepare you for a procedure. It's tailored to an intrauterine insemination (IUI, see page 59), but you can adapt it to any procedure by replacing the details of the IUI with the specifics and ideal outcome of the procedure you are having. You might find it easier to do the exercise by listening to an audiotape. You can make one of yourself or ask someone with a soothing voice to read either this particular exercise or an adaptation of it that's appropriate for you and tailored to the procedure you're having.

The day of the procedure, carve out about fifteen minutes for yourself. Find a quiet place where you won't be disturbed. Sit or lie down in a comfortable position, and start to focus on your breath. Use the belly breathing technique described above: Breathe in through your nose, out through your mouth. Let the inhaled air go deep into your belly, filling it up, and then exhale completely. Feel that as you inhale, you're drawing in what you need, and as you exhale, you're releasing what you don't. You're breathing in energy and breathing out fear. You're breathing in strength and breathing out apprehension.

Start to focus on the procedure. Focus on the procedure helping you reach a place where you want to be; helping you bring a life into your world. Keep inhaling and exhaling slowly; in through your nose, out through your mouth. Begin to imagine the procedure: You're in the room, surrounded by a bubble of white light, and as you lie back, you are calm. Soon the sperm will enter your womb. They're strong and healthy and vibrant. Imagine the sperm meeting up with your egg. Imagine the sperm that's just right for you meeting your egg that is ready to accept it and create a new life. Don't worry about being technically or scientifically accurate; simply let your visions of the procedure float before you. Focus on feeling the positive energy move through you along with your breath (whatever that might mean to you). Take the bubble of white light that surrounds you and move it inside of you to surround the newly formed union of sperm and egg. Keep breathing slowly and consciously throughout, focusing your attention on your newly fertilized egg as it becomes filled with the energy of new cells and new life. When you feel complete with the exercise, slowly open your eyes.

Later that day, while you're waiting for the procedure, try to sit comfortably and breathe deeply, using the breath to fill you with serenity. During the procedure, close your eyes and imagine the energy of the white light enveloping you, moving inside of you to surround the sperm, the egg, and the bright new embryo they'll form. When it's over, let the light dissipate throughout your body like a gentle shower. Slowly open your eyes, and turn your attention back to the room.

REAL VOICES
We had this little ritual after each IUI—we had six of them. The doctor would leave and tell me to rest for twenty minutes. Then Nathaniel, my husband, would sing, "Swim, Sonya, Swim!" I did have a girl, and I think she heard him.

Sarah, mom of one

Exercise four: daily meditation

Meditation gives you respite from fear or anxiety about the future and anger or regrets about the past by focusing your attention completely on the present moment. From a medical perspective, daily meditation has been shown to improve hormonal balance, immune responses, and general mood.

There are literally hundreds of ways to meditate. Most fall into one of three categories: concentrative, expressive, or awareness. A concentrative meditation generally involves sitting quietly and focusing on something, for example the breath, as with the belly breathing exercise, or the flame of a burning candle, or a mantra (a repeated word or phrase, like "peace"). Expressive meditations involve movement, like dancing. Awareness meditations allow you to focus completely on your experience in a certain situation, during a walk, for example, or chopping vegetables for soup.

Quiet meditation—taking five, ten, twenty minutes each day to sit while paying attention only to your breath—has both concentrative and awareness elements. It can be a powerful relaxation tool, and over time it can help you gain perspective on many different aspects of your life.

To practice a seated, quiet meditation, find a place where you won't be disturbed. Turn off the ringer on your home and cell phones. Sit on a comfortable chair with your feet flat on the ground and your palms resting gently on your thighs. Then, slowly shut your eyes. Next, breathe in through your nose and out through your mouth at a natural pace, focusing your attention on each inhale and exhale. Thoughts will come; let them do that. Just be sure to let them go, too. Try not to hold onto any one thought; allow your mind to let each thing pass, and keep coming back to your breath. To start, you can sit like this for five or ten minutes, and then, if you find it sustaining, work your way up to as long as thirty minutes.

Feel free to modify this meditation—or any of these exercises—to fit your own needs. Try to keep up a daily meditation, even if you feel like "nothing's happening." Something is definitely happening, but it may be just below your level of awareness. All religious and spiritual traditions emphasize that practice and patience will have their reward. Meditating consistently, particularly during stressful times, is ideal, but whenever you get the chance to sit and meditate, even if you can't do it on a regular basis, you will reap its benefits.

A Mind-Body Fertility Support Group

✦ For several years now, I've run mind-body groups for women dealing with fertility issues, and I've seen firsthand how helpful they can be. A mind-body group may differ from a general fertility support group because participants learn a range of relaxation and meditation techniques while sharing and exploring their feelings in a safe environment, supported by those going through a similar experience.

In the groups I run, everyone has been trying to conceive for six months to a year, depending on their ages. We meet for two-hour sessions once a week for ten to twelve weeks. Some participants have had medical testing or interventions, some have started alternative treatments, and for some, joining the group is their first step.

We begin each session with a short relaxation meditation (similar to belly breathing), after which everyone shares how she's feeling, how the week went, etc. Then I describe the theory and practice of a specific mind-body technique. We practice the technique and discuss any insights that people may have had from it. Combining peer support with mind-body exercises is a powerful way to access the subconscious mind; the group becomes a venue for safe self-discovery, and the exercises offer techniques for exploring and relaxing the mind that wouldn't otherwise be available. Ultimately, the women who participate not only have a range of mind-body exercises to choose from, but they also develop a better understanding of themselves, their lives, and their motivations.

Mind-Body Medicine: The Power of Movement

Beyond the day-to-day stress that builds when it takes longer than six to twelve months to conceive, the delay may trigger many layers of complicated feelings about your body, to which you may be paying exquisite attention. Every cramp ("Am I ovulating?"), every twinge ("My breasts are sore—what does that mean?") may seem like a sign of "something." And then there's the fact that even with all your attention, your body hasn't yet done what you expect. There's a gap between what you want your body to do and what is actually happening—a painful situation that can leave you feeling disappointed in and disconnected from your body.

To help reconnect and establish a more positive relationship with your body, I recommend moving your body. Though this recommendation might seem peculiar at first, it is based on the experience of the many women I've worked with over the years. With physical movement, you can reconnect to your body without judging it and without scanning it for signs that you're pregnant.

When I speak about moving the body, I'm not only talking about a cardiovascular exercise like jogging. Exercise is wonderful, but it can often feel like something you are "supposed" to do. I think it's important to find something you *want* to do, some way to move that simply expresses your pleasure in being. For many of the women I work with, that means dancing. Not necessarily in a class, but maybe in your own room. No matter how long you have been trying or what kind of treatment you have sought out, dancing freely simply feels great. All you have to do is give yourself ten or fifteen minutes *every* day when you're alone, put on your favorite songs, and go!

If you do exercise regularly, you may still want to try dancing every day, either in addition to your regular exercise or as a substitute, because it offers a completely different way to experience your body.

I've gotten so much positive feedback from my patients about dancing that even if thinking about dancing around your bedroom seems silly to you, I'd still recommend trying it every day for a full week as an experiment just to see if it feels too odd to be worthwhile.

Mind-Body Medicine: Energy Work

Though we don't often think about it this way, the body is electrically charged. For example, an electrocardiogram records the electricity the heart produces with each heartbeat, and an electroencephalogram measures the electric activity of the brain. Electricity—energy—keeps the body going. So the questions spring up: If there's a flow of electricity, of energy, in the body, does it flow differently in people who are healthy versus those who are sick? Could a change in energy flow be a contributing factor in a physical illness, or the result of an illness? Can improving the flow of electricity—of energy—affect health?

As of now, those of us who practice conventional medicine don't have definitive answers, but I can't ignore the potential impact that the flow of energy in and around the body might have on overall health.

In alternative medical systems such as traditional Chinese medicine (TCM) and

Treating Fertility Problems with Acupuncture

✦ Jacques Depardieu, MSOM, L/Ac, is a colleague and member of my practice who treats patients with acupuncture, Chinese herbs, diet, and qi gong.

Q: How do you approach a patient coming to you for fertility treatments?

Jacques Depardieu: It depends on the patient. If a woman comes to me and says, "We've been trying for a year, and I want to try to get pregnant naturally. I don't want to do IVF," I'll still recommend that she and her partner get tested. She might have some problem like a blockage of the tubes, or there could be a sperm problem. There are all kinds of issues that could affect fertility, and I try to rule out or understand every identifiable medical issue before we start working together.

For women who are in treatment or have dealt with fertility issues for a long time, I really try to work on the emotional side of things. I've learned so much about that over the years—every month when a woman gets her period, it's devastating. So even though treatment totally depends on the individual, one thing that's consistent with every patient, along with balancing their qi (energy), is to go as deep as we can to find some harmony in the present moment, some kind of acceptance of what's going on in order to move to a different place in her experience of fertility problems.

I'll give you an example of an actual patient. A woman came in, she's forty years old, she's tried IVF six times, and her last FSH levels were so high that they told her there's nothing they can do for her and she was referred to me for depression. I felt her pulses, looked at her tongue (key diagnostic tools for acupuncturists), and got a history. I told her that she had certain types of deficiencies—the energy in her body was depleted. So I gave her herbs for the energy deficiencies while at the same time talking through and treating her for the depression. I treated this patient for a couple of weeks, and she really felt a lot better, a lot happier. She felt at peace with what had happened, and she said she reached a place where she felt like her fertility issues didn't matter. And then she got pregnant the next month. This doesn't happen every time, but the work is about supporting the patient and tapping into the body's wisdom to heal and restore itself.

ayurveda, good health is intertwined with the flow of energy in the body (for example, through meridians in TCM or chakras and nadis in ayurveda). While I don't practice what's known as energetic medicine myself, I believe that by improving the flow of energy in your body, you can get closer to optimal health, which boosts your fertility simply because the body is working better. To this end, I encourage the women I work with who are trying to conceive to have some kind of "energy work." There are many types to choose from; I work consistently with acupuncture combined with herbal medicine (especially with fertility issues) as well as reflexology, Reiki, and craniosacral therapy. (For a description of each, see the CAM glossary on page 525.) In certain situations, I do recommend a particular modality (see "Elevated FSH" on page 53), but usually, after describing the different types of energy-healing modalities, I encourage my patients to pursue the treatment that they feel best suits them.

Part Two

Part Two

7

The First Trimester

The great journey of pregnancy begins! The first trimester is a time of tremendous physical and emotional intensity. As your body adjusts to the flood of hormones, you have time to adjust to the idea that you're actually pregnant. Over the course of these twelve weeks, the embryo, which started out as just two cells, will develop into a recognizable little human with arms, legs, and all her internal organs. As these changes happen, make time for yourself—to rest, take long walks, and connect with the idea that you're nurturing a new life.

◆ ◆ ◆

In this chapter you'll find:

- Confirming a Pregnancy
- Prenatal Caregivers: Working with a Doctor or Midwife
- Caregivers and Their Practices
  - Medical doctors
  - Midwives
  - Finding a caregiver

Confirming a Pregnancy

Pregnancy announces itself in about as many ways as there are women. You may experience some of its symptoms even before you miss your period—for example, your breasts may be tender or your nipples sensitive; you may be nauseous, especially sensitive to smells, or hungrier than usual; you may have strong cramps or bloating, have to urinate frequently, or find yourself feeling moody. You might experience some of these symptoms, all of them, or none of them—a late period may be the only indication that you're pregnant.

If you suspect you're pregnant, either take a urine test at home or a blood test through your practitioner once your period is late. Both tests measure the levels of HCG (human chorionic gonadotropin), a hormone produced by the developing embryo.

Q: When should I take a pregnancy test?
Dr. Evans: A blood test of HCG levels may be taken as early as two days before you expect your period (for example, day 26 of a twenty-eight-day cycle), but until you've missed a period, you may get a negative result when in fact you're pregnant, because the pregnancy hormone hasn't yet reached a measurable level. A blood or home pregnancy test taken a day after your period is due is most likely to be accurate.

If you take a blood pregnancy test, anything over 5 IU/L (international units per liter) of HCG would be considered positive. Depending on the laboratory, you should be able to get the results the day of the test. After a positive test, HCG levels should *roughly* double every forty-eight hours until around the eighth week of pregnancy.

REAL VOICES
The very first time I got pregnant, I completely intuited it. I was getting dressed and I looked at myself in the mirror and I said, "I am pregnant." We'd only been trying about a month, but I just knew. I ran out and got a test, and sure enough I was. That was really strange because I don't think of myself as an incredibly intuitive person. The second time I figured it out quickly—because I tend to get a great deal of nausea during pregnancy. The third time, I had no idea. My kids were maybe six and ten. I had a very large fibroid—my doctor had even talked to me about having a hysterectomy about a month

earlier. One weekend I was really nauseous. I called a friend and said, "It's really weird, my fibroid is mimicking pregnancy symptoms." She said, "That's not possible," and came over with a pregnancy test. Such is the power of denial—delighted to have her but not really planning to.

Andrea, mom of three

I just always thought because I had never gotten pregnant, I must not be able to get pregnant. So I was shocked when it happened right away.

Asha, mom of one, pregnant

With the first pregnancy, I had no idea but took the test because my period, which was incredibly predictable, was a matter of a few hours late. When the test came out positive, I was completely surprised . . . I didn't think it could read a pregnancy on the same day my period was due. It's such an amazing feeling and so foreign, too.

Kate, mom of one, pregnant

• *Figuring out your due date:* Even though less than 5 percent of women deliver on their actual due date, figuring out a reasonably accurate due date is important. With it, a caregiver can assess your pregnancy's progress, and make better-informed decisions as delivery nears. Obstetricians and midwives typically use a wheel to calculate a due date; it matches up calendar dates with the 266 days of pregnancy. You can figure out your due date using something called Nagle's rule. If you have a twenty-eight-day cycle, add a year to the date of your last menstrual period (LMP), subtract three months, and add seven days. If you have a thirty-day cycle, add a year, subtract three months, and add nine days. (For example, if your LMP is October 1, and you have twenty-eight-day cycles, your due date would be July 8 of the next year. If you have thirty-day cycles, your due date would be July 10.) The due date you calculate may be a few days off from the one you get from your caregiver, because the "wheel" counts the actual number of days as opposed to rounding off by months like Nagle's rule.

If you don't know the date of your last menstrual period or you have very irregular periods, you'll probably need bloodwork and/or an ultrasound, depending on your situation, to help figure out when you're due. Newer, more sophisticated ultrasound machines can date a pregnancy as early as five weeks; these machines are mostly available in a hospital or a high-risk obstetrician's (perinatologist's) office.

You've Got Time

✦ If this is your first pregnancy, you may be feeling a little overwhelmed. Go ahead and set up a first prenatal appointment, and if you don't feel like talking to your doctor or midwife about their prenatal care philosophy or birthing practices now, simply wait until you're ready. Take time to get comfortable with the idea of being pregnant and gather information from books (you're off to a great start with this book!), Web sites, and other women you know who've recently had children.

Q: Why does my doctor say I'm about six weeks pregnant when I only found out I was pregnant a week and a half ago?

Dr. Evans: Modern obstetrics calculates forty weeks in a pregnancy, but in fact pregnancy is closer to thirty-eight weeks. Why the two-week difference? Since it's almost impossible to pinpoint exactly when a woman becomes pregnant, conventional practice tacks on two weeks to standardize pregnancy's length. Therefore, the first four weeks of your pregnancy include the two weeks before you actually conceived. As you read about pregnancy, you may come across references to embryonic age; because it's calculated from conception, it'll be two weeks behind the obstetric calendar.

Prenatal Caregivers:
Working with a Doctor or Midwife

Establishing the kind of relationship *you want* with your doctor or midwife is an important step toward caring for yourself and your growing baby. For some, this may mean finding a new caregiver or practice; others may not want to change caregivers or, because of insurance constraints, may not be able to.

Whether or not you're planning to change practitioners for your pregnancy, *when you feel ready,* take some time to figure out what's important to you in your prenatal care. (To help you get started, check out the list of questions on pages 79–80.) Then, set up a meeting with your current or new caregiver during which you can discuss the caregiver's prenatal philosophy to get a sense of how you can work together.

Going from Gyn to OB

✦ If you plan to use your longtime gynecologist or midwife during your pregnancy, keep in mind that routine gynecologic care is very different from prenatal care. This may seem odd, but once you shift into prenatal care, you may discover that you have different expectations of your caregiver or that your caregiver approaches you in a new way. Often women find themselves changing caregivers in their first pregnancy—either within a practice, or changing from a doctor to midwife or vice versa—even though they had not anticipated doing that while preparing for pregnancy. Whether you decide to go or stay, what's important is feeling empowered to get the kind of prenatal care you want.

If you're interviewing a potential practitioner, tell his administrative person when you call to set up the appointment that you'd like a preliminary prenatal interview. Find out what kind of coverage you have from your insurance carrier for this type of visit, and if it's limited, discuss the charges with the receptionist when you call to schedule the appointment.

Here are some questions to help you figure out your priorities in prenatal care. Use them as a blueprint for talking with your caregiver, interviewing a potential caregiver, or as a jumping-off point for yourself:

- *Questions about practical matters:*
  1. Is your practitioner's office close to where you work or where you live? Is it relatively easy for you to get there? Is the waiting room clean and comfortable?
  2. With what hospital or birthing center is the doctor or midwife associated? Is the facility relatively close to you? Is it a teaching hospital (which usually means the physicians are affiliated with a medical school and the hospital is equipped with the latest technology)? If so, ask if there will be medical students or residents (physicians-in-training) at your delivery. (*Note:* If you're interested in a home birth, it's important to establish what hospital will serve as your backup birthing location in order to create a contingency plan in case of emergency.)

3. Can you call in advance to find out if the office is running on schedule? When the doctor or midwife runs late (for example, if there's a delivery or emergency), how will the practice handle it?

4. What's the schedule for prenatal care visits and how long does each visit typically last? Do you prefer long or short visits? Do you like to get a lot of information and really talk with your care provider or would you rather be in and out? (If you prefer more time with your care provider, a midwife might be a better choice.)

5. Does the office take your insurance—or any insurance? If not, what are the financial policies? Do you pay up front for a pregnancy care package and then submit to your insurance company? Are you okay with the extra paperwork?

• *Questions for a prenatal caregiver (and yourself) about being pregnant:*

1. What do you think you want and need from your relationship with your care provider?

2. What makes you nervous about being pregnant and what are you comfortable with? For example, are you nervous about your body changing or what birth will be like? Can you talk about your concerns with your caregiver?

3. Do you exercise? Do you want to continue to exercise? What is your caregiver's opinion on exercise during pregnancy? (See chapter 14 for information on exercise during pregnancy.)

4. How involved do you want your partner to be in your prenatal care and delivery preparation? How involved does your partner want to be?

REAL VOICES
In my first pregnancy, I had mild preeclampsia and a C-section. That experience, and wanting to have a VBAC (vaginal birth after Cesarean), made me really want to enlist the OBs and midwives and get them to know me and my story in case anything happened, because my awareness that stuff can happen was heightened. So in my second pregnancy I was more aggressive in establishing what kind of relationship I wanted to have with them. I wanted them to be my advocates, and that really paid off in the end.

Jill, mom of two

From My Office

✦ Jennifer came to my office to interview me as a caregiver for her pregnancy. She had heard good things about me from other patients, but after visiting my Web site (*www.centerforwomenshealth.com*), she was concerned that I was too "alternative" for her. Would I force any "natural stuff" on her? Could she have an epidural? She said that her father was a physician, and she didn't trust the holistic approach.

We had a long discussion, during which I reassured her that I never force the women I work with into any treatments—conventional or alternative—and that she could have whatever kind of pain medication during labor she wanted.

As we were finishing, I politely asked what had given her such negative feelings about holistic medicine. Did she know someone who had a bad experience? Much to my surprise (and I think hers, too), Jennifer got a little teary. She explained that when she had first heard about my practice, she was excited by the possibility of a holistic approach to her prenatal care, but her father had filled her with dread about holistic medicine without explaining why. She then apologized for "wasting my time" and got up to leave. As she was gathering her things, I asked if she had time to talk a little more and then asked how she was feeling right at that moment. She said she was frustrated that her father's opinions had made her give up on her own enthusiasm and curiosity about holistic medicine. We then talked about how hard it can be to parent when your children have very different ideas from yours, and she described feeling excited about the chance to support, not dampen, her own child's interests and ideas.

Again she got up to leave, but this time she was clearly excited. As she herself said, she was excited about the possibilities of parenting, and a holistic approach to her pregnancy might be just the right thing for her as she follows the example she wants to set for her child—doing "what feels right."

• *Labor and birth:* These questions are meant to help you start thinking about your delivery, and they're here for you whenever you're ready for them. If you're newly pregnant, it may feel like it's too early to think about labor. It does come into play, however, when you're choosing a caregiver, because how she thinks about labor and birth will have a strong impact on your childbirth experience and, to some degree, your prenatal care. (For a full discussion of how to prepare for child-birth, see chapter 19. For a discussion of the stages of labor, turn to chapter 21.)

- *Questions for you about labor and birth*
  1. What image pops into your mind when you think about birth? Where are you? Who's with you?
  2. Are you worried about pain in labor? Do you have specific ideas about it, or do you feel confident when you think about it?
  3. What kind of support do you imagine getting from your partner during labor? Is it the support you want? Can you talk about it?
  4. How do you see your doctor or midwife's role in labor? Can you talk about your ideas and expectations with your care provider?

- *Questions for a doctor or midwife about labor and birth*
  1. How would you describe your role in labor?
  2. What kind of childbirth education do you recommend?
  3. What's your take on pain medication? Do you consider it routine? Do you look down on it? Do you offer it? Do you offer pain medication besides an epidural? At what point in labor would you give an epidural? (For a description of pain relief medication, turn to page 461.)
  4. How often do you perform Cesarean sections? (For a doctor.)
  5. How do you feel about a vaginal birth after a Cesarean (VBAC)?
  6. How often and under what circumstances do you induce labor?
  7. What's your episiotomy rate in first-time deliveries? Do you take any steps during labor, such as perineal stretching, to avoid them? Do you consider them routine or perform them as needed? (For more on episiotomies, see page 474.)
  8. How do you feel about working with a doula (professional labor assistant)? (See page 445.)

REAL VOICES

I changed from a doctor to a midwife when I found out I was pregnant, largely because I called up my doctor, and I wanted to make an appointment to make sure everything was okay. He was so blasé about the whole thing. He said, "Well, if the test says you're pregnant, I'm sure you're pregnant." I'm asking questions—like should I be eating anything different? Should I be doing anything? He said, "Well, if all you can get down is a strawberry milkshake, then just drink strawberry milkshakes." And I'm thinking: I can eat anything! I don't have nausea. I'm fine, but you're giving me no guidance! So I switched to a midwife and had a really good experience.

Rochelle, mom of three

• *Using complementary therapies in pregnancy:* If you're interested in using any complementary therapies during your pregnancy—especially herbal remedies—it's important that your doctor or midwife know. By talking it over first, you ensure that: (1) you've taken necessary precautions for yourself and your baby; (2) your prenatal caregiver knows about the variables that may affect your treatment; (3) you and your caregiver each have a better understanding of how the other feels about complementary therapies that may be considered unorthodox by the medical establishment.

Similarly, if you've been working with a complementary practitioner like an herbalist, acupuncturist, or chiropractor, talk with your caregiver about how these therapies have helped improve your health and well-being.

Here are some questions you could use to start a discussion with your prenatal caregiver about complementary therapies:

1. What's your take on complementary therapies? Are you open to using them? Which ones?
2. Are there specific circumstances under which you would be uncomfortable using a complementary approach? What are they?
3. If you've never tried something in your own practice, say using acupuncture for back pain or moxibustion to turn a breech baby (see page 430), would you be open to me trying it?
4. Will you consult with my complementary practitioner if necessary?
5. What, if any, are your general concerns?

Tip: Keep a little notebook handy to jot down questions for your caregiver as they pop into your head. By the time you get to an appointment, you may have forgotten what you wanted to ask, and no issue is too small to discuss.

Caregivers and Their Practices

Medical doctors

• *Obstetrician/gynecologist (ob-gyn):* These doctors are trained in women's health and pregnancy care. They may specialize in different aspects of women's health (not all gynecologists practice obstetrics). An obstetrician can manage both low-risk and, depending on the individual doctor, more complicated pregnancies. During labor, an obstetrician will check in with you periodically to see how you are progressing, until close to the delivery itself, when he will be there full-time.

• *Family practitioner (FP):* These doctors are trained in fields like primary care obstetrics and pediatrics. They care for whole families, and look at the interpersonal dynamics that affect the health of each member. A family practitioner is trained to manage uncomplicated, low-risk pregnancies.

• *Perinatologist:* Also known as high-risk specialists, perinatologists are ob-gyns who have gone through two to three additional years of training in order to manage more serious medical complications that may arise in the course of a "normal" pregnancy, or to care for women with high-risk pregnancies—for example, when a woman has a history of pregnancy complications, a preexisting

---

WHAT TO LOOK FOR

Whatever kind of caregiver you work with, and whatever kind of birth you're planning, here are some basics to keep in mind:

• *Experience:* When you meet with a caregiver—family practitioner, obstetrician, or midwife (see page 86)—ask how long he's been working and about how many babies he's delivered. If your caregiver is relatively inexperienced, ask if he has a more experienced professional partner or mentor, and what role this professional partner plays in his practice.

• *Responsiveness:* Every practice has emergency contact guidelines; make sure they're absolutely clear. You need to know how you can get in touch with your caregiver at all times, and how quickly you will typically get a callback.

• *Reliability:* You need to know that someone will be there for you when you need it. Whether you're working with a group or solo practitioner, find out how your caregiver will be covered in case she's unavailable.

medical condition, or a history of pregnancy loss. In addition to practicing obstetrics, they can perform special procedures, such as advanced anatomy ultrasound scans and amniocentesis. (See chapter 15 for test descriptions.) Often perinatologists function as consultants to OBs and family practitioners, offering additional expertise either in performing or interpreting the results of certain prenatal tests.

Practices

• *Solo practice:* The great advantage of a solo practitioner is the relationship that can develop between doctor and patient. The disadvantage is no doctor can be available 24/7, 365 days a year, so there's a chance your doctor won't be there for your labor. Typically, a solo practitioner will have a covering physician, whom you can meet if you choose, especially if your due date is around your doctor's scheduled vacation.

• *Group practice:* Any practice of two or more doctors is considered a group practice, but each group functions differently. Some allow you to select a primary OB, and then have you meet with every doctor in the practice at least once over the course of your pregnancy. Other groups have you see all the physicians for an equal number of visits. In most groups, your doctor for the delivery will be the doctor who is on call that day or night. A group of two doctors would typically provide a more intimate experience, closer to that of a solo practice.

• *Combination practice:* In these groups, midwives and doctors work together to provide general health and pregnancy care.

Q: I've heard if I'm over thirty-five, I'm automatically a "high-risk" patient. Is that true, and would I need to work with a high-risk obstetrician?

Dr. Evans: Technically speaking, a mother's age at the time of delivery is considered a risk factor in pregnancy. But there's a big difference between having a risk factor and being high-risk. If you are over thirty-five and in good health, there's no reason to think your pregnancy will be anything but low-risk. In my experience, most pregnancies progress smoothly regardless of a woman's age. A woman who's over thirty-five can choose to work with a midwife or doctor depending on her preference—not her age.

REAL VOICES
We had just moved, and I didn't have an OB. I got referred to a large practice, all women, and it was kind of impersonal. I was hoping for something a little more intimate, especially in my first pregnancy. But I just thought, "Okay,

I'll go with this." And then I was in the locker room in the gym one day and I heard a woman who was older, her kids are grown, raving about her OB, who's a male, who she said is just the most sensitive, warm person, and he's a solo practitioner. I got his number, and Alexander and I went to meet him, and we just loved him—and so we went with him.

Mary, mom of two

Midwives

• *Certified nurse midwife (CNM):* Certified nurse midwives are registered nurses who have received special training in general women's health care, prenatal care, and childbirth management. They're licensed in nursing and midwifery, and they have passed a national certification exam administered by the American College of Certified Nurse Midwives. Since 1999, certified midwifery programs require a bachelor's degree and confer a master's degree (68 percent of all midwives have master's degrees; 4 per-

---

Male Doctors, Women's Issues

Q: Do you feel as a man there are any barriers in treating women?

Dr. Evans: I'm always asked, "Do your patients have a problem with you being a man?" And the answer I always give is they don't because they've decided to see me. In reality, I don't think the fact that I've never given birth or had a Pap smear is important. Doctors and midwives often effectively treat patients experiencing a medical or physiological event that they have not experienced. To me, the emotional issues are more important than the physical questions. As a doctor, I need to be able to identify with my patients emotionally. For example, self-care is a constant theme in holistic medicine. I've experienced the struggles that come with trying to take care of yourself. I've faced loss and a major illness, and I've grappled with the issues that those circumstances brought up. So I can be effective talking with someone about the barriers they're facing with self-care, because I've faced some of those barriers myself. Ultimately, for doctors to help their patients, they must have not only professional expertise but also life experiences that they can draw on to relate to people emotionally.

cent have doctorates). They can provide primary gynecologic care as well as prenatal care, and typically manage low-risk pregnancies and deliveries in hospitals, birthing centers, or at home. Unlike a doctor, a midwife will stay with a laboring woman through her entire labor. They're trained to recognize developing emergencies and can manage them until help is available. A CNM works with a consulting doctor in the event of a serious complication, certain prenatal tests, or emergency.

Note: If you're working with a midwife either in a group practice or in a birthing center (see "Midwifery Practices," page 89), ask if you can meet with the consulting physician at some point in your pregnancy. That way, if there's a situation in which you need a doctor, she won't be a total stranger.

• *Certified midwife (CM):* A certified midwife has met the certification requirements established in 1996 by the North American Registry of Midwives. This means that a CM has passed the same certification exam as a CNM, but she's not a registered nurse. Since 1999, all CMs are required to have an undergraduate degree. CMs follow the same standards and practices established for CNMs, and a medical doctor will serve as a consultant in case of emergency. The designation CM is relatively new, and isn't yet accepted in all states. Check with your insurance company to see if CMs are covered in your state.

• *Direct entry (or lay) midwife:* Like a CM, a direct entry midwife (DEM) is not necessarily a nurse. Unlike a CM, she is neither certified nor regulated. DEMs do not have to use a medical doctor as a backup, but many do. In rural areas, where a medical doctor may not be close by, a DEM should have a working relationship with a doctor who's relatively close, which would speed the process of reach-

---

WHAT'S A DOULA?

There are two kinds of doulas: those who attend births and those who help women postpartum. A birth doula may also be known as a *professional labor assistant, labor support specialist,* or *labor companion.* She'll have been trained to support a woman and her partner during labor and childbirth, helping with breathing, relaxation, and massage, and providing support and advice throughout the entire labor. Studies have shown that having a birth doula present throughout labor results in fewer interventions, particularly in women who don't have other family members present. Postpartum doulas care for new mothers in their first days after giving birth. (For more on birth doulas, see page 445. For more on postpartum doulas, see page 505.)

Working with a Midwife

✦ An interview with Elizabeth Parr, CNM, coauthor of *Choosing a Nurse-Midwife* (John Wiley & Sons, New York, 1994) and faculty member of Philadelphia University's certificate program in nurse-midwifery.

Q: What's most important in choosing a prenatal care provider?

Elizabeth Parr: Whether you work with a midwife or an obstetrician, it's important that you feel comfortable and secure in the care you receive. First, you have to have confidence in the quality of the medical care; second, it's important to feel psychologically safe, especially as labor approaches. Depending on her practice, a midwife may be able to spend more time with a patient during each prenatal visit, partly because she may not have the same time constraints as a doctor, and also because a central value of the midwifery profession is developing a relationship with the client. This happens whether the midwife is lucky enough to know the client over the course of her pregnancy, or just meets her in labor, when a midwife would stay with a laboring woman throughout.

Q: Who can work with a midwife?

Elizabeth Parr: Midwives are trained to care for women having normal, low-risk pregnancies—over 90 percent of pregnancies. We're also trained to recognize and deal with complications should they arise. Depending on the situation, a midwife may continue to work with a woman who's developed a complication and co-manage her pregnancy with a consulting physician.

Q: What's the biggest misconception you regularly encounter about midwives?

Elizabeth Parr: Culturally in the U.S. we're not oriented toward working with midwives, so women don't have regular contact with what we do. For example, many women think working with a midwife means having a home birth or not using pain medication. In fact, most midwife-attended births occur in a hospital setting. Midwives are trained in the use of pain medication during labor, as well as having a large repertoire of natural comfort measures for labor.

ing a doctor in case of emergency. If you choose to work with a DEM, I would recommend that she be very experienced and have a consulting physician in place. (I've served as a consultant to both CNMs and DEMs.)

Midwifery practices
Certified nurse midwives and certified midwives are licensed to attend births in all fifty states and the District of Columbia. They have prescription-writing authority in forty-eight states, the District of Columbia, American Samoa, and Guam. As with doctors, a midwife may be in a solo or group practice. If you choose a group practice, as with doctors, you might have one primary midwife and meet the others intermittently, or you might see each midwife an equal number of times throughout your pregnancy. Birth-attending practices will likewise vary—in some practices "your" midwife will attend your birth, while in others, whoever is "on call" will be there.

Group midwifery practices with MD consultants typically staff birth centers associated with hospitals. Independent birth centers are most often owned and operated by a midwife or a midwifery practice and also offer MD consultants.

Questions to ask a midwife
While midwifery is thousands of years old, in the twentieth century it fell out of favor in the United States until the mid-1970s. Since 1975, the number of midwife-attended births has risen steadily. They now account for around 10 percent of all births in the U.S.; 96 percent of those births take place in a hospital setting. Here are additional questions to consider when interviewing a midwife about prenatal care (for a discussion of labor and birth, including creating a birth plan, see chapter 19):

1. If she's in solo practice: Who are your backup midwives? What kind of certification and experience does each have?
2. Who's your consulting physician? May we meet or are there practical constraints to that? Under what circumstances would you call for help from a doctor or would I consult with one? Do we make that decision together?
3. What kinds of tests are routine in your practice for someone my age? What if I want additional tests?
4. Do you ever co-manage pregnancies with a doctor? If complications develop, can I work with you and a doctor?
5. At what point in labor will you join me? Do you usually stay the whole time? What happens if you have more than one patient in labor?

6. How do you feel about pain medication? Can I have an epidural?
7. Can I work with you if I had a C-section in my first delivery?
8. Will you stay with me if I need a C-section?
9. Do you work with doulas?

Q: I just found out I'm having twins—can I still see my midwife?
Dr. Evans: If you're in good health and your midwife is experienced, there's no reason not to use a midwife in a twin pregnancy. That said, test results from twins, particularly in the third trimester, can be difficult to interpret. For this reason, I always co-manage twin pregnancies with a perinatologist. You may want to discuss the co-management option with your midwife.

Finding a caregiver

Just as you would in looking for any specialist, start looking for a prenatal care provider by gathering a list of names:

- Talk to women who have recently given birth—a friend, a friend of a friend, or a relative. Find out about their experience and if they would recommend the caregiver they worked with.
- Ask your doctor. If you see a general practitioner, or if your gynecologist no longer delivers babies, ask whom he recommends and why.
- If there's a birthing center that you're interested in, call and ask about their practice and if you can meet staff members and tour the facility.
- If there's a nearby hospital that you've heard about or that's known for its birthing facility, call and ask for a list of doctors and midwives associated with it.
- To find a midwife, you may turn to professional organizations. The American College of Nurse-Midwives (*www.midwife.org/find*) is a professional organization for CNMs and CMs. Midwives Alliance of North America (*www.mana.org*) includes direct-entry midwives in its membership and listings.

8

First Things: Early Prenatal Care

When you'll have a first prenatal visit depends on the practice you work with. You may have a visit right after you call to say you're pregnant, or you may have it at eight or twelve weeks. No matter what week you end up going in, the basics of the care and the information you receive should be fairly consistent. Here I discuss what you can expect to happen, why, and the first steps you can take in prenatal self-care.

◆ ◆ ◆

In this chapter you'll find:

- • What Happens at a First Prenatal Visit?
  - – Bloodwork
  - – Genetic counseling
- • First Steps: Lifestyle Changes for Early Pregnancy
  - – Foods to moderate
  - – Foods to avoid
  - – Alcohol
  - – Recreational drugs
  - – Smoking

What Happens at a First Prenatal Visit?

During the first prenatal visit, you'll have a physical exam and give blood and urine samples. The urine sample will be tested for sugar levels, protein, and bacteria which can lead to a urinary tract infection, a very common problem in pregnancy. Your blood will be analyzed for its type, immunities, and certain diseases (see "Bloodwork" below). You'll also begin to get to know your caregiver in the context of your pregnancy.

If you're seeing a new caregiver, she'll take a complete medical history of you, your family, and the father. You'll then have a full physical exam including a Pap smear. (I do a Pap smear if it's been more than three months from a woman's last Pap.) You'll also be weighed and have your blood pressure taken. (For a description of what happens at each prenatal visit and why, see chapter 15.)

Note: In my practice, the first "official" prenatal visit is at eight weeks. But when a woman calls to say she's had a positive pregnancy test or suspects she's pregnant, we have her come in within the next two days for what we call a "pre-OB" visit. This appointment lasts about fifteen minutes. We calculate her due date based on her last menstrual period, then we may take a blood test to make sure that her hormone levels (specifically HCG and progesterone) are where we'd expect them to be based on when she last menstruated. This is very important if she's miscarried or if her periods tend to be irregular. At the end of the pre-OB visit, we briefly review foods that are important and those she needs to avoid (see page 98). We have a more thorough discussion of nutrition during pregnancy at the eight-week visit.

Bloodwork

The blood drawn at a first prenatal visit will be analyzed for its type and, depending on your history, the following:

- *Immunity to German measles* (aka rubella): Even if you were vaccinated for German measles as a child, you need this test because the vaccine can become less effective over time, and the illness is very dangerous to a developing fetus.
- *Immunity to chicken pox* (aka varicella): Your blood may also be tested for immunity to chicken pox. If you've had chicken pox or even been exposed to it by coming

in contact with someone who had it, you are likely to be immune and may not need the test. If you can't remember if you've had chicken pox or if you're in regular contact with small children, let your caregiver know, because your immunity should be tested.

Note: If you're not immune to either virus, your provider will review basic precautions you can take, such as checking with the parents of small children to see if they've recently been exposed to either virus and always washing your hands before and after spending time with small children.

• *Rh factor:* Your blood will be tested for a protein known as Rh. If you have it, your blood is considered "Rh positive"; if not, it's "Rh negative." Most women (and men) are Rh positive (if you know your blood type and it's "positive," as in B positive, then you're Rh positive). But if an Rh-negative woman is carrying an Rh-positive child (which is likely since most people are Rh positive), then her blood is incompatible with her baby's. If mother and baby's blood mingle, a common event during labor, then the mother's blood could become "Rh sensitized." This wouldn't affect the baby she's giving birth to, but in a subsequent pregnancy with an Rh-positive baby, a mother's immune system would attack the fetus's blood. This can be prevented by an injection of an immunizing drug called Rh immunoglobulin, which is typically given around twenty-eight weeks and then again within three days of a full-term delivery or miscarriage or abortion.

• *Antibody screen:* There are certain antibodies that could endanger the pregnancy. These are usually, but not always, the result of previous blood transfusions. If they are present, a pregnancy is closely monitored for danger signs, particularly as labor nears.

• *Transmittable diseases:* The blood sample will be tested for type and then run through a standard set of screens that include anemia, sickle-cell anemia, hepatitis, syphilis, and HIV.

Genetic counseling

If you didn't have a chance to discuss genetic testing with your caregiver before you conceived, you'll talk it over during your first prenatal visit. Certain families and ethnic and racial groups have a higher incidence of specific genetic disorders, which are passed to a fetus by either a recessive or dominant gene. When a *recessive* gene carries a condition, then both parents have to carry the gene for the fetus to have an increased risk. When a *dominant* gene carries a condition, the disease will be passed on

An Eight-week Ultrasound

✦ At an eight-week prenatal visit, you may have a transvaginal ultrasound (also known as a sonogram). If you don't have an ultrasound at eight weeks, it's likely you'll be offered a transabdominal ultrasound between weeks 16 and 20. (For more on ultrasounds, see page 303.) To perform the test, a long, fairly narrow wand (a transducer probe) is inserted into the vagina. It transmits inaudible sound waves that bounce off the uterus and the baby to make an image—a sonogram. At eight weeks, a sonogram can detect a fetal heartbeat and confirm a due date based on the size of the embryo and the pregnancy sac.

Not everyone has transvaginal sonograms in the first trimester (while safe and standard in some practices, they're expensive and not always covered as part of routine early pregnancy care). You might have one if you don't know when you last menstruated, because the results of the sonogram can help date the pregnancy. You'd also have a sonogram if you have spotting or bleeding (as about 20 percent of women do in their first trimester; see "Spotting," page 123). Finally, if you became pregnant after in vitro fertilization or if your pregnancy is considered high risk, your pregnancy will be closely monitored until around ten weeks, and you're likely to have at least two sonograms in that time.

if only one parent (and it could be *either* parent) carries the gene. However, even if only one person in a couple is a member of one of these groups, it's worth being tested on the off chance that both are carriers for the same disease.

If you and your partner *both* test positive for one of these conditions, it doesn't mean that your child will automatically have the condition. It only means that there is an increased risk for it. (For example, if both parents are carriers of the Tay-Sachs gene, there's a 25 percent chance the child will be affected.) If this is the case, you'll meet with a genetic counselor to get a clearer picture of your situation.

Blood tests are usually given to those of Eastern-European Jewish descent (primarily for Tay-Sachs, but also for several other diseases), Mediterranean and Latino descent (for a type of anemia called thalassemia), and African-Americans (for sickle-cell anemia). *All couples* should be tested for the gene that carries cystic fibrosis, which is more prevalent among Caucasians. (For more information about these genetic tests, see pages 16–18.)

Pregnancy and Survivors of Childhood Sexual Abuse

✦ If you are a survivor of childhood sexual abuse, pregnancy and childbirth may present many challenging, and potentially healing, moments. Simply being pregnant—managing your shifting hormones, making changes to your diet, experiencing a rapidly changing body—can lead to feeling out of control. It can also bring aspects of your past that you've dealt with back to the surface in new ways. These reactions can offer new insights into your emotional world, but they can be very difficult. Having to work with and trust a medical authority figure—a doctor or midwife—can be difficult in and of itself, since an authority figure may be the least trustworthy person for you. And the medical aspects of pregnancy, such as blood tests, weigh-ins, and labor and childbirth itself, can trigger a flood of difficult memories or fears.

While it's impossible to anticipate how you'll respond to pregnancy, it's important to try to stay connected with all the emotional changes you may be experiencing. Just like it's important to listen to your body throughout pregnancy, and identify what feels "off," it's equally important to pay attention to the emotional signals you may be getting. Allow yourself to name what's going on. Be compassionate with yourself in every way you can, and take the time and space you need to take care of yourself. If it's appropriate for you, seek help from an experienced therapist or a support group.

If you feel safe with your caregiver, share your history and your concerns—it may be helpful in ways you don't anticipate. (For example, when working with a survivor of childhood abuse, I try to shift the language I use during labor and childbirth to give her more control.) Whether or not you wish to share your history with your caregiver, bring a support person with you to your office visits. He or she can probably stay in the room with you while you're being examined and during any conversation you choose to have with your caregiver about your past. As your pregnancy progresses and you begin to prepare for birth, think carefully about who you want present when you're in labor, who will help you feel safe, supported, and loved as you welcome your child to the world.

First Steps: Lifestyle Changes for Early Pregnancy

During the first trimester, your baby is growing by leaps and bounds; this is when organogenesis, or organ development, takes place. (For details of fetal development, see chapter 10.) With essential growth happening daily, it's important to try to eat as clean a diet as you can, and limit toxins by not drinking or smoking. (For a discussion of how to limit your exposure to environmental toxins throughout pregnancy, see pages 320–328.)

Foods to moderate

• *Caffeine:* There's an ongoing debate over how much, if any, caffeine is safe in pregnancy. As with sugar, moderation is the key. If you have to have that first cup of coffee in the morning, go ahead and drink it guilt-free. Simply limit your overall caffeine consumption (including the caffeine in tea, colas, and chocolate) to about 300 mg, the equivalent of two brewed eight-ounce cups of coffee, per day. In large doses, caffeine can interfere with the absorption of iron and calcium, plus it's a diuretic, and during pregnancy you need more fluid. (For a chart of caffeine in foods and drinks, see pages 239–240.)

• *Processed sugar:* During pregnancy, it's important to eat a balanced diet, doing your best to ensure that the foods you eat are nutritious. Sweet foods are typically high in calories and low in nutrients, so while there's no reason to deny yourself cookies or chocolate, it's a good idea to try to be moderate in your portions and how often you eat sweets. (For more on food, diet, and nutrition during pregnancy, see chapter 13.)

Note: Many of the women I work with find keeping a food journal for a short period of time a helpful way to identify and adjust trends in their eating habits. For more on keeping a food journal, see pages 217–218.

Red Raspberry Leaf and Pregnancy-Blend Tea

✦ We offer the women we work with an herb tea blend to support their pregnancies. The tea is made up of red raspberry leaf, squaw vine, nettle leaf, alfalfa, oat straw, lemon balm, spearmint, and burdock root.

Red raspberry leaf is the foundation of this blend. It's high in vitamin C, potassium, and other nutrients; it can help soothe nausea; and it's thought to tone the uterus (that is, help it work more efficiently). You can drink red raspberry leaf tea daily, combine it with some of the herbs listed above, or mix the complete blend. Here's a rundown of what each element is known for:

- *Red raspberry leaf* and *squaw vine* both strengthen and tone the muscles of the uterus.
- *Nettle leaf* and *alfalfa* are both rich in important vitamins and minerals. Alfalfa helps balance the stomach's pH (alkaline) levels, keeping acid levels in check. Nettle leaf helps maintain normal fluid balance and prevent bloating.
- *Oat straw* and *lemon balm* both soothe the nerves. Lemon balm also aids digestion and eases nausea.
- *Spearmint* adds flavor and relieves nausea and vomiting.
- *Burdock root* helps digestion.

To make: For a simple daily serving of red raspberry leaf tea, mix one teaspoon per eight-ounce cup of cold filtered or spring water in a glass, porcelain, or stainless steel pot. Heat until the water just begins to boil, remove from heat, cover with a tight-fitting lid, and allow to steep for fifteen minutes. Strain the tea and reheat it slowly on the stovetop (do not microwave), or drink it cold.

To make a batch of tea: Mix one to two tablespoons of herbs with a quart of cold filtered or spring water. Follow the instructions above. The tea will keep for up to two days in the fridge. You can drink up to four eight-ounce cups of red raspberry leaf tea daily.

Note: If you notice that you feel at all "off" after drinking an herb tea, stop drinking it. Purchase organic wild-crafted herbs at a reputable health food store or Web site and store them in airtight containers in a cool, dark cabinet. (For recommendations of herbal sources and a pregnancy tea blend, turn to Resources, page 521)

(Richard Mandelbaum consulted on the uses of herbal medicine throughout this book. The tea blend described here was created by herbalist Kimberly DuBois.)

Foods to avoid

For a discussion of foods to avoid throughout pregnancy, see pages 246–248.

Q: I've heard some herb teas aren't safe during pregnancy. What's the story?

Dr. Evans: Pregnant women should avoid *medicinal doses* of some common herbs, like lemongrass, rosemary, and basil. What comprises a medicinal dose varies depending on the herb, but small amounts, such as those used in cooking or in teas bought in the supermarket, are safe. Similarly with peppermint oil—medicinal-strength peppermint oil should be avoided, but peppermint tea is absolutely safe to drink and soothing for nausea. Drink up to four eight-ounce cups daily.

I would avoid teas that are given for a specific reason or a nonpregnancy–related condition, like ginseng or St. John's wort, unless you're under the care of an experienced herbalist who's in contact with your doctor or midwife. Herbal teas that are safe for treating pregnancy-related discomforts are included in chapter 11.

Alcohol

Throughout pregnancy, but especially during the first trimester, you can think of your body as a space that needs to be kept clean by limiting the toxins that enter it. Giving up alcohol is an important step in that process. No one knows how much, or how little, alcohol can affect a growing baby during the first trimester. Studies have shown that two alcoholic drinks in a row or in the same day (one drink = 1.5 ounces of hard alcohol, one twelve-ounce beer, or one five-ounce glass of wine) can have a negative effect on a developing fetus. Certainly, heavy drinking in pregnancy is damaging. Children of women who drink excessively during their pregnancies are at risk for fetal alcohol syndrome (FAS); a child with FAS could be small, fail to thrive after birth, and/or have a small or abnormally shaped brain and/or facial abnormalities.

Because there's no information about how little alcohol will interfere with proper embryonic development, it's best to give it up entirely during the first trimester.

In the second and third trimesters, I feel it's acceptable to have an *occasional* drink (*one* glass of wine or beer with a meal every one to two weeks). This is what I advise the women I work with, and what I suggested to my wife when she was pregnant with our two children, but there's no scientific evidence to support this.

Note: Approximately 50 percent of pregnancies are unplanned. Therefore, some women worry immediately because they had a big night out and drank before they knew they were pregnant. This is not a cause for great concern. However, as soon as you find out you're pregnant, it's important to stop drinking.

> REAL VOICES
>
> I'm embarrassed to say that I drank a few tequila shots and smoked some cig-
> arettes at a party before I knew I was pregnant. Once I knew I was having a
> baby, I stopped caffeine, drinking, everything . . . except the occasional glass
> of red wine!
>
> Jennifer, mom of one

Recreational drugs

Smoking marijuana before you conceive hasn't been shown to harm a fetus. But whether you look at it holistically or conventionally, when you smoke marijuana, you breathe in toxins, something you want to avoid at all times, and especially when you're pregnant.

While there have been no major studies of the effects of marijuana once you're pregnant, some studies suggest that regularly smoking pot during pregnancy puts you and your baby at risk for serious complications such as premature labor.

If you're struggling with an addiction to illegal drugs and use them during pregnancy, it's unfortunately likely that your child will be addicted when she's born. In addition to addiction, heroin, cocaine, crack, LSD, and PCP can cause, among other things, miscarriage, stillbirth, complicated labor, mental retardation, low birth weight and failure to gain weight after birth, premature labor, and can increase the risk of sudden infant death syndrome (SIDS).

Smoking

After more than twenty years of research into smoking and pregnancy, there's no doubt that smoking is bad for you and bad for a developing baby. Smoking increases the risk of miscarriage, preterm delivery (see page 363), and placental abruption (when the placenta separates from the uterus prematurely; see page 349 for details). Nicotine reduces blood flow to the fetus, and carbon monoxide reduces the amount of oxygen the fetus receives, meaning that the children of women who smoke have an increased risk of low birth weight, which in turn increases the risk of other serious complications for a newborn. There's more: A recent study conducted at Brown University Medical School showed that the newborns of women who smoke six cigarettes a day throughout pregnancy seem to suffer from nicotine withdrawal. The newborns are tense, hard to soothe, and need more handling to rest calmly. There's no doubt that from a health perspective, it's now crucial to quit smoking as quickly as you can—for your own safety and your child's.

If you smoke, talk to your caregiver about safe, effective ways to quit during pregnancy. Everybody is different. Some women can quit cold turkey; others succeed by tapering off over the course of a week or two; still others find hypnosis helpful. The jury is still out on the safety of nicotine patches and gum, but they're better than smoking since they have no carbon monoxide and fewer chemicals than cigarette smoke. If you think using either will help you quit faster, talk it over with your doctor or midwife.

The good news about quitting: If you quit in the first trimester—the earlier the better—you can significantly reduce the risks smoking poses to your baby and yourself. In fact, when you quit in the first trimester, the risks to the baby are the same as for the baby of a nonsmoker.

Note: Secondhand smoke is just as dangerous to you, a developing fetus, and a newborn baby. If your partner smokes, he or she should quit when you become pregnant. If that isn't possible, ask that your partner not smoke in the house, in the car, or anywhere around you and/or the baby.

Q: I got pregnant unexpectedly and take Prozac. Is it safe to keep taking it?

Dr. Evans: Prozac was the first of a group of antidepressants known as SSRIs (selective serotonin reuptake inhibitors) that are now widely prescribed. Of all the SSRIs (they include the drugs Paxil, and Zoloft), Prozac is generally considered the best understood and safest to use in pregnancy. Whether or not you should continue taking Prozac, or a different antidepressant, is a personal decision you need to make after talking with your psychiatrist and obstetrician. If your antidepressant is

---

Creating a Smoke-free Routine

✦ No matter what technique you use or how motivated you are, it's very, very hard to quit smoking. Smoking is not only an addiction, but also a habit—when and where you smoke may be deeply ingrained into your daily routine. Taking steps to change your routine can be a small but powerful addition to any smoking-cessation plan you're following. For example, if you always come home from work, sit in the same chair, and have a cigarette, don't sit there. Don't even stay in when you get home. Instead go for a walk around the block. Walk slowly and savor each breath. When you get home, sit in a different spot, a different room—or even rearrange the furniture. If you're at work and you're ready for a cigarette break, try to either go for a brisk walk or find a place to do a simple belly breathing exercise. (See page 63 for a description.)

You know best how you can shake up your own habits. What can be hard is actually recognizing a habit for what it is—something you're used to as opposed to something you need.

---

prescribed by your GP, talk to her about your situation or ask for a referral to a psychiatrist who has experience working with pregnant women.

Q: Is it safe to continue taking St. John's wort now that I'm pregnant?

Dr. Evans: If you've been taking St. John's wort, you need to evaluate how well you're feeling when deciding whether or not to continue taking it. You also need to discuss your situation with your doctor or midwife. There isn't much data on the use of St. John's wort during pregnancy. Personally, I'd recommend tapering off St. John's wort and taking up to three grams (3,000 milligrams) of DHA, an omega-3 essential fatty acid that's been shown to help stabilize mood in general and improve depression in particular.

Q: Is it okay to take Advil in the first trimester?

Dr. Evans: Advil, and any other drug whose active ingredient is ibuprofen, ideally should *not* be taken at all during pregnancy or while trying to conceive. Instead, take two regular or extra-strength acetaminophen (Tylenol) tablets. If the acetaminophen doesn't work, talk with your caregiver about trying ibuprofen or another remedy, but don't take it without consulting with your caregiver first. Ibuprofen has been linked to miscarriage early in pregnancy and labor complications in the third trimester.

Note: Because organs and limbs develop throughout the first trimester, when it comes to taking over-the-counter (OTC) medication or herbal or homeopathic remedies, I counsel women to err on the side of caution and avoid taking anything for minor aches and pains. (This doesn't apply to women taking prescription medication for an ongoing condition.) That doesn't mean you can't take some acetaminophen for a headache or to lower a fever. It simply means to be careful, conscious, and cautious in your choices. (For more on herbs and medications that are safe, and those that must be avoided during pregnancy, see chapter 12.)

Q: I had acupuncture for some pain in my neck a few days before I found out I was pregnant. Is that okay? Can I keep going?

Dr. Evans: The treatment you had shouldn't affect your pregnancy. Acupuncture is safe throughout pregnancy, and it's useful for treating many pregnancy-related symptoms, but talk to your acupuncturist about continuing your treatment now that you're pregnant. There are some acupuncture points that can cause premature labor, and not all acupuncturists are comfortable working with pregnant women. The same holds true for shiatsu, a form of Japanese massage that also uses pressure points. It's safe, but the practitioner needs to know you're pregnant as well as what points to avoid during pregnancy.

Q. I just found out I'm pregnant, and I have a massage scheduled next week. A friend told me I should cancel. Should I? Is it safe to have a massage in the first trimester?

Dr. Evans: Absolutely keep the appointment! Massage is safe throughout pregnancy. In fact, a massage can help relieve pregnancy-related nausea in the first trimester. Just let your massage therapist know you are pregnant, and don't be shy about letting her know if the massage is too deep or intense. If you've gotten massages before, you may respond differently to touch now that you're pregnant. If your massage therapist uses aromatherapy oils, or if you're feeling nauseated, ask if she would use either an unscented oil (in case the scent triggers worsening nausea or vomiting) or an oil known to be safe and mixed appropriately for a pregnant woman. (See box, page 103.)

Later in pregnancy, when your abdomen is bigger, you can have a massage either on a special table that has a cut-out area for your stomach, or on your side supported by pillows. The latter is likely to be more comfortable, because the uterine ligaments can be strained when your belly hangs down.

Essential Oils and Aromatherapy in Pregnancy

✦ Essential oils are used in two ways: (1) rubbed on the skin in massage oil; (2) as pure aromatherapy, when the oil is heated (such as over a candle or an electric device) and doesn't touch the body. When essential oils are used in pregnancy, compounds in the oil may get into the bloodstream and cause harm. This is a greater concern with massage, since the skin will absorb more of the oil than the nose, but the worry doesn't disappear entirely with aromatherapy. Therefore, it's important to be cautious. While there haven't been any clinical trials in the obstetrical medical literature on the use of essential oils in pregnancy, it's discussed in nursing and midwifery literature. In fact, a recent survey of midwives in North Carolina showed that over 32 percent used aromatherapy with their pregnant patients.

For prenatal massage, essential oils should be mixed at a concentration that's about half the standard usage, or three to five drops of essential oil to each ounce of carrier oil.

Here are the oils that are likely to be safe when used for prenatal massage and those that should be avoided:

Popular essential oils to avoid in prenatal massage
Note: The primary concern with these oils is that they can trigger uterine contractions. For this reason, midwives and other practitioners may use them during labor.

Rosemary	Basil
Thyme	Juniper
Peppermint	Oregano
Pennyroyal	

Essential oils that are considered safe for prenatal massage

Rose	Tangerine
Lavender	Neroli
Chamomile	Ylang Ylang
Jasmine	

9

The Emotional and Physical World of Early Pregnancy

There are as many emotional and physical responses to pregnancy as there are women—feelings can run the gamut from joy and excitement to trepidation and anxiety. Likewise, symptoms can range from the minor to the persistent. There's no one way you're supposed to feel—emotionally or physically—but there are all sorts of things you might feel.

◆ ◆ ◆

In this chapter you'll find:

- The Ups and Downs of Early Pregnancy
  - Telling your partner the news
  - Emotional patterns
- Typical First Trimester Symptoms
  - Breast changes and tenderness
  - Constipation
  - Cramps
  - Depressed mood or mood swings
  - Excess saliva
  - Fatigue
  - Lack of libido
  - Food aversions, cravings, and appetite changes

- Nausea, vomiting, and sensitivity to smells ("morning sickness")
- Spotting or bleeding
- Urinary frequency

The Ups and Downs of Early Pregnancy

Even with the delight the news of pregnancy brings, some women describe early pregnancy as an emotional roller coaster. On a purely physical level, the body is producing more hormones than ever before, and they can affect everything—your mood, energy level, appetite. You may find you feel wonderful one minute, and the next you're weeping because you can't find your car keys.

Sometimes, the women I work with are surprised when they feel ambivalent or apprehensive about a pregnancy (even a long-planned one). These are feelings they think of as "negative" or "inappropriate." But having a child means going through enormous changes—many of them wonderful, a few of them, frankly, less appealing. It only makes sense that your emotional responses could run the gamut from thrill to fear and back. As your body slows down in the first trimester, give yourself a chance to slow down emotionally as well. Let yourself experience your emotions on their own terms and try to avoid judging whether you "should" or "shouldn't" feel whatever it is you're feeling.

Telling your partner the news

Whether you take a pregnancy test alone or with your partner, at some point, you'll tell your partner either that you think you're pregnant or that you are. No matter how he or she learns of it, whether you are both in the bathroom staring at the pregnancy test or you ceremoniously pour sparkling apple cider for a toast to your baby, the news of your pregnancy is momentous, marking a major milestone in the life-long journey two people take together.

But the fact that *two* people are doing this can spark some friction along with joy. You and your partner may respond very differently to the news. For example, your partner, who has not experienced any symptoms yet, may need time, or a test result from a doctor, to feel like the pregnancy is "real." Or you may be worried about miscarrying, while your partner is busy investigating college savings plans. The point is that each of you will have your own response in your own time—and it's important to let each other have the space to feel whatever comes up, while at the same time finding a way to meet each other's emotional needs. While you're each adjusting to the news, make time to spend together—to take a walk or just lie around and talk about what you're each feeling: hope, fear, joy, anxiety, exhilaration—whatever it is.

If you already have children, you and your partner will have to decide when to tell them. Kids don't keep secrets, so once you tell them, everybody else in your life (and even some people you didn't realize were in your life) will know pretty soon, too.

REAL VOICES
I knew something was strange when my nipples were unusually hard one day. I took a pregnancy test at work, without telling my husband, Dan. When Dan picked me up from work, he called up from the security desk to my office to tell me that he was in the building and I just blurted out: "I am pregnant." Dan shared soon after that he was thrilled but thought that maybe there was a more romantic way to share that news. I was shocked and terrified, though—we'd only had unprotected sex once—and I needed to tell him immediately.

Katie, mom of one

I knew right away that I was pregnant (the second time). I was very happy about it, but it was a little surprising because I had just started a business, my husband and I had been married less than a year, and it was sooner than we had planned. We were like, "Oh my god! It's happening!" My husband had just started a new job and he was sort of in disbelief. He said, "Oh, we have to wait until we go to the doctor." And I said, "The tests are 99.9 percent accurate." It was a little frustrating actually, but after a couple of days, he realized it was true. I think he was just sort of scared.

Shawn, mom of two

Emotional patterns

As wide-ranging as the emotional responses to pregnancy are, my colleagues and I have noticed some common reactions among the women we work with during their first trimesters. Here are a few of them:

• *Mixed feelings:* You may be caught off guard by your ambivalence or even lack of feeling about being pregnant. It may be hard to connect your physical symptoms (which may be very mild) with having a baby or motherhood. Or you may find that because you feel bad physically (tired, nauseated), you feel resentful of the baby, and

Keeping a Journal

✦ If you can, take time out of your regular schedule to focus on what's going on inside of you. Keeping a journal of your emotional journey—for no one to read but yourself—is a wonderful way to do this. On those pages, you can really let down your guard and say whatever you want without feeling judged or fearing that you'll hurt someone (like your partner, your mother, your best friend, or, down the road, your child). Set aside a half hour at intervals that are reasonable for you (daily, three times a week, every Sunday) and at a time of day when you know you can be undisturbed.

We often think of a journal as something written, but it can take many forms. You can write, but you can also draw pictures or create collages. Or you may notice that you want to listen to—or if you play an instrument, play—different types of music as your pregnancy progresses. Take notes on what your ear is craving. Whatever medium you choose—words, images, music—gives you a window into your emotional world. Use it to learn about your pregnant life.

then guilty about feeling resentful! If you have been trying to get pregnant for a while, you may be surprised that your excitement is tinged with ambivalence. Any of these is a "normal" response to a complex situation.

REAL VOICES

I didn't feel ready to get pregnant when I did. It happened the second month we tried, and I was expecting it to take a year. I talked to my husband a little bit about it, but it was hard for him to understand. He was beside himself with excitement—but it affects men differently. His body's not changing; he doesn't have the hormonal ups and downs; he's not going to be judged at work except in a positive way. So he sympathized, but he didn't quite get it. Mostly I reached out to girlfriends. As it turned out, six of my very good friends from college were all pregnant and all had babies within two months of each other, which was kind of weird but an amazing support.

Suzanne, mom of two

• *Anxiety about changes in your life:* While you may not know exactly how your life will change with a baby, you know it will change, and even though you want to have

Uncertain Times

✦ One of the most challenging (and wonderful) aspects of being pregnant is that you simply don't know what's going to happen. Even though we often assume we know what the future holds, more often than not we don't, and pregnancy brings that uncertainty into sharper focus. You can look at this as an invitation to develop a way of believing—in yourself, the universe, God—that acknowledges life's uncertainty but suspends some of the anxiety and allows you to fully experience, and rejoice in, your life now.

When I work with a pregnant woman, especially if she or someone she's close to has had a difficult experience such as a miscarriage or a serious illness, I try to help her to cultivate a more accepting attitude toward life's uncertainties by shifting her focus toward what each day brings and away from what happened in the past or what may happen in the future. How we can be comforted in the face of the unknown is one of life's great questions—and an important issue to think about as we journey into parenthood. Finding an answer is a very personal project that warrants taking time to investigate what feels right for you. It may be praying in an organized religious service, creating a daily ritual upon waking up or going to sleep, repeating an affirmation throughout the day (such as "I trust in the universe and that all will be as it should"), or meditating (see page 67). The point is to set aside time to acknowledge where you are right now and find comfort for what concerns you about the future.

a baby, you may not want your life to change just yet. Maybe you've started a new job or an exciting new project at work and you're concerned about having the energy to complete it. Maybe you and your partner have planned a big trip and you're worried you won't be able to go. (Odds are you will; see page 317 for travel during pregnancy.) Or maybe you're simply worried about what it'll be like to live with a baby.

REAL VOICES
I was very self-conscious at my job and worried that I might not be holding my own. I missed a few days of work, which was unlike me. Fortunately, I was able to function in meetings, but if they lasted more than forty-five minutes, I would become more nauseous, and I'd get nervous if I wasn't able to snack.

Then there were times where I would just sit at my desk and stare at the computer . . . doing nothing because I couldn't focus. Overall, I managed, but I didn't give any more than I needed to.

Beth, pregnant

I had only been at my job for four or five months when I got pregnant, so all of a sudden I was like, wait a minute—it'll be just a year that I've been at this job and then I'm having this baby and how does that reflect upon me as an employee? Do I get put into that mommy track now? How will this affect me as an employee? How will I tell my boss . . . All those things went through my head. Confusing is I guess the right way to put it.

Suzanne, mom of two

• *Changing body image:* While you're pregnant, your body will change dramatically—and those changes can provoke anxiety or bad feelings. Many women we work with are concerned that they'll look "fat" while they're pregnant, that their partners will no longer find them attractive, and that their bodies won't return to "normal" afterward.

Your body will change during your pregnancy and afterward. But change can mean so many different things. When you eat a well-balanced, healthy diet, your body will gain the weight it needs and you'll lose weight after you give birth. (For a rundown of where pregnancy weight goes, see page 243.) If you're very concerned about changes to your body, I'd recommend talking with a therapist who specializes in food-related issues. Likewise, if you're very concerned about your relationship, individual or couples counseling may help.

REAL VOICES
One thing that people did that drove both me and my husband crazy was constantly "warn" us about taking advantage of our sleep and our free time and all of that before the baby came along. People kept saying how our lives would change and we should appreciate the freedom before we lost it, yadda, yadda. It was so annoying! Nobody said how—despite the drastic change in lifestyle—amazing it would be and all of the good things that were to come.

Kate, mom of one, pregnant

When I found out I was pregnant, it just was surreal to me—you know, the idea of pregnancy is so abstract if you haven't really gone through it. I couldn't relate to what it meant because it was so new. Then it began:

What's this going to mean for my life? Is it going to change my relationship? How is it going to impact my body? How is it going to impact my self-identity? Answering those kinds of questions was a major process for me not just over the nine months of being pregnant but also, I'd say, the first nine months of having my child.

Lisa, mom of one

Tall Tales

✦ For some reason, when people find out you're pregnant, they think they can tell you any horrible pregnancy or labor tale. I'm not sure what makes people tell pregnant women these stories, but in our practice we've seen how they can contribute to the normal anxiety of a newly pregnant woman. Keep in mind that these stories circulate because they are the *exceptions,* not the rule. No one tells you about a first cousin's best friend who had a straightforward pregnancy and delivery—why would they? It happens every day.

• *Fear of childbirth:* From very early on, many of the women we work with express concern about the physical demands of childbirth. Often, in the back of a woman's mind is the idea that a woman can die in childbirth. This is true, but it's very, very rare in developed countries. An experienced caregiver (doctor or midwife) can help you maintain a healthy pregnancy, give birth, and prevent tragedy. However, talking with your caregiver about any fears you may have about labor is useful because it gives your caregiver a chance to better understand your needs, and it'll help you establish a venue to work through your fears over the course of your pregnancy, so you can approach childbirth with excitement rather than trepidation. (For more on preparing for childbirth, see chapter 19.)

• *Questions about motherhood:* Aside from the physical challenges, being pregnant means becoming a mother, a thrilling, and possibly unnerving, idea. Many women I work with talk about wanting to parent differently from their own mothers. They start to see their pregnancies as a time to develop more insight into their relation-

---

From My Office

✦ The question of how to parent can come up strongly both for women who are newly pregnant and for those trying to conceive. I run mind-body groups for women dealing with infertility. (See chapter 6.) One exercise we do is to draw a family tree (the relationships on these trees are familial, not genetic) to get a picture of how each woman sees her extended family, its relationships, and her place in it. After doing the drawing, Elizabeth saw that what she had always thought of as individual feuds were actually a pattern of severe rifts between all the women in her family—mothers and daughters as well as sisters—including a rift in her relationship with her mother. She didn't want to replicate the conflict in her relationship with her child, so she began to work with a therapist to investigate her own role in the disagreements and to improve her relationship with her mother. When Elizabeth eventually became pregnant, after IVF, she felt closer to her mother and better prepared to parent.

---

ship with their parents, as well as a time to learn more about how they see themselves as parents—and how they hope to mother their children.

• *Fear of miscarriage:* It's normal to be concerned that you'll miscarry—miscarriages are, unfortunately, relatively common in first pregnancies. (The overall miscarriage rate is 15 to 20 percent of all pregnancies.) Fear of miscarriage can be especially strong if you've miscarried once, but because most miscarriages are caused by a chromosomal problem that occurs spontaneously, second miscarriages are relatively rare. Still, it's easy to worry. Even something as natural as shifting symptoms—for example, if you feel very nauseated for several days and then feel better for a day or two—can trigger concern. You may worry that there's something wrong with the pregnancy instead of thinking, "Well, I'm having a good day." This is challenging to go through, but normal. It might sound like a cliché, but simply trying to focus on each day as it comes can help you manage your anxiety. (For more about miscarriage, see chapter 18.)

Telling Friends and Family

✦ When is the right time to tell friends and family? It used to be that people kept this news a secret until at least the first trimester was over. Now many couples share their news after an eight-week sonogram detects a heartbeat and confirms the health of the pregnancy. You should not feel pressure to tell people at a certain time or to keep it private—you and your partner can decide whom to tell when. One rule of thumb that may be helpful is to tell only those people whom you would want to know in the unlikely event you miscarried.

REAL VOICES

We did wait until after twelve weeks. I've watched so many people have miscarriages, and I didn't want that to be a public pain. If that's going to happen, I want it to be something that happens just between us. Or the people with whom I'm close, and that's it.

Asha, mom of one, pregnant

Are you kidding me? I was on the phone with twenty of my closest friends, starting with my mom, the night we found out. It took me two years to get pregnant, and I kept saying to my husband, "If I miscarry, I want the fun of having been pregnant, and I want the support of those people."

Katherine, mom of two

My husband and I talked a lot about this. His thing was not to tell for the first three months, and my philosophy was I had to tell because I was so excited. If I was going to lose the baby, I would want my friends to know that I had lost a baby so they would be with me on it, whereas he's much more private about things. So I told my closest friends, but I was very careful about not telling the people I worked with or anyone in the art scene—I'm an artist—until after the first trimester.

Glenda, mom of two, stepmom to one

Typical First Trimester Symptoms

Overall, the first trimester is an exciting time—the beginning of a momentous life experience. But the physical symptoms of early pregnancy can be uncomfortable. Try to think of them as guides, there to let you know how you can take care of yourself. Listen to what your body tells you. Rest when you need to, eat well, drink lots of water, take walks, and give yourself over to your daydreams.

Q: I just found out I'm pregnant, but I really don't feel very different at all. Is that a problem?

Dr. Evans: Some women experience many, many symptoms from the day their pregnancies are confirmed; others experience very few. Most often, the absence of pregnancy symptoms doesn't mean there is anything wrong with a pregnancy. But I do take note when a woman says she really feels nothing out of the ordinary after eight to ten weeks, and I watch her a little more carefully, so let your doctor or midwife know how you are feeling.

Q: I just found out I'm pregnant for the second time. Can I expect to have the same symptoms as last time?

Dr. Evans: There's no clear-cut answer to this question. In my practice, I would say about half of the women I work with have similar symptoms from one pregnancy to the next. There's an old wives' tale that says if the second baby's a different sex from the first, the mom will have different symptoms—and I have found there's some truth to that. All you can do, though, is wait and see. Don't be concerned if your symptoms turn out to be very different, because each pregnancy, just like each child, has its own unique characteristics.

Here's an alphabetical list of pregnancy side effects that are most common during the first trimester. (For a discussion of symptoms that occur throughout pregnancy, see chapter 11.)

Breast changes and tenderness

• *What happens:* Even before you know for sure that you're pregnant, your breasts may feel heavy and tingle, and you may notice pronounced blue veins lining them. Your breasts may continue to be quite tender throughout the first trimester, after which the tenderness tends to be less noticeable. Because you're retaining fluids and your breasts are preparing to produce milk, they'll grow throughout your pregnancy—about one cup size the first trimester and possibly that much again over the course of the second and third trimesters combined. As your breasts grow, you may have some shooting pains; these are normal and they should pass fairly quickly (lasting no more than a couple of minutes). In addition to expanding breasts, your nipples will get bigger and may move more easily, while the areolae, the circles that surround the nipples, will darken and may get bumpy.

• *What you can do:* A good support bra will help relieve sore breasts; it's a good idea to wear one throughout your pregnancy, even if your breasts don't bother you. Good, consistent support helps prevent your breasts from stretching too much, which in turn can help reduce the drooping that often follows a pregnancy. If your breasts are especially tender and swollen, you may find it more comfortable to sleep in a bra.

Constipation

• *What happens:* Progesterone, which keeps the uterine lining rich and full of nutrients throughout the first trimester, relaxes everything, including the muscles in your small intestine and colon. Because the intestinal muscles are relaxed, food moves more slowly through them, making bowel movements less frequent. Plus, if you aren't drinking enough water (you need more fluids even early in pregnancy), your body will get the water it needs from your food, which will make your stools harder. The combined effect of sluggish intestines and hard stools causes constipation early in pregnancy. (Later you may become constipated for another reason: The growing uterus pushes up against the intestines, compressing them and making it harder for them to move stool along.) The extra iron that you're getting from foods or supplements can also aggravate constipation.

Keep in mind, however, that there's no experience in pregnancy that applies to everyone: You may find that you aren't constipated at all, or that you have much more frequent bowel movements.

• *What you can do:*
  – *Stay hydrated:* Drink as much as one eight-ounce glass of water or clear fluids (like herbal teas or broth) every hour.
  – *Exercise:* Physical activity helps to keep your digestive tract moving. If you feel up to it, exercise moderately for twenty-five to thirty minutes as often as you can (ideally daily). Try walking, yoga, or swimming.

- *Small dishes:* Frequent, small meals won't stress the colon too much and will keep it relatively active all the time.
- *Increase fiber:* Raw vegetables and fruits such as prunes, dates, and figs (not bananas, which are binding) are excellent sources of dietary fiber. Eat them as often as you can. If eating more fruits and vegetables combined with the other suggestions does not work, try a fiber supplement.

Flaxseed is the ideal fiber; in addition to relieving constipation, it's high in omega-3 essential fatty acids, an excellent nutrient for you and your growing baby. Buy raw, whole organic flaxseeds and a new coffee grinder (you don't want flax to mix with your coffee beans). Every day, grind one tablespoon for twenty seconds and sprinkle it on cereal, salad, yogurt, cottage cheese, or soup. Store whole seeds in an airtight container and don't grind seeds in advance. They become rancid after about a half hour.

If you don't like flaxseeds, one tablespoon of wheat germ every day is another good choice. Metamucil, which is fiber with sugar added, is also safe and effective. Try it for one night; if it works, try it again a few days later. If you still need it, gradually increase to nightly doses. It's safe to take throughout pregnancy, but as with any over-the-counter medication, be sure to check with your caregiver before taking it and to confirm dosing.

If you're taking a fiber supplement like flaxseed or wheat germ, be sure to stay well hydrated.

Caution: Do *not* take mineral oil; it can deplete vitamins A, D, and E, and may cause contractions.

Cramps

• *What happens:* As the uterus grows, you may experience some cramping; it's completely normal. Usually women feel it early on, but you may have some cramping up to week 10 or even 12.

• *What you can do:*

- *Apply heat:* Use a heating pad set to medium heat, not high, or a hot water bottle to soothe cramps.
- *Chamomile tea (Chamaemelum nobile):* Chamomile tea can be soothing. Drink up to four eight-ounce cups a day.
- *Red raspberry leaf tea (Rubus idaeus):* It's full of nutrients, helps tone the muscles of the uterus, and soothes cramps and nausea. Drink up to four eight-ounce cups a day.

— Either *Wild yam (Dioscorea villosa)* or *Blackhaw (Viburnum prunifolium):* Both can be taken as teas, and both have mild agents that effectively relieve muscle spasms. (Dose: one eight-ounce cup of tea up to three times a day. Don't drink more; while both are widely considered safe during pregnancy, and blackhaw is even used to prevent miscarriage, there's no information about very high doses of either in pregnancy. Mix one teaspoon of either ground herb in eight ounces of hot water and let it steep for ten minutes. You may add a pinch of fresh ginger, which will make the herbs taste and work better.

— *Acetaminophen (Tylenol):* Two extra-strength acetaminophens can relieve the discomfort of cramping.

Caution: If your cramps are nearly as painful as bad period cramps, or if you only have them on one side, call your doctor or midwife that day. If you have severe cramping or it's accompanied by spotting, call your doctor right away.

Depressed mood or mood swings

• *What happens:* All the emotional and life changes pregnancy brings, combined with the extra progesterone your body produces, may provoke mood swings or leave you feeling unusually blue.

• *What you can do:*

— *Be open about your feelings:* Try not to focus exclusively on what you think you *should* feel. Let yourself express exactly what you *are* feeling. Being pregnant is exciting, but it can be physically demanding and emotionally complicated. Find someone you trust with whom you can share your feelings. This may be your partner, a dear friend, a therapist or pastor, or any combination of these people. Also, your doctor or midwife will be able to either help you or guide you to someone who can.

— *Exercise moderately:* If you have the energy—or even if you don't think you do—try to exercise. Even a fifteen-minute walk can be helpful. If you exercised regularly before you were pregnant—jogging, swimming, walking, biking—try to keep it up. You may have to be more moderate when you exercise, but it's important to make the effort. Physical movement can lift the spirits because during exercise, the body produces chemicals that elevate mood. This is true for aerobic exercise as well as for quieter activities like stretching, prenatal Pilates, yoga, and qi gong. (For more information on exercise in pregnancy, see chapter 14.)

— *Connect with nature:* In addition to shorter walks, when you have time, go to a nature preserve or park. Take a long walk on an easy trail. Even if you think you should be running errands instead, taking time to get out of your routine and connect with the bigger, natural world can soothe the soul, especially when you're nurturing new life.

— *Omega-3 essential fatty acid supplements:* Omega-3 fatty acids have been shown to stabilize and improve mood, plus they support fetal brain growth, so taking them early in pregnancy is a double win. For depression and mood swings, take up to 3 grams (3,000 milligrams) of DHA daily with food. Tell your caregiver you're taking this supplement and why. *Only take a supplement that's guaranteed free of PCBs and heavy metals.* (See page 522 for sources.)

— *Massage:* Our skin and muscles are densely packed with nerves, which connect to our central nervous system. The extended soothing touch of massage can help improve mood while relaxing and calming the body.

— *Acupuncture:* Acupuncture may help alleviate depression throughout pregnancy. Seek an experienced acupuncturist who regularly works with pregnant women.

Excess saliva

• *What happens:* You may feel like you have too much saliva in your mouth, especially if you're already nauseated. When you swallow, if the saliva hits an empty stomach, you'll feel even more nausea—an unpleasant cycle, to say the least.

• *What you can do:* Nibble away at snacks and small meals to keep your stomach from getting empty and triggering the saliva-nausea cycle. You may also want to carry around a small container to use as your personal "spittoon." (For more, see "Nausea, vomiting," page 120.)

Fatigue

• *What happens:* From pregnancy's start, a woman's body works hard. Progesterone, that all-important hormone, relaxes the central nervous system, which slows down the body's metabolism, and may leave you feeling sluggish. Frequent urination, another side effect of early pregnancy (see page 124), also hinders rest. Many women find themselves going to the bathroom throughout the night, interrupting sleep and adding to fatigue.

- *What you can do:*
  - *Rest:* As much as you can, sleep when you need to. Take naps and go to bed as early as you want.
  - *Pace yourself:* Don't take on extra projects for friends, at home, or at work. Ask for help with housework or do not do it as frequently. Give yourself permission to take things slowly, because that's what your body needs and what it's asking for.
  - *Exercise:* It may seem counterintuitive, but moderate exercise can be refreshing. If you didn't exercise regularly before you became pregnant, start by taking fifteen- to twenty-minute walks as often as you can manage. If you exercised regularly before you got pregnant, try to get some moderate exercise now. Go for a slow, gentle swim or take a walk after dinner. If you practice yoga, keep doing so, only more gently, avoiding twists and poses that put pressure on the abdomen and uterus. Let your teacher know you are pregnant, drink water if you sweat a lot, and avoid heated classrooms. (For more on exercise and yoga in pregnancy, see chapter 14.)
  - *Eat small meals often:* Don't eat too much at any one time and also avoid very sweet processed foods, which are high in calories. When the body has to metabolize a lot of calories at any one time, it can leave you feeling fatigued and light-headed.
  - *Energy work:* Many of the women we work with have found that energy work such as acupuncture, shiatsu, Reiki, and reflexology helps improve their energy levels and manage the fatigue that early pregnancy often brings. There's no minimum number of treatments that are required to help fatigue—everyone responds differently. (For descriptions of each, see the CAM glossary in appendix 2.)

Note: While all of these therapies are safe during pregnancy, if you do have acupuncture, reflexology, or shiatsu sessions, see an experienced practitioner who regularly works with pregnant women and tell her that you are pregnant. There are certain pressure points in each modality that shouldn't be used during pregnancy.

Lack of libido

In the first trimester, many women find that they are completely uninterested in sex. The other side effects of early pregnancy—like fatigue, nausea, and moodiness—can really dampen the libido. The situation is not permanent, however. During the second trimester, sexual desire often rebounds, and women report being extremely interested in, and satisfied by, sex.

Note: Once again, the pregnant body resists any hard-and-fast rules. Even though decreased libido is common, some women find their sex drives increase in early pregnancy. (For more on sex during pregnancy, see page 309.)

Q: I'm about eleven weeks pregnant and my symptoms have become weaker over the last few days—does that mean something's wrong?

Dr. Evans: By this time in your pregnancy, it's most likely that your body is adjusting to the hormones and their effects are becoming less noticeable. But give your caregiver a call—she may have you come in just to reassure both of you that everything is okay.

Food aversions, cravings, and appetite changes

• *What happens:* Along with nausea and vomiting (see page 120), you may find that certain foods repel you, while others appeal strongly to you. You also may find

---

Hyperemesis Gravidarum

✦ Relatively few women (between 0.5 and 2 percent) experience a severe form of morning sickness known as *hyperemesis gravidarum*. When it occurs, nausea and/or vomiting are particularly intense and can continue throughout pregnancy. Vomiting can be so frequent that it requires hospitalization for dehydration. There is no threat to the baby when a woman has hyperemesis; the baby will take the nutrients it needs from the mother. But a woman with hyperemesis has to do whatever she can to maintain a minimum of nutrients for her own health and well-being. If your nausea and vomiting are debilitating, talk to your caregiver about the risks and benefits of medical intervention. In general, if you're vomiting frequently, call your doctor or midwife if you:

1. Feel light-headed or weak, or have abdominal pain or a headache.
2. Begin to produce copious amounts of saliva that then makes you vomit.
3. Feel terrible and think you're vomiting too often.

that your appetite swings wildly: One minute you're ravenous, and the next you can't imagine eating a thing.

- *What you can do:*
  - *Use common sense:* Eat what appeals to you, and don't eat what makes you sick, even if it's "good for you." When your body adjusts to the hormones and your appetite is more regular, you can focus on balancing your diet. The one exception here is protein; it's important throughout pregnancy, so try to eat as much as you can even when you're not feeling great. Good sources of protein include salmon, chicken, cottage cheese, health bars (like a Luna or Clif bar), or even a smoothie made with low-molecular-weight whey protein (which you can get at a health food store). Don't drink supplement shakes like Ensure, because they're very high in sugar.
  - *Eat small meals:* Small, frequent meals and snacks will keep food in your stomach, so your appetite won't swing from famished to nauseated.

REAL VOICES

Mostly what I had was food aversions. For example, my partner would cook chicken for me, because I asked for it. And then she'd put it in front of me and I'd think, "I cannot eat this." But if you were biting into a pickle I'd think, "Man, that looks good!"

Laura, mom of one, pregnant

I get really sick when I'm pregnant. If I don't eat every two hours or so, I throw up—and that means I wake up in the middle of the night to eat, especially in the first trimester. I keep some bread, cheese, and some fruit by my bed at night so I have some choices about what to eat. The cracker thing never cut it for me.

Stephanie, mom of one, pregnant

Nausea, vomiting, and sensitivity to smells ("morning sickness")

- *What happens:* About 70 to 85 percent of all pregnant women experience some nausea and vomiting. No one can say for sure why pregnant women are nauseated and throw up, but it's not specific to any one country, culture, or historical period (there are reports of pregnancy-related nausea from ancient Greece). The symptoms aren't limited to mornings, but they can be very intense when you first wake up. There's a fair amount of variety with these symptoms: Some women are nauseated all day but never vomit; others experience both nausea and vomiting. Morning sickness typically begins between the fourth and sixth weeks of pregnancy, peaks around week 9, and goes away by week 16, at the latest.

While you're pregnant, you may also find you're more sensitive to odors, meaning you can pick them up more easily, and they may trigger nausea—another side effect of progesterone.

- *What you can do:*
  - *Eat small meals often:* Have frequent small meals with complex carbohydrates like bread, rice, pasta (if you can, eat whole-grain versions). Eat slowly and chew your food completely.
  - *Keep snacks handy:* Keep crackers by your bedside, so if you wake up very hungry or nauseated, there's something right there to settle your stomach. (Look for whole-grain crackers that don't have saturated fats or hydrogenated oils.) Keep snacks like pretzels or almonds in your bag or desk so you have something to nibble on if you're stuck in traffic or tied to your office. You don't want to have an empty stomach.
  - *Avoid strong smells and strong foods:* Spicy, fried, and fatty foods are difficult to digest, so avoid them. Also, strong smells can trigger both nausea and vomiting. If smells bother you, try to prepare simple meals or ask your partner or a friend to prepare them for you.
  - *Sip liquids:* Water, ginger tea, peppermint tea, red raspberry leaf tea, lemonade, clear soup, even cola or a sports drink like Gatorade. If you're vomiting, it's important to make sure you're getting enough fluids.
  - *Eat what you can:* The baby will get the nutrients she needs, so eat what appeals to you. If that means you are living on bagels and cucumbers for a couple of weeks, so be it.
  - *Take prenatal vitamins strategically:* If your prenatal vitamin triggers nausea, take it with your biggest meal of the day, every other day, or before you go to bed, so you sleep through the nausea.
  - *Vitamin B–rich foods:* Some women find B vitamins help relieve nausea; they're in whole grains, avocados, corn, nuts, liver, fish, and chicken.
  - *Vitamin B6 supplements:* If vitamin B foods don't appeal to you, you can try taking 100 mg of vitamin B6 (50 mg twice a day) in addition to your prenatal vitamin.
  - *Combine vitamin B6 and doxylamine:* If B6 alone doesn't work, combine it with doxylamine, an antihistamine frequently used to treat insomnia. (For example, it's in Unisom.) Take 10 mg of vitamin B6 and 10 mg of doxylamine

three to four times a day. A pharmacy where they mix compounds can prepare a capsule containing both substances for you. Keep in mind that it will make you drowsy.

— *Acupressure bands:* Recently approved by the FDA and known commercially as Seabands, these are one of the best-studied complementary therapies for any pregnancy symptom. They've been shown to relieve nausea by stimulating an acupuncture point on the inner wrist, about two inches above the crease. Available at most drugstores, you can use them whenever you are feeling nauseous.

— *Massage:* Massage can be very soothing and refreshing, and some women find it provides relief from persistent nausea.

— *Craniosacral therapy:* We've found that women with moderate to severe nausea feel much better for a few days after a craniosacral therapy session. (For a description of craniosacral therapy, see the CAM glossary in appendix 2.)

— *Seated meditation:* Use this mind-body technique to turn your attention away from the nausea, which may bring relief. Sit in a comfortable chair with your feet on the floor and your hands resting lightly on your thighs. You want to feel supported and at ease. Lower your eyelids and start to breathe slowly and gently, in through your nose, out through your slightly open mouth. Let the breath cool and calm you. Focus only on the breath and let thoughts come and go. Sit like this for ten to fifteen minutes each day.

— *Dried gingerroot capsules:* Take three capsules when you wake up and every four hours thereafter, or take during the day as needed.

— *Fresh (not dried) ginger tea:* Peel the skin off the fresh ginger with a veg-

Acupressure for Morning Sickness

✦ According to Jacques Depardieu, MSOM, L/Ac, and the acupuncturist in my practice, the acupressure point that can relieve nausea is called "pericardium 6." To find it, bend your hand forward and put three fingers on your wrist starting at the crease. Notice the two tendons in the wrist, and probe gently between them until you find a tender spot—that's the point. For acupressure to work, you must press the point so hard it hurts. When you release the point, you should feel some relief from the nausea.

CHECKLIST: STOMACH-FRIENDLY FOODS

Here are some foods that may appeal to you and settle your stomach:

- Citrus: lemons and tangerines in any form—drinks, sucking candies, the fruits on their own
- Cucumbers
- Frozen banana smoothies (made with low-fat milk or soy milk)
- Frozen grapes
- Ginger: candies, tea, ginger ale, even pickled
- Licorice
- Mint or peppermint: tea, candies, breath fresheners
- Pasta
- Saltines or soda crackers
- Salty snacks like pretzels and potato chips
- Toast and bagels
- Tomatoes
- Watermelon

---

etable peeler, then slice it thin and steep it in eight ounces of hot water. Dose: a half cup two to three times daily.

- *Chamomile tea:* Drink up to four eight-ounce cups per day. Some women find chamomile combined with ginger very effective at alleviating nausea.
- *Red raspberry leaf tea (Rubus idaeus):* Steep two teaspoons in eight ounces of water. Drink up to four eight-ounce cups per day.

Spotting or bleeding

• *What happens:* Spotting or bleeding occurs in about one out of five pregnancies, and while either can be nerve-racking, neither necessarily signals a problem. Spotting may be the result of what's known as implantation bleeding. As the embryo digs into the uterine lining, it must connect to the mother's blood supply; sometimes that process can cause light spotting, typically around six weeks. Heavier bleeding may have a number of causes.

• *What you can do:* Spotting or bleeding always warrants a phone call to your caregiver. If light spotting—a few drops on a pad—occurs in the middle of the night, you can usually wait until the morning to call. If you notice light spotting during the day, call the same day. If you feel that the spotting is light but something is not right, call as soon as you can. If you feel pain with spotting, particularly lower abdominal pain or pain that is focused on one side, call your doctor or midwife immediately; he will want to make sure the pregnancy is not ectopic. (See box, page 125.) *If you experience heavy bleeding—if you need to use a maxi pad or tampon or you see some clots—call your doctor or midwife immediately.*

At your first prenatal visit, be sure to ask your caregiver for his guidelines for after-hours calls and how quickly you can expect a callback.

REAL VOICES

I used to bring orange peels to work and sort of squirt them at my nose to relieve nausea. I would sit in meetings and hold the orange peel to my nose and breathe in.

Eileen, mom of two

I had heard that pineapple helps with nausea, so I would eat it after meals, which sometimes actually helped.

Martha, mom of two

At six weeks it hit me like a brick. I smelled everything from miles away; my olfactory senses were in superhigh gear. I threw up everything. And living in an apartment building, there are smells everywhere. So I would carry around a pack of fruit-striped gum, its very lemony flavor, and sniff it. It really helped!

Sarah, mom of one

I had a lot of bleeding around six weeks in my first pregnancy, and I was terrified that I was miscarrying. I had a brand-new OB and went in that day for a sonogram. It was implantation bleeding.

Allison, mom of two

Urinary frequency

• *What happens:* Early in pregnancy, progesterone causes stomach muscles to relax and slump into the bladder, which makes you feel like you have to pee. Plus, the uterus is quickly expanding and you're retaining more fluids, both of which also make you have to urinate—during the day and throughout the night. Don't try to hold it in, and don't try to drink less. You need a steady supply of fluids in pregnancy, and you want to prevent urinary tract infections, a common problem in pregnancy. (See page 209.)

Ectopic Pregnancy

✦ When an embryo implants outside of the uterus, it's known as an ectopic pregnancy ("ectopic" literally means "out of place"). About 2 percent of pregnancies are ectopic, and most of these—about 96 percent—occur in one of the fallopian tubes, and are the result of some kind of blockage within it. (Rarely, ectopic pregnancies are located on the cervix, ovary, or abdomen.) Fortunately, ectopic pregnancies can be diagnosed as early as four and a half to six weeks, which greatly reduces the potential for serious complications.

Risk Factors

1. If you've already had an ectopic pregnancy, your risk for a second is higher.
2. If you've had surgery on or near your fallopian tubes, scarring may put you at risk.
3. A history of pelvic inflammatory disease (PID)
4. Endometriosis
5. Exposure to DES (diethylstilbestrol)

Symptoms

An ectopic pregnancy may be accompanied by one or several of these symptoms:

1. Lower abdominal pain or tenderness, possibly on one side; if an ectopic pregnancy ruptures, it creates sharp pain or cramping.
2. Spotting (brown) or light bleeding
3. Shoulder pain
4. Dizziness
5. Nausea and vomiting (although this could also be morning sickness)
6. Tenderness on one side or pain during a pelvic exam
7. You have a follow-up blood pregnancy test and your HCG levels have not risen to the expected levels.

If you have any of these symptoms, call your doctor or midwife immediately. Ectopic pregnancies can't be carried to term, and the earlier an ectopic pregnancy is diagnosed, the safer it will be for you.

10

A Pregnancy Timeline

Every woman will have her own, unique experience of pregnancy, its symptoms and emotions, and every baby will grow at her own pace in utero. But even with the enormous range of what's considered "normal" in pregnancy, pregnancies in general follow a relatively predictable course. Here I review how a pregnancy unfolds: how an embryo becomes a baby, the typical physical and emotional changes you may experience, and the standard elements of the prenatal care you'll receive along the way.

❖ ❖ ❖

In this chapter you'll find:

Note: There are two ways to count the weeks in pregnancy: the obstetric calendar and the embryonic calendar. Throughout this book, I follow the obstetric calendar and count the weeks from the first day of your last menstrual period. The embryonic calendar begins around two weeks after the first day of your last menstrual period, when fertilization most likely took place.

Also, you'll notice as you go through this timeline that pregnancy isn't actually nine months, but nearly ten. (This reflects how we, as a culture, typically use imprecise terminology when it comes to determining age.) When caregivers refer to weeks of pregnancy, we mean completed weeks—in the same way that chronological age refers to completed years. You turn thirty on your thirtieth birthday, when you've completed thirty years on earth, but you're technically starting your thirty-first year. In the same way, when you're thirty weeks, four days, you're *in* your thirty-first week of pregnancy, but you're not said to be thirty-one weeks until the seventh day of your thirtieth week. Since the total time of pregnancy is forty completed weeks (or almost ten months), when you're between thirty-six and forty weeks you are nine months plus X days or weeks.

Weeks 1–4

• *The baby:* The miraculous moment that makes a baby—the fertilization of an egg by a sperm—comes during the five days of peak fertility leading up to, and including, ovulation (see page 39). A fertilized egg (or zygote) spends the next week dividing into many cells and traveling from the outer part of the fallopian tubes down into the uterus, which has prepared itself for this arrival, as it does every month, by fortifying its walls with extra blood and nutrients. If you conceived on day 14 of a twenty-eight-day cycle, around day 21 the embryo (now technically in its *blastocyst* stage) arrives in the uterus and begins to bury itself in the uterine wall in the process known as implantation. (At this point, the embryo has so many cells clumped together that it looks like a blackberry.) Within the next few days, the early placenta starts to form, establishing the life-sustaining connection between uterus and embryo through a myriad of interconnecting blood vessels.

Once implanted, the embryo begins producing a hormone called human chorionic gonadotropin (HCG, also known as "the pregnancy hormone"), which builds up in a mother's blood and is excreted in urine. HCG does two things: (1) It helps the uterine lining nurture a developing embryo; and (2) it helps the body figure out that it shouldn't prepare another egg for ovulation. HCG is the hormone pregnancy tests measure, and by day 26, some sensitive tests can detect enough of it to diagnose a pregnancy.

By day 28 of a twenty-eight-day cycle, the embryo, while tiny, is visible to the naked eye—it's about the size of the period at the end of this sentence.

Note: Scientists refer to an "embryo" until obstetric week 10, at which point the embryo becomes a "fetus."

• *Mom:* Some women suspect they're pregnant from the very first days after conception, well before their periods are due. Other women have no idea they're pregnant until they're looking at a little plus sign on the end of a plastic stick. Regardless of when or how you know you're pregnant, by the time your period is late, your hormones are surging and you may begin to notice some of the changes of early pregnancy: Your breasts may feel heavier or sore; you may be tired; you may have to urinate frequently. Then again, you may not have any symptoms of pregnancy other than a missed period. (For more on early signs of pregnancy, see page 76.)

Whether this pregnancy is a surprise or planned, a positive pregnancy test marks a new beginning of what can be an exciting and confusing time. As you're adjusting to the fact that your body, life, and identity will change dramatically over the next year, your hormones are running wild to support the pregnancy—and changing hormones can have a big impact on emotions. To complicate matters even more, you may be worried about a miscarriage. Considering everything that happens physically in early pregnancy, it's perfectly normal to feel both happy and overwhelmed when you first learn you're pregnant. (For more on the emotional world of early pregnancy, see chapter 9.)

• *Prenatal care:* If you learn you're pregnant after taking a home pregnancy test, call your gynecological care provider to let him know. He'll explain when he'd like to see you and any lifestyle changes you should make right away. (For more on early prenatal care, see chapter 9.)

REAL VOICES

With my second pregnancy, I knew right away—the second day after we conceived—because I knew what it was like to be pregnant. This was before I missed my period. I just felt it—and I was exhausted immediately.

Glenda, mom of two, stepmom of one

Weeks 5–8

- *The baby:* Over these weeks, all of a baby's body parts form. The embryo's thousands of cells split into three groups. One will become the brain, central nervous system, skin, and hair; a second group will grow into the gastrointestinal system; and the third will become the circulatory, musculoskeletal, and genitourinary systems.

At the start of the fifth week, an embryo measures about 2 mm long (about the size of a pea) and has an enormous head compared to a relatively small body. By the end of the sixth week, a rudimentary heart is beating—something that an early ultrasound may pick up—and there are the beginnings of ears and eyes. (The embryo's eyes are all the way on the sides of the head, and the ears are set quite low.)

In week 7, the heart has four chambers, and the embryo has nostrils, lips, a tongue, and arms and legs, which begin to move spontaneously as the connections between the brain and nerves improve.

By week 8, the baby's own blood circulates, her heart beats strongly, and all of her major internal organs have formed. She has knees and elbows, and she now measures about an inch long from head to rump.

- *Mom:* These weeks can be physically and emotionally intense. First-trimester symptoms like morning sickness/nausea (see page 120), fatigue (see page 117), and aversion to smells (see page 120) are likely to begin around week 6. Your breasts could be bigger and heavier, and you may notice other subtle changes in your body. (For more on first-trimester symptoms, see chapter 9.)

Emotionally, this can be a complicated time as you get used to the idea of being pregnant and begin to contemplate the many joys and responsibilities that are part and parcel of the transition into pregnancy and parenthood. (For more, see chapter 9.)

- *Prenatal care:* It's not unusual to have a first prenatal appointment by eight weeks. When you go in, remember to bring the date of the *first day* of your last menstrual period (LMP), which will be used to calculate your due date (for how to calculate your due date, see page 77). During the appointment, you'll have blood and urine tests, your blood pressure will be taken, and you'll be weighed.

Depending on how far along you are, your caregiver may use a small device called a Doppler to listen to the baby's heartbeat. (The Doppler has a small wand, or transducer, that's about the size of a pen and attached to a handheld monitor. It can pick up a heartbeat through your abdomen.) Or, if it's appropriate, you'll have an ultrasound exam to measure the baby, confirm your due date, and locate the heartbeat. (For more on first trimester (early) ultrasound exams, see page 303.)

Early Miscarriage

✦ Amid all the emotion and excitement of a new pregnancy lies the hard reality of miscarriage. Estimates vary, but anywhere from 10 to 20 percent of pregnancies end in miscarriage, with the great majority of losses occurring before twelve weeks (typically by eight weeks). Most of these early losses are the result of a problem with the embryo's chromosomes. They are *not* the result of anything a mother did, with the possible exception of abusing certain illegal drugs or drinking quite heavily. The impact of an early pregnancy loss shouldn't be minimized by anyone. A common complaint among women who've miscarried is that a care provider seemed dismissive of their loss because all she said was, "Not to worry. You should get over it quickly because many women experience this and go on to conceive again and carry healthy babies to term."

The medical facts of this statement are correct: After a first miscarriage, most women do go on to have a healthy baby. But the emotional significance of a loss is different for each woman. If you've miscarried, give yourself the time and space to fully grieve and try not to ignore your sadness. By letting yourself feel your feelings, you'll give yourself the chance to move through the sorrow and start to think about getting pregnant again. If you feel you need professional help, pursue it. There's no need to "tough it out" on your own. (For more on early miscarriage, see chapter 18.)

A first prenatal visit typically lasts longer than subsequent visits in order to give you time to ask any questions you might have about how the practice works and the doctor or midwife's approach to prenatal care and birth. (For more on the first prenatal visit and questions you might ask a care provider, see page 82.)

Weeks 9–12

• *The baby:* By week 10, your little embryo has graduated to fetus status. The body starts to lengthen and grow rapidly in relation to the fetus's head. The brain structure is in place and the muscles of the fetus's digestive tract become functional, even though your baby won't eat any actual food until after being born. The fetus's

Making the Connection:
Breathing Through the First Trimester (Weeks 4–14)

✦ The first trimester is a time of constant change. Your body must adapt to all the hormonal changes that allow you to nurture this new being. You may have had to change your eating, drinking, and even cooking habits (maybe you suddenly can't stand the smell of garlic, or the look of chicken, or the idea of tomato sauce). You may feel exhausted or energized, sexually supercharged or totally lacking in libido. Whatever you're feeling, odds are it's different from how you felt before you were pregnant.

To help you adjust to your evolving pregnant body and expanding emotional world, try breathing. Even though we breathe all the time, we usually do so without bringing any awareness to what we're doing. We don't think about how deeply we're breathing, where the breath is going in our bodies, what sensations the breath brings, or how it makes us feel. But in many traditions around the world, it's breath that carries the life force; in addition to its physical purpose of bringing oxygen into our bodies, it carries spirit with it. During the first trimester, try to tap into the spiritual and energetic potential of the simple act of breathing. By spending five or ten minutes focusing on your breath, you practice quieting your thoughts, making time for yourself, and getting in touch with your inner world. In doing so, you can foster a sense of calm and a connection to the life that's blossoming inside of you.

To focus on your breath, you can practice the calming "belly breathing" exercise (described on page 63) in which you simply inhale deeply, letting the breath fill your abdomen, and then slowly exhale, saying to yourself the word "soft" (or "peace" or "trust" or "love," etc.) on the inhale and "belly" (or "calm" or "present," etc.) on the exhale. This breathing exercise is particularly useful if you're anxious, if you're coping with pregnancy-related headaches, nausea, and/or vomiting, or if you're new to meditation or breathing exercises.

Alternatively, you can practice any breathing exercise that you know helps you slow down and focus on your breath. For example, breathing in for a count of four, concentrating on feeling the breath move through the top of the lungs, the middle of the chest, the diaphragm, the belly, and into the womb. Hold there for four counts, and exhale on a count of four, observing the breath making the reverse journey out. Or just breathe slowly, directing the breath into your womb with each inhalation, using your imagination to bring in a calm, loving energy to support your baby, and using the exhalation to release any anxiety or fear. Whatever breathing method you choose, you're creating time to nurture yourself, your changing body, and your growing baby.

pancreas starts producing insulin, the liver makes bile, and the intestines move from the umbilical cord into the abdominal cavity.

During week 11, the baby starts producing sterile urine, which will surround him and, in the second trimester, become amniotic fluid. By twelve weeks, he starts opening and closing his mouth; he's practicing sucking and beginning to swallow. He can open and close his fists and move his thumb in opposition to his other fingers, and his finger- and toenails start to grow. His sex organs are now visible. By the end of the twelfth week, he'll be three inches long.

• *Mom:* If you've had morning sickness, you may find it eases up over the course of these four weeks. While many women experience some nausea through sixteen weeks, it's typically at its most severe through week 11 or 12, after which it usually becomes much less intense.

At some point over these weeks, either after you first hear the baby's heartbeat or when you pass the twelve-week mark, you may decide it's time to tell people you're pregnant. If you've already told some close friends and family members, you may feel ready to tell a wider circle of friends, acquaintances, and maybe even coworkers. (For more on "when to tell," see page 112.) Then again, you may not be ready to tell anyone, particularly if you know you're going to have an amniocentesis (see page 287). Many women who plan to have the test decide to wait to "go public" until they get their amnio results.

Finally, don't assume anyone can guess you're pregnant. While you may have experienced a wide range of physical and emotional changes over the last eight to ten weeks, you still may not look all that different to people who don't know or wouldn't suspect you're pregnant.

REAL VOICES
Right after I got pregnant, it was so funny, my breasts got a little bigger and I thought, "Okay, everyone knows I'm pregnant." I thought I had this arrow pointing at me. I remember saying to my husband, "Oh my gosh! My breasts are

so big. Everybody must know I'm pregnant." And he just looked at me and said, "I hate to break it to you, but they're still not that big." A great reality check.

Suzanne, mom of two

• *Prenatal care:* If you didn't have your first prenatal visit at eight weeks, you'll have had it by twelve weeks. If you've already had a first visit, it's likely you'll head back to the office for a second visit in the twelfth week. In your eleventh week, two prenatal screening tests become available:

— *Nuchal translucency test (also known as the ultra-screen or early screen):* This noninvasive test evaluates your risk for Down syndrome and certain other chromosomal abnormalities by taking the results of ultrasound and a blood test and plugging them into a specific formula. The test, combined with the quad screen (see "AFP/Multiple Marker Screen" on page 281), is affecting how many couples think about prenatal testing. Women under thirty-five who have no risk factors for a chromosomal abnormality but would still like the security of an amnio, are choosing to have this test and a quad screen instead since neither poses any direct risk to the pregnancy, as amnio does (see "Amniocentesis" on page 287). The two tests provide very good information about the likelihood of having a baby with a chromosomal abnormality. (For more on the nuchal translucency screen, see page 300.)

— *Chorionic villus sampling (CVS):* During this procedure, a doctor extracts a piece of the chorionic villi, a part of the placenta. Because the placenta has the same genetic material as the baby, these cells can be

RED RASPBERRY LEAF TEA

In the second trimester, you may want to start drinking four eight-ounce cups of red raspberry leaf tea daily (earlier if you've had morning sickness). Red raspberry leaf tea is not only full of nutrients, but it also "tones" the uterine muscle. Drinking it daily could help you at the end of your pregnancy and in labor because the toning work of the herb makes contractions more productive, which in turn could make your labor shorter overall. (For brewing instructions, see page 97; for sources of herbs, turn to "Resources," page 521.)

A PRENATAL CARE SCHEDULE

Here's a *sample* schedule for routine prenatal care. Not every caregiver will follow the same schedule or do the same tests.

- *Singleton:* Prenatal visits are every four weeks until thirty weeks; then every two weeks until thirty-six weeks; then every week until the birth.
- *Multiples:* Prenatal visits are every three weeks until twenty weeks; then every two weeks until twenty-eight or thirty-two weeks; then every week until birth. After twenty weeks, ultrasounds every four weeks measure fetal growth.
- *Standard tests:* These are done at every prenatal visit: weight measured, urine tested for protein and sugar, blood pressure taken, fetal heart rate checked (with a Doppler).
- *8 weeks:*
  First prenatal visit (see page 92)
  Q&A with care provider
  Counseling about diet and lifestyle (see page 96)
  Prenatal bloodwork, including immunity and genetic screens (see pages 92–94)
  Pap smear
- *10–12 weeks:*
  Nuchal translucency test if requested (see page 300)
  CVS if requested (see page 291)

analyzed for chromosomal abnormalities and certain genetic diseases. The test can also tell you the baby's gender with 99 percent accuracy. (For more on CVS, see page 291.)

Weeks 13–16

- *The baby:* The baby is still quite small, just three to four inches long from crown to rump. If she's a girl, she now has between six and seven million eggs in her ovaries; by the time she's born, she'll have two to four million eggs (and by the time of her first menstruation, she'll have about 400,000). Starting at fourteen weeks, her body grows at a faster rate than her head. At sixteen weeks, her body is covered by translucent skin; the fine, silky hair known as *lanugo* begins to appear. By now, the baby's eyes have moved from the sides of her head to the front of her face (she's been blinking since around fourteen weeks), and her ears are in their final position. At the end of these weeks, your baby will have grown to four and a half inches long and will weigh a little more than three ounces (about the size of a pear or avocado). Amazingly, she can make faces—like squinting or frowning—in response to outside stimulation.

• *Mom:* The second trimester begins! If you're still feeling nauseous or vomiting, the odds are good that you'll start to feel much better by the end of your sixteenth week. Over these weeks you may also begin to feel more energetic, more sexual (if your libido waned in the early months of your pregnancy), and, in general, more comfortable in your body and with the idea of being pregnant.

As you start to feel better and more secure in your pregnancy, you may turn your attention to planning a vacation. The second trimester is a good time to travel because your symptoms have eased, your energy level is probably higher, and your belly is still small enough that it's relatively easy to get around. (For more on travel during pregnancy, see page 317.)

Even though you may feel much better, you may not know exactly what to wear. These are the weeks when you can't quite button your

---

A PRENATAL CARE SCHEDULE (CONTINUED)

• *15–20 weeks:*
AFP/Multiple Marker Screen (see page 281)
Amniocentesis if requested (see page 287)

• *18–22 weeks:*
Level 2 ultrasound (see page 303)
Begin to explore childbirth education (see page 407)

• *25–28 weeks:*
Sign up for childbirth education
Iron levels checked (see "Anemia" on page 339)
Glucose Screening Test (1 hour; see page 296)
Glucose Tolerance Test if necessary (3 hours; see page 297)
If Rh-negative, Rh immunoglobulin treatment (see page XX)

• *32 weeks:*
Iron levels rechecked if low in first test

• *36 weeks:*
Group B Streptococcus Screening (see page 298)

---

pants and your blouses may tug around your breasts, but you may not be quite ready for maternity clothes. (For maternity fashion advice from real moms, see pages 315–317.) To complicate the "what to wear" situation further, instead of feeling beautifully pregnant, you may just feel large and mushy. Your belly (and possibly other fashion-sensitive body parts) may be bigger, but your body doesn't yet announce "baby on board."

• *Prenatal care:* Between fifteen and twenty weeks, prenatal tests become available. First, there's the AFP/multiple marker screen (aka triple screen or quadruple screen). This blood test assesses your risk of having a baby with Down syndrome or other health problems. The newer quadruple screen, which, as of this writing, is rapidly becoming the standard of care, is widely considered more accurate than the triple screen, which has a reputation for "false positives." (For a discussion of the AFP/multiple marker test, see page 281.)

You could also have an amniocentesis, which is usually performed between weeks 15 and 20. The test involves drawing some amniotic fluid out of the uterus and testing the chromosomes in the fetal cells it contains. It's recommended to women who will be thirty-five or older when they give birth and those with specific reasons (family history, personal, etc.) to have the test done. An amnio can tell you with 99 percent accuracy whether there's a chromosomal abnormality, a problem like spina bifida, and whether you're having a boy or a girl. (For a discussion of amniocentesis, see page 287.)

REAL VOICES

The first time I was pregnant we didn't find out if it was a boy or a girl, but we convinced ourselves that we were having a girl—and I really wanted to have a girl. Then, right at the moment of birth, when someone said, "It's a boy!" I felt this moment of "Huh?" and a little disappointment. Of course that faded in a few seconds, and I was thrilled to meet my son and have been madly in love with him ever since. This time, I thought, "I really want a girl, and if I'm going to raise two boys that's fine, but I want to know in advance so I can have time to prepare myself" . . . My partner at first was really into finding out, and then he wavered. At the last minute, he took a poll at a gathering of his rather large extended family, and they suggested he find out. So he finally agreed, and we found out—I'm having a girl.

Michelle, mom of one, pregnant

I had such a strong feeling that I was having a boy from very early on that I wanted to know just because I didn't want to have that strong a feeling and then be wrong. I thought I'd just rather get used to the idea now than have to do an about-face on the day I give birth.

Lisa, mom of one (boy)

The first time it wasn't even a question; we knew we didn't want to find out. We felt like there was no better surprise in the world, and we really didn't care.

The second time, I really cared. I really wanted a girl, and so I tried to rationalize all these different maps in my head, like, "If I don't find out, it'll be like thirty seconds of disappointment if it's a boy, and then I'll be so happy I have this baby." But then I thought, "If I find out, I'll be wishing for the opposite the entire time." We had a lot of talks about it, and we decided not to . . . Then, after our ultrasound, they gave us an envelope, and in the envelope was the answer. We hung the envelope on the refrigerator, and it just stayed there. Once I had the envelope I stopped caring, which was very strange. *Then,* I had to have a follow-up ultrasound, which was in 3-D—it was amazing—and the technician slipped and said "he." We weren't 100 percent sure, though, so we finally opened the envelope, and it's a boy. I realized afterwards that what I really wanted from a girl was to be able to buy the clothes . . . and that's stupid. I totally let go of it. Now I think having two boys will be great.

Asha, mom of one, pregnant

For me whether to find out came back to being surprised that I was pregnant in the first place. I'd gotten pregnant a lot faster than I thought I would, and I thought that if I knew the sex, we could settle on a name and I would feel a connection sooner. And that definitely was the case. Once I knew, I stopped thinking of the baby as an abstract "it." From that minute I could touch my belly and think "my daughter." It definitely helped me feel more positively towards being pregnant.

Suzanne, mom of two

Weeks 17–20

• *The baby:* At seventeen weeks, the baby is about five inches long; by the end of twenty weeks he'll be eight to ten inches from crown to rump. He's not only gaining height, but also weight, and by twenty weeks he'll tip the scales at three quarters of a pound. His legs are becoming more muscular, and he's using them more—you might feel his kicks as little bubbles. The baby regularly swallows and urinates amniotic fluid, a process that helps both his lungs and digestive system mature, and he may even be sucking his fingers or thumb. But the baby isn't active all the time; he now has relatively consistent sleep patterns.

Because he's swimming in liquid, the baby's skin needs protection. Over these weeks his oil glands will secrete a waxy substance known as *vernix caseosa,* which builds

Feeling the Baby Move

✦ Between sixteen and twenty-two weeks, you'll probably feel the baby move for the first time. When exactly you feel movement depends on a number of things: if this is a first pregnancy (first-time moms tend to feel movement a little later); where the placenta is located (if it's lying against the front of your uterus—anterior—you'll probably feel movement later, when the baby's stronger and bigger, because the placenta absorbs some of the sensation); if you're having more than one (moms of multiples tend to feel movement earlier); and your baby's personality (some babies move a lot, others less so).

Let your caregiver know when you first feel your baby move, because it's a good sign of fetal well-being. As I've noted, many women describe those first movements, which are sometimes called "quickening," as being like "little bubbles." Because every baby and every pregnancy is different, it's hard to predict when and how often you'll feel the baby move *after* that first time. Generally speaking, babies are active after you eat or when you lie down. Early on, the movements may be fairly subtle, but as your pregnancy progresses, they'll get stronger and more defined. The kicks and pokes and dragging feet will get pronounced (in the third trimester, a strong kick can even hurt!), and you may see your belly move along with a hand, foot, or elbow.

By early in your third trimester, around thirty to thirty-two weeks, a baby's movements usually follow a predictable pattern. At that point, your caregiver may recommend that you start keeping track of the baby's movement, setting aside some time each day to count between six and ten movements in an hour (or two hours—instructions vary among care providers).

Shortly before you give birth, it might seem like the baby's moving less (she's got less room to maneuver), but you should still be able to feel six to ten movements in an hour or two at any time of day or night when she's typically active.

Because babies tend to move less at the end of pregnancy, and decreased fetal movement can be a sign of a problem with the baby, every care provider will advise his patients about what to pay attention to when it comes to fetal movement. Talk with your care providers about their guidelines. If you're at all concerned about your baby's movement, call your care provider. (For instructions on how to count fetal movement, turn to "How to Track Fetal Movement" box on page 347.)

up in the lanugo (the fine hair that now covers his body) to form a protective coating. Sometimes the vernix is shed before birth; sometimes babies are born with it.

Fine hair forms on the baby's scalp, and eyebrows are beginning to take shape over eyes that now blink in response to light coming in from the outside.

REAL VOICES

With my twin daughters, I remember it was a really stressful day at work, and I was running around like crazy. Then at the end of the day I felt this thing shift in my stomach. That was awesome. When they were older, I would be at my desk, and I would try to catch one of their hands. One of my daughters loved to pull her hand across my stomach—it would look like the Loch Ness monster moving. I'd try to catch it, and she'd duck out of the way, and she'd come back up—we'd play games.

Rochelle, mom of three

I think you're supposed to say exciting and thrilling, but it just seemed weird. It just seemed, I don't know alien—like Wow, this is *real* that someone other than me is *in* me.

Andrea, mom of three

I felt very connected (to my kids) once I felt movement. My daughter Sasha was a tiny baby, but I could feel where she was in my body. She'd always poke out in the same place, and she'd always get hiccups at ten-thirty at night. Oliver was a really big baby, and he was all over and everywhere! I mean legs and arms . . . It was a really different experience with him because he was really active and Sasha was sort of this gentle little thing inside of me that sort of poked around every once in a while.

Mary, mom of two

• *Mom:* These weeks can be both exciting and a little fraught. You may start to feel the baby move, and you'll probably have a chance to take a good long look at her during a level 2 ultrasound, which is given between weeks 18 and 22. (Also known as an anatomy scan, see page 303.) Usually, if you want, you can find out whether you're having a boy or a girl during an anatomy scan. But sometimes the baby's in a funny position and the doctor or technician can't tell.

Many women feel the ultrasound is a real highlight of pregnancy—but waiting to have the test can be a little nerve-racking for some moms-to-be since the test

The Importance of Sound to Your Baby

✦ Reports of the sophistication of a baby's sense of sound in the womb are amazing. For example, researchers have shown that fetuses can react to a sound as early as sixteen weeks. By twenty-four weeks, they can move in rhythm to the mother's speech, and after birth, babies calm down when they listen to lullabies they first heard in the womb. For all these reasons, starting at twenty-two to twenty-four weeks, I recommend talking, reading, singing, and playing music to your baby. These activities give you a concrete way to connect with and focus on your baby. In addition, there's a device called Baby IQ that I find very exciting because I believe it can enhance the experience of communicating with your baby. It has speakers that you strap over your uterus to safely and gently transmit your voice to your baby.

Both the high-tech speaker system and the low-tech hands on the belly and talking out loud or singing method are great ways to spend "quality time" with your baby when he's still in the womb. (For more on sound and the womb, see page 208. For more on prenatal psychology, go to *www.birthpsychology.com.*)

could reveal an anatomical problem. (After all, it's given to make sure that the baby's anatomically healthy.) Also, if you've had or are planning to have an AFP/multiple marker test or an amniocentesis, you may be anxious about either how the test itself will go or what the results will be.

Once the prenatal tests are over, the results are in, and you hopefully have learned that all is well with your baby, you may find yourself embracing being pregnant in a whole new way. You may even start to look more obviously pregnant. Even with symptoms that can crop up in the second trimester, like round ligament pain (see page 183) or a bloody or stuffy nose (see page 176), many women find these next months to be relatively comfortable, sexy, and exciting. It's not for nothing that the second trimester is called "the honeymoon trimester."

• *Your prenatal care:* Starting at twenty weeks, caregivers begin to keep track of fetal growth by measuring the distance from the top of the pubic bone to the top of the uterus (also known as the *fundus*). In a singleton pregnancy, this distance should roughly correspond in centimeters to the length of gestation (e.g., twenty weeks = twenty centimeters). Your caregiver will measure fundal height at every prenatal visit from here on out. It's a simple way to make sure that your baby is growing consistently and that your amniotic fluid level is appropriate, which is a sign that the baby is doing well. (For more on measuring fundal height, see page 346; for more on changes in amniotic fluid levels, see page 334.)

If you've having multiples, however, your fundal height isn't a reliable way to track fetal growth. Therefore, it's likely you'll have ultrasounds every four weeks after your level 2 ultrasound to keep track of fetal growth and amniotic fluid levels.

Weeks 21–24

• *The baby:* Over these next few weeks, the bones of your baby's middle ear will harden, and at around twenty-one weeks, she can hear. (Sound is the first sense that a fetus develops.) She can make out your heartbeat and breathing, your voice and your partner's—soon she'll even recognize specific pieces of music. In addition to hearing, she'll also start to practice breathing. Her nostrils will open up, and her lungs will develop little air sacs called alveoli, which, after she's born, will help deliver oxygen from the air into her bloodstream. And, of course, the baby keeps on growing. By week twenty-four, she measures about 12 inches, and she's adding weight in muscle, bone, and organs, tipping the scales at around a pound and a half.

• *Mom:* Not only is your baby growing, but your breasts are, too. They're getting ready for the work of breastfeeding, and from time to time you may notice some fluid, known as colostrum (or "pre-milk") leaking out of them. If you don't catch the leaking, you may find some dried colostrum on your nipples or in your bra (it's whitish or yellowish).

Unfortunately, breasts aren't the only things that could start leaking. You may notice that a little urine trickles out when you sneeze or laugh hard. While you might find this a bit disconcerting, it's totally normal. When you sneeze or laugh, the diaphragm contracts, pushing your abdomen and uterus down onto your bladder with more force than usual. This can strain your bladder, and urine can seep out. If you notice this happening—it's more common after a first pregnancy or with multiples—do five sets of ten Kegels, or vaginal muscle squeezes, each day. (For more on Kegels, see page 415.)

Other symptoms that may crop up include hemorrhoids (see page 170), leg cramps (see page 173), and some tingling in your hands (see page 179). (For a complete discussion of pregnancy aches and pains, see chapter 11.)

Moving from body to mind and heart, having had the big prenatal tests, possibly finding out the sex of your baby, and feeling her move more often, you may find yourself thinking more concretely about becoming a parent and having *this particular* baby. What's she going to be like? What kind of personality will she have? What does being a mom mean to you? What kind of parent do you want to be?

These questions may float in and out of your head from time to time, or you might find yourself preoccupied with them. Fantasizing about life with your baby, nurturing ideas about being a parent while you're nurturing the baby herself, feeling excited, nervous, amazed by the prospect of mothering—emotions like these are all a basic part of being pregnant.

• *Prenatal care:* If you haven't yet talked about labor and birth with your care provider, now's a good time to do so. Bring up any questions you have, share your thoughts and preferences about labor and childbirth, and find out if he has any recommendations for a childbirth class. (For questions to ask your care provider about labor and birth, see page 82.) As always, if you have any pregnancy side effects that are especially nagging, worrying, or uncomfortable, bring those up, too.

Preparing for Childbirth

✦ Once all the tests are back and you feel well on your way into the second half of your pregnancy, you might be ready to turn your thoughts toward your birthing experience. It's still a little early to make any concrete plans, but if you have strong feelings about the birth itself (for example, if you have specific desires, concerns, or fears), by starting now to think about them, you can give yourself time to explore your questions, communicate your desires, establish your priorities, and work through any fears, so you can embrace the birth experience with excitement and love. Some elements of preparing for birth include:

• *Classes:* A childbirth class should help you understand how your body works, how birth is handled in different settings, and the choices you'll have in labor. There are a few different types of childbirth preparation classes from which to choose. Hospital-based classes tend to take place over the course of one day or several evenings. Classes in a particular approach to birth tend to require a bigger time commitment—up to twelve meetings. (For more on choosing a childbirth class, see page 407.)

• *A birthing team:* Who will be with you when you are in labor and giving birth is a crucial, and often overlooked, element of the birth experience. Your birthing team can be made up of just you and your primary support person (many women choose their partner, but it doesn't have to be your partner) or your partner and any number of other people—for example, a birth doula (see page 445), a close friend, or a family member. Two things to keep in mind when you create a birthing team: (1) Choose people you trust to support you in ways you'll be comfortable with, and (2) talk with your partner about each of your expectations and needs in labor—they don't always align. (For more on creating a "birthing team," see page 397.)

Note: If you decide you want to have a doula for labor, or even if you're just considering it, start asking around for names. Talk to other women who've worked with a doula and ask your care provider if there's anyone he'd recommend.

• *A mind-body visualization exercise:* There is a specific mind-body exercise that I ask all the pregnant women I work with to try after twenty to twenty-two weeks. It takes about twenty minutes, and when you're ready to do it, turn to page 63 for instructions/description. If you read the description before you're prepared to do the exercise, it will be less effective.

• *Talking with your care provider:* Whenever you start thinking about giving birth—whether it's now or later in your pregnancy—it's important to figure out what's right for *you*. If in this process you begin to have doubts about whether your care provider is a good match for your needs, try to talk to her about it. Your concerns may be well founded and you may want to find another care provider, or the discussion can help you deepen your confidence in the one you have, her care and overall approach. Either way, you'll be in a better position to trust your care provider when you're in labor and really need to depend on her. (For a discussion of the emotional preparation for labor, please see chapter 19. For a discussion of what happens during labor, including the stages of labor and some of the standard medical procedures, please see chapter 21.)

Weeks 25–28

• *The baby:* The baby's brain is developing rapidly. A fatty substance called myelin coats the outside of nerve cells, making them more efficient at transmitting information, and the nervous system can control some movement (so those kicks

THE TWENTY-EIGHTH WEEK HURDLE

At twenty-eight weeks, the baby's lungs are not yet fully mature (that happens around thirty-seven weeks), but they're developed enough to breathe air. Therefore, you've now passed into the viability zone. This means that if a serious complication occurs or preterm labor begins and the baby must be born prematurely, his chances of survival are very good.

you're feeling aren't just reflexes!). His senses are coming alive: in addition to hearing things, he can turn toward or away from outside sources of light. And by twenty-eight weeks, the baby's lungs, which continue to mature daily, could breathe air if necessary.

At the end of these weeks, many babies flip into a head-down position in the pelvis (known as the vertex position), which is best for a vaginal birth. If your baby doesn't turn—meaning she's breech (buttocks first) or transverse (lying across your uterus), don't worry. There's plenty of time and room for her to change position; in fact, at twenty-eight weeks, 25 percent of babies are breech, but babies in the breech position account for only 3 to 4 percent of all labors. (For more on breech babies and how to encourage them to turn, see page 430.)

As of twenty-eight weeks, 2 to 3 percent of a baby's body is composed of body fat; she'll be about fifteen inches long and weigh close to three pounds.

• *Mom:* At twenty-eight weeks, the third trimester begins! Because your baby is bigger and stronger, but there's still some room for her to maneuver in the uterus, you may notice that her kicking is more . . . enthusiastic. Start to pay attention to when your baby tends to move around and when she's quiet; knowing when she tends to move will help you keep tabs on her movement overall. (For tracking fetal movement, see page 347.)

Your ever-expanding uterus displaces other organs to make room for the baby (see page 113). This can bring on side effects like constipation (see page 158) or heartburn (see page 166). And as the baby gets heavier and settles into your pelvis, you may also notice some sciatica (see page 182).

After twenty-eight weeks, you may either start having Braxton Hicks contractions, or you may find they're more frequent. (For more on Braxton Hicks, see page 193.) Braxton Hicks help the uterus prepare for labor, but they're different from "real" labor contractions because Braxton Hicks don't get more intense, don't come closer together, and may not even come at consistent time intervals. Keep drinking clear fluids, because dehydration is associated with Braxton Hicks. Call your care provider if you have more than six painful contractions in an hour.

If you have a fibroid, you may have some sharp pain from it around this time as your uterus is now big enough that it can cut off the fibroid's blood supply. If you have some pain, let your care provider know. The discomfort usually passes in a day or so, and acetaminophen and a heating pad should help. (For more on fibroids during pregnancy, see page 184.)

Two steps you can take in preparation for your birth: (1) Finalize your choice of a childbirth education class (see page 407 for a discussion of various class options), and (2) if you want to work with a birth and/or postpartum doula, ask for recommendations from your care provider, childbirth instructor, or friends who've recently had children. Then set up some interviews. With either a birth or postpartum doula, it's important to find someone who's a good fit for your personality, your dynamic with your partner and family, and your needs. (For more on birth doulas, see page 448; for more on postpartum doulas, see page 505.)

• *Prenatal care:* Between weeks 25 and 28, you'll probably have an initial test for gestational diabetes and a blood test for anemia (see page 339). The gestational diabetes test is known as a glucose screen. It involves drinking a sugary liquid, waiting an hour, and having your blood taken to test blood sugar (glucose) levels. (For a full description, see page 296.) If the results of the first test show your blood sugar levels are high, even marginally so, you'll be asked to take the follow-up test, known as the glucose tolerance test (see page 297). Only 15 percent of women who take the glucose tolerance test are eventually diagnosed with gestational diabetes.

Weeks 29–32

• *The baby:* That rhythmic thumping in your belly may have told you that your baby hiccups on a regular basis. But she also breathes rhythmically (amniotic fluid, not air) and has dream (REM) sleep and non-dream sleep. When she's awake, her eyes are open. Her brain continues to develop at a fast clip, and she has even more control over her movements. The fine hair, or lanugo, that once covered her body is starting to fall off, and by thirty-two weeks, she could weigh between three and four pounds.

• *Mom:* The baby is big, you're big, and you may start to feel like the experience of being pregnant is changing. You may tire more easily. If so, honor that and rest as much as you can. You may also find that you're more distracted and forgetful. This isn't unusual at any time in a pregnancy, but it tends to be more pronounced in the third trimester as the final hormonal surges set in.

Over these and the coming weeks, you may also notice that your emotions are even more intense than they've been (which is saying something) and your dreams may become extremely vivid. In my practice, we've found that women are very receptive to imagery exercises in the third trimester, and we use them to help moms work through any persistent fears or emotional blocks they have about birth. (For example, see "From My Office: Using Guided Imagery and Creating a Birthing Team" on page 399.)

• *Prenatal care:* Depending on your care provider, if you've had a low-risk pregnancy, you may start having prenatal appointments every two weeks starting around thirty weeks. (Women with higher-risk pregnancies and multiples may already be going every two weeks.) In the third trimester your caregiver will want to keep closer tabs on how you're progressing and catch any potential red flags as soon as they show up.

Your caregiver will continue to monitor fundal height, urine, weight, and blood pressure to see if there's any major change that could indicate a problem such as low, or high, levels of amniotic fluid (see pages 334–339) or preeclampsia (see page 357).

Note: Now's a good time to start thinking about a pediatrician. Once again, ask around for recommendations. Some pediatricians schedule prenatal visits during which you have a chance to meet the doctor, discuss his approach, and figure out if he's a good fit for you and your family.

Weeks 33–40

• *The baby:* These weeks are all about weight gain for the baby. She continues to move around, which could feel more like jabs as she has less and less room to maneuver. She spends her waking hours practicing movements like turning her head, grasping, and, of course, sucking and swallowing, which she's been doing for months. Most important, at thirty-seven weeks, her lungs are mature (or nearly so) and lined with surfactant, a substance that keeps the lungs expanded after each breath.

Meconium, the dark green waste product that will be baby's first bowel movement, accumulates in her intestines. Babies usually pass meconium within twenty-four hours of their birth, but *occasionally* they pass it in the womb or during labor. (Meconium is found in amniotic fluid in 5 to 10 percent of births.) If there's meconium in your amniotic fluid when your water breaks and it's before your due date, it

Making the Connection: Breathing with Your Baby

✦ As childbirth nears, you may be busy wrapping things up at work, preparing your house, running errands, etc. No matter how busy you are, starting six or eight weeks before you expect to give birth, think about setting aside a little time each day or every few days to slow down and connect with your baby. Use the time to prepare for the birth experience you'll share with your baby and practice being in the present moment together. You can talk to your baby about the birth and/or sit quietly with your hands on your abdomen and simply *be* together. (For a description of simple ways you can connect with your baby before birth, see page 405.)

might be a sign of distress, because babies sometimes move their bowels when they're stressed. However, if you're postdate and you have meconium in your amniotic fluid, it's more likely to be normal, because the baby's digestive system could be mature and simply passing meconium because it's ready to.

Either way, if your water breaks at home and there's meconium in it, let your caregiver know. You'll be able to tell if meconium is present if it's at all green and/or at all thick; normal amniotic fluid is usually thin and clear or straw-colored. The amount of meconium in amniotic fluid determines its color and consistency. With less meconium in it, the amniotic fluid can be "light," meaning it's light green and still fairly thin. With more, it can be described as "thick," meaning it's dark green and has the consistency of pea soup. Thicker, pea soup–like meconium is more worrisome because it may indicate that a particularly stressful event either has happened or is ongoing. No matter the consistency or color of the fluid, if meconium is present, the baby will need some extra attention and suctioning at birth to make sure she hasn't breathed in any of it, which could irritate her lungs. ("Pea soup" meconium is also a bigger concern because it's more irritating to a baby's lungs if she breathes it in.)

Note: Eight-five percent of babies are born two weeks before or two weeks after their due dates.

• *Mom:* In the final stretch, you may feel the weight of time on your hands . . . and your hips. Your uterus will probably reach its highest point by week 36, after which the baby may "drop" down into your pelvis at any time (usually, this happens about two weeks before labor starts). Once the baby drops, your uterus will measure a little smaller. You may find it's easier to breathe and eat because there's more room at the top of your abdomen. But you may also find that you have to go to the bathroom even more often because there's more pressure on your pelvis. The urge to go to the bathroom, along with general excitement/anxiety about the upcoming birth and your growing size, can make it hard both to get comfortable and to sleep. (For insomnia in the third trimester, see page 185.)

Your emotions at this stage are likely to be fairly intense. You may be short-tempered or preoccupied. You may be simultaneously excited and nervous about the birth. You may find you're more introspective and spending a lot of time thinking about the transition to motherhood or imagining childbirth.

And you've heard of the famous nesting instinct? Not everyone experiences it, but many do. Women talk about needing to scrub all the light switches or reorganize home offices with a particular zeal that they've never experienced before. (See "Signs of Labor" on page 435.)

• *Prenatal care:* After thirty-six weeks, you'll probably start seeing your caregiver once a week. During these last weeks of your pregnancy, your care provider will keep an eye out for symptoms of late-developing complications such as a change in your blood pressure or weight (see preeclampsia on page 357), as well as any signs that labor may begin sooner as opposed to later, for example if your cervix begins to thin (efface) or open (dilate). (For a discussion of signs of labor, see page 491.) If your care provider is at all concerned about how the baby's doing, or if you reach forty-one weeks, you may have a biophysical profile (see page 288) or non-stress test (see page 299) to make sure the baby continues to do well.

11

Pregnancy's Effects

Every pregnant woman notices her body changing as it adapts to the flood of hormones and makes room for a growing baby. These changes may be uncomfortable or surprising, but they're all part and parcel of the extraordinary physical journey through pregnancy.

◆ ◆ ◆

In this chapter you'll find:

- Acne/Skin Changes
- Back Pain
- Bleeding Gums
- Breast Leakage
- Changes in Libido
- Constipation
- Darkening Skin
- Fatigue
- Gas and Bloating
- Hair and Nail Growth
- Headaches

- Heartburn (acid reflux) and Indigestion
- Hemorrhoids and Varicose Veins
- Itchiness in General and Heat Rash
- Leg Cramps
- Nosebleeds and Stuffy Noses
- Pimply Rash
- Pink/Red Palms
- Pins and Needles in the Hands
- Pins and Needles: Carpal Tunnel Syndrome

- Rib Pain and/or Pain in the Middle Back
- Sciatica
- Sharp Pain or Dull Ache in Lower Abdomen or Groin
- Skin Tags
- Sleep Problems
- Sore Tailbone
- Soreness at the Top of the Belly

- Stretch Marks
- Swelling
- Swollen Labia
- Tightening of the Abdomen
- Umbilical Hernia
- Urinary Frequency
- Vaginal Discharge
- Vaginal Pain

Note: For pregnancy side effects specific to the first trimester, see chapter 9.

Bear in Mind

✦ Throughout this chapter, I give specific recommendations for herbal remedies and over-the-counter medications. Every doctor and midwife will have his or her own opinion of what works and, for herbs and medications, what's safe. The recommendations I give here are the ones I give to my patients. To the best of my knowledge and understanding of the latest scientific literature as of this writing, they're safe during pregnancy. But the effects of many conventional and herbal medicines during pregnancy haven't been well studied, and new research is being published all the time. Therefore, I advise following these guidelines before taking any conventional or herbal medication:

- Avoid taking any conventional or herbal medication during the first trimester, when organ and limb development occurs.
- Don't take conventional medication, even over-the-counter, unless it's prescribed or approved by your caregiver. Don't take herbal medications or supplements without checking with your caregiver first.
- Purchase all herbal supplements from a reputable source. (See appendix 1 for recommendations.)
- *Call your caregiver before taking any over-the-counter medication or herbal remedy.*

Acne/Skin Changes*

- *When it happens:* Throughout pregnancy.
- *What happens:* While you're pregnant, rising hormone levels can either clear up your skin or trigger acne. If you experience pregnancy-related breakouts, take good care of your skin. Oral antibiotics for acne are generally *not* prescribed during pregnancy. Topical, over-the-counter acne medications that contain salicylic acid or glycolic acid, and various prescription topical antibiotics, particularly topical erythromycin, are safe to use. Most often, pregnancy-related acne clears up after delivery.
- *What you can do:*
  - *Keep skin clean:* Wash your face twice a day and after exercising. You may want to add a gentle exfoliant once a day, especially if your skin is oily, and use a light moisturizer. You may find it helpful to use facial acne masks with glycolic or salicylic acid once or twice a week, especially if your face is oily.
  - *Eat and drink well:* Avoid greasy, sugary, and salty foods and continue to drink plenty of water, which keeps skin from drying out.
  - *Treat as needed:* Use topical, over-the-counter creams that contain glycolic acid or salicylic acid.

Note: Facials are a good idea for acne and safe during pregnancy. From around twenty-four weeks on, lying flat on your back for the duration of a facial (usually sixty to ninety minutes) may make you dizzy, faint, or uncomfortable because your uterus may press against the vena cava, a major blood vessel that runs along the right side of your body, and reduce blood flow. To counter that, prop your left hip and low back up on a pillow (your hip should be at least on a fifteen-degree angle above the table), which will shift the uterus off the vena cava. (For more advice on beauty treatments during pregnancy, see page 311.)

Cautions:

1. *Never take Accutane while pregnant or trying to conceive.* It's extremely dangerous to a developing fetus. If you discover you're pregnant while taking Accutane, call your caregiver immediately.

---

*Dr. Robin Evans, dermatologist (and wife of Dr. Joel Evans), contributed to all material related to skin and hair.

2. Retin-A, a topical prescription acne medication, is *not* safe to use during pregnancy, nor are over-the-counter medications with retinol.
3. Over-the-counter topical acne ointments are not necessarily safe during pregnancy. Avoid creams with benzoyl peroxide. Over-the-counter sulfur-based ointments may be used safely during the *second* and *third* trimesters.

Q: I'm pregnant with twins. Will my symptoms be different?

Dr. Evans: It's impossible to predict what symptoms any pregnant woman will experience, but there aren't any pregnancy symptoms that are unique to a multiple pregnancy. When you're pregnant with more than one baby, your symptoms aren't necessarily any different, but they may be stronger because the demands made on your body are that much greater. And if you're carrying triplets, your symptoms could be that much more significant than those of a woman carrying twins.

Back Pain (especially low back pain)

• *When it happens:* Second and third trimesters.

• *What happens:* When you're not pregnant, your low back supports you with the help of your abdominal muscles and round ligaments, which stretch from your pelvis to your spine. As your pregnancy progresses, your abdominal muscles stretch and weaken while the pregnancy hormones relaxin and estrogen loosen the ligaments around your pelvis, leaving much more work for your low back. In addition, your growing belly shifts your center of gravity forward, which can create a "sway," a more pronounced curve in your low back. As your pregnancy progresses, you may even start walking differently. All of these changes strain your low back and contribute to low back pain, which can range from very mild to quite severe.

• *What you can do:*

— *Pay attention to your posture:* When you find yourself standing somewhere (on a line, waiting to cross the street, chopping vegetables), check in with your tailbone, the nub on the very end of your spine. Is it swaying far out behind you? If so, try to tuck it in by bringing your pubic bone forward. The goal is to *lengthen* your low back, *not* straighten it, and the movement is fairly subtle. As you extend your spine, try to keep your chest open and shoulders back. (Shoulders tend to fall forward when the pubic bone moves forward.) Finally, try not to squeeze your buttocks as you make these adjustments.

— *Sit and stand with support:* Sit with both feet on the ground and, if you can, with a little pillow behind your low back. If you know you'll be on your feet for a while, see if you can put one or the other foot up on a low footstool.

— *Lift from bent knees:* When you lift something up, put one foot forward, bend your knees, use both hands, and lift up by straightening your knees. (Don't ever lift from your hips or a bent back.)

— *Wear comfortable shoes:* Wear shoes with a wide heel and arch support. Avoid high heels.

— *Exercise:* Both prenatal yoga classes and swimming can help build up abdominal muscles, which will relieve back pain. Daily walks can relieve stiffness in your back. If you jog or go for "power walks," do so on soft surfaces like a tartan track, sand, dirt, or grass. Avoid pavement as much as you can and remember to stretch before and after a workout. (*Note:* Some women find swimming during pregnancy strains their backs; if you find this to be the case, don't keep trying to swim.)

— *Hot and cold compresses:* Apply heat and cold each for fifteen minutes at a time. If one is more soothing, stick with it instead of switching.

— *Warm baths:* A warm bath with some lavender in it can be relaxing and soothing to sore muscles and back. The water shouldn't be above 102 degrees F. In other words, when you stick your toe in the water, if the water is comfortable, the bath is a good temperature. If you need to pull your foot back and get used to the water, it's too hot.

— *Sleep with extra pillows:* Place a pillow between your legs when you sleep or even when you are lying on the couch.

— *Home massage with herbal rubs:* Ask your partner or a friend to massage your low back with Tiger Balm or White Flower Analgesic Balm. Both are available in health food stores. Tiger Balm may also be available in hardware stores. Begin by sensitizing the skin and body to the effects of the massage: Gently massage the length of the spine without the rub. (You may want to use some lotion or massage oil to reduce friction.) After a few minutes, apply the herbal rub into the low back by making wide circles over the area that's uncomfortable. "Dig" gently with thumbs to make smaller circles while pressing into especially sore spots.

— *Acupuncture:* For some women, one acupuncture session relieves back pain; for others, it takes several sessions for the pain to improve. Be sure to work with an acupuncturist who has experience with pregnant women. If you don't feel a difference after a few treatments, consider finding a different practitioner. (For more on working with an acupuncturist, see chapter 1.)

- *Chiropractic:* Chiropractic therapy, performed by an experienced practitioner who has worked with pregnant women, can offer relief for pregnancy-related back pain.
- *Massage:* Swedish or shiatsu massage can relax and soothe muscles that are working overtime.
- *Extra-strength acetaminophen (Tylenol):* A safe option when the pain is bad. Take 1,000 mg every six hours as needed. See your provider if the pain isn't getting better or if you have taken acetaminophen for more than fourteen days.
• *Herbal remedies:*
- *Valerian (Valeriana officinalis):* Take thirty drops of a standard tincture mixed into hot water about an hour before bedtime. It calms muscle spasms and will help you sleep through the night. Don't take for more than seven nights in a row. (For more on valerian, see "Sleep Problems" on page 185.) It's available at health food stores, natural markets, and online. (For herbal medicine resources, turn to page 523.)

Using Herbal Tinctures and Teas

✦ Using herbal medicine means locating reliable brands for teas and tinctures and using them appropriately. According to herbalist Richard Mandelbaum, keep the following in mind when mixing tinctures and teas:

• *Herbal tinctures:* Tinctures contain alcohol, but because they're taken in very small doses over a limited period of time, their alcohol content should not cause concern in pregnancy. To burn off about half of the alcohol, drop the tincture into water that has been brought to a boil and allowed to cool slightly. Then, let the mixture steep for ten to fifteen minutes. If you drop the tincture directly into boiling water, you'll burn away most of its medicinal properties along with the alcohol.

Caution: If you're a recovering alcoholic, avoid herbal tinctures and use herbal teas instead.

• *Herbal teas:* For the most part, commercially sold herbal teas are weak. To produce a more potent infusion from store-bought teas, try using two tea bags at once.

From My Office

✦ Low back pain in pregnancy has clear biomechanical causes. But low back pain is a physical symptom that's known to be aggravated by stress and anxiety—whether or not you're pregnant. When I'm working with a pregnant woman who has persistent low back pain (or headaches, which also can have a stress component), first we explore all the physical causes through various tests and consultations with specialists. If nothing unusual appears and her back pain doesn't get any better with physical therapy and appropriate exercise, I may ask the woman to think about what the symptom is telling her. In other words, I'll suggest that she ask the pain directly why it's there.

For example, Julie was in her late thirties and pregnant with her first baby. Her back pain, which was severe, had started in her second trimester. She had seen a neurologist and back specialist, and both attributed the pain to "pregnancy." Nothing they suggested, other than strong medication that Julie didn't want to take, eased the pain. During an office visit early in her third trimester, we were talking about her low back pain—when it was really bad, when it eased. I said to her, "The next time the pain gets intense, ask it what it's telling you." To be honest, she looked quite skeptical about doing this.

At her next office visit, she told me she had tried talking to her pain and what happened amazed her. When she asked the pain "Why are you here?" she got an answer: "You're trying too hard." She realized she was exhausted from trying to make sure she got everything for the baby "right"—the perfect stroller, the perfect paint color for the nursery, the most detailed birth plan. As we talked, it became clear to both of us that Julie thought by controlling everything she could, she would protect her son, and herself, from everything she couldn't control.

We then talked about how she could nurture a belief that the baby would be fine even if everything wasn't "perfect." I recommended that she begin and end each day by repeating an affirmation three times. She agreed to try saying the following: "I trust in the universe, and that everything will be as it should." She used the affirmation to help her focus her attention on the idea that loving her child was the most perfect thing she could do to help him be safe and happy. In the last phase of her pregnancy, Julie slowed down considerably, preparing less and concentrating more on what it meant to her to be there for her son. As she did, her back pain improved quite a bit.

Note: While valerian is generally considered safe in pregnancy, a small percentage of people find it works as a stimulant. If you're trying it for the first time, particularly at night, take a smaller dose—about half the normal dose—as a trial.

Tip: Massage is a relaxing, appealing treatment for many of the side effects of pregnancy, but frequent massages can get expensive. An electric or manual massage device, available at drugstores and specialty shops, can give you some of the benefits of a massage at a fraction of the cost.

Alternatively, if there's a reputable massage therapy school in your area, you can get relatively inexpensive massage treatments from its students. To get licensed or accredited, students need to spend a certain number of hours providing massage therapy, and they usually offer low rates to those who are open to massage from a student. When you set up your appointment, be sure to let the school and the massage therapist know that you're pregnant. See if they train students in prenatal massage, and ask for a student who already has prenatal massage experience.

REAL VOICES

I had prenatal massage almost weekly throughout my first pregnancy. It was fabulous and luxurious. I really couldn't do it the second time around, working full-time with a kid. But it was great.

Martha, mom of two

Bleeding Gums

- *When it happens:* Typically begins in the second trimester.
- *What happens:* The hormones of pregnancy can make your gums tender and inflamed. In addition, the veins throughout your body, including in your mouth, swell when you're pregnant. The combination of inflamed gums and swollen veins means that your gums may bleed more than normal. If you notice this happening, go to the dentist to have your teeth and gums cleaned and examined. Switching to a soft-bristle toothbrush may help reduce the bleeding, but it's no substitute for a visit to the dentist.

Note: Be sure to brush and floss well throughout your pregnancy, and see your dentist for at least one cleaning while you're expecting. Advanced gum disease (gingivitis) has been linked to preterm labor, so you need to make sure your gums stay healthy.

Caution: If you experience heavy bleeding from your gums, call your doctor or midwife.

Breast Leakage

• *When it happens:* Typically begins around twenty weeks; may begin in first trimester.

• *What happens:* From about twenty weeks until delivery, you may notice liquid leaking from your breasts from time to time—it may also happen when your nipples are stimulated. While relatively unusual, breast leakage is absolutely normal. The liquid is colostrum, the "pre-milk" that the breasts produce. (For more on colostrum and breastfeeding, see page 499.) If the leaking becomes heavy, you can put a breast pad in your bra, and let your caregiver know.

> ### SUDDEN BREAST LUMPS
>
> Breast cysts form as a response to hormones, which are at dramatically high levels during pregnancy. Therefore, you may notice a lump that seems to have appeared suddenly in one or both breasts. This isn't a common side effect of pregnancy, but it's not unknown. If you find a lump, let your caregiver know immediately so you can have it checked out. But keep in mind that it's most likely there because of the hormones of pregnancy.

Caution: If you notice that the liquid from your breasts is pink or red, notify your doctor or midwife. The most common cause of a reddish or bloody nipple discharge is a noncancerous growth that should be checked out by your caregiver or a specialist.

Changes in Libido

• *When it happens:* Throughout pregnancy.

• *What happens:* Early in pregnancy, you may be tired, nauseated, or simply uncomfortable in your changing body—all of which can lower sex drive. But there are no hard-and-fast rules here. You may find your libido to be the same or increased during the first trimester. During your second trimester, it's entirely normal to experience a sharp increase in your libido. We don't really know why this happens, but more blood flow in the pelvis and vagina may be responsible for some of the enhanced sensation. Whatever the reason, some women say they have the most intense orgasms of their lives during this period. Once the third trimester rolls around, you may once again be more tired, less comfortable, and less interested in sex. This is absolutely normal.

REAL VOICES

My sex drive went from one extreme to the other . . . sometimes I was very horny, and sometimes I couldn't imagine anything less appealing!

Kate, mom of one, pregnant

I definitely wasn't one of those women who felt erotic during pregnancy, even though I felt great about my body . . . I was kind of scared to have an orgasm—not what would it do to the baby but I had so many contractions in both of my pregnancies that the one time I did have an orgasm I had a lot of contractions and it was scary. I knew it wouldn't put me into labor, but I definitely shied away.

Mary, mom of two

Constipation

• *When it happens:* Typically in the first and third trimesters, but it can happen at any time during pregnancy.
• *What happens:* Like gas and bloating, in the first trimester, constipation is a side effect of slowed digestion. In the third trimester, the baby presses against the colon, slowing it down. (For what you can do about it, see first trimester symptoms on page 114.)

Darkening Skin (hyperpigmentation)

• *When it happens:* Typically in the second trimester, though it can happen earlier or later.
• *What happens:*
  – *Dark patches and darkening skin:* Dark patches may appear on your breasts, nipples—especially the areolae—vulva, and abdomen because of hormonal

changes. (Actually, this can happen at any time in a woman's life, but especially during pregnancy or when taking a birth control pill.) Similarly, you may notice that overall your skin looks darker. After you give birth, your skin and the dark patches should slowly return to their pre-pregnancy color.

— *Darkening freckles and moles:* This is a result of the same hormonal shifts that bring on hyperpigmentation. As you would whenever you notice a change in a freckle or mole, ask your doctor, midwife, or dermatologist to take a look. After delivery, your freckles and moles may or may not return to their pre-pregnancy color.

— *Linea nigra:* A dark line, the linea nigra, is likely to extend from the center of the pubic bone to just below the ribs; it will become more and more obvious as your pregnancy progresses. In fact, you've always had a faint white line from your pubic bone to your navel—when it's white, it's called the linea alba—but it's darker now because of hyperpigmentation.

— *The mask of pregnancy:* Very often, dark patches will develop across a pregnant woman's cheeks and face in a butterfly pattern. Commonly called "the mask of pregnancy," this phenomenon, technically called "melasma," is also the result of hyperpigmentation that may develop during pregnancy. Typically the discoloration will fade slowly after the baby's birth. If your "mask" doesn't fade entirely before you become pregnant again, your skin may darken in your next pregnancy. It may also darken if you take birth control pills or after even slight exposure to the sun.

• *What you can do:*

— *Protect yourself from the sun:* If your skin or freckles are darker or if you have the mask of pregnancy, use a light moisturizer that contains at least SPF 15 every morning. SPF 30 is a better choice during the summer. On sunny days wear a hat or visor, and avoid prolonged exposure to the sun. (Spending hours in the sun tanning isn't a great idea during pregnancy. The heat isn't good for the developing baby, and a sunburn, uncomfortable in the best of circumstances, is especially annoying during pregnancy, when your skin may already be sensitive and itchy.)

— *Treatment:* After delivery, if the dark patches don't fade, or don't fade quickly enough, a dermatologist can treat them with bleaching creams, Retin-A (a topical medication available by prescription only), or skin peels.

Fatigue

• *When it happens:* First and third trimesters.

• *What happens:* In the first trimester, progesterone floods your body, relaxing muscles, slowing your metabolism, and leaving you with less energy. At the same time your baby is growing at a very fast clip, which you may find draining as well. As a result, you'll probably feel more tired than usual (and possibly more tired than ever before). In the second trimester, your energy levels should rebound, but they may dip again in the third trimester because you're carrying so much more weight around. Also in the third trimester, your sleep may be frequently interrupted for three reasons: (1) the baby's moving; (2) you need to urinate; (3) it's difficult to get and stay comfortable.

• *What you can do:* The most important thing you can do for fatigue is honor it, not fight it. Sleep as much as you need to—take naps and go to bed early—but try to balance sleep with movement. Take walks, swim, or go to a tai chi or prenatal Pilates class. (For more on fatigue and how you can manage it, see first trimester symptoms, page 117.)

Caution: If you're very tired all the time at any point in your pregnancy, but especially in the third trimester, let your doctor or midwife know; you may need to have a blood test for anemia, a common problem in the third trimester. (For more on anemia, see page 339.)

REAL VOICES
I was tired (in the first pregnancy), but not like this. I mean, on Saturday, I must have slept six hours during the day, and then I went to bed at nine-thirty. I'm just so low energy.

Asha, mom of one, pregnant

Gas and Bloating

• *When it happens:* Throughout pregnancy.

• *What happens:* From early in your pregnancy, you might find that you're burping and passing gas more often. Because progesterone relaxes the muscles of the small and large intestines, your digestion slows down. Slower digesting produces more gas, which means more burping, flatulence, and general bloating. In the second trimester, when your body has adapted to the progesterone and the baby is not that big, you may find you're more comfortable and less gassy. But in the third trimester, as the baby gets bigger and pushes against the intestines, the movement of the intestines slows down again, which leads to more constipation and bloating.

• *What you can do:*
   — *Exercise:* Moderate activity, like walking or swimming, can help keep food moving through the digestive tract. Since gas develops when food stalls, this limits gas production to some degree.
   — *Try not to swallow extra air:* We all swallow air when we eat and drink. But more air means more gas. To reduce the amount of air that you swallow, sip when you drink and avoid using a straw. Eat slowly and chew thoroughly. Drink before and after a meal, but limit how much you drink while you eat. Try to avoid or limit carbonated drinks—those little bubbles are all gas.
   — *Eat small meals sitting up:* Always eat sitting up—even if it means sitting up on the couch to have a cookie or apple when you're watching TV. Also, try to eat small meals throughout the day. If you have to digest a big meal, food will stagnate in your slow-working digestive tract, which produces gas.
   — *Limit gassy foods:* Cabbage, brussels sprouts, beans, asparagus—these are foods that can make you gassy. If you can cut back on them while maintaining a well-balanced diet, do so. Similarly, fiber-rich foods (fruits, vegetables, whole grains) may cause gas. With fiber-rich foods, you have to balance your need to alleviate constipation and maintain a balanced diet with your gassiness. If you want to cut down on fiber-rich foods, try wheat germ or ground flaxseed for constipation. (For details, see page 114.) Wheat germ passes through your system without being digested (which is why it helps with constipation), flaxseed, which is high in omega-3 essential fatty acids, has some elements that pass right through and others that are absorbed, but it may make you gassy. The only way to figure out if it works is to try it.
   — *Try acidophilus:* You can buy acidophilus and bifidobacter in one capsule; it's sold at health food stores, some organic markets, and online. Choose a brand that guarantees between 2.5 and 5 billion live bacteria per capsule up through the expiration date.
   — *Antacids:* Try an over-the-counter antacid like Maalox, Mylanta, or Tums.
• *Herbal remedies:*
   — *Fennel seed (Foeniculum vulgare):* Taken either as a tea or tincture, fennel seed is an excellent remedy for gas and bloating, and except in rare cases of allergy,

it's widely considered safe in pregnancy. You can also chew fennel seeds any-time. (Fennel seed is also known to stimulate lactation.)
Dose:

- ○ *Tea:* Drink three eight-ounce cups of tea per day.
- ○ *Tincture:* Take 2–4 ml (typically between 50 and 120 drops, depending on the viscosity of the tincture; the instructions on the bottle will guide you) in eight ounces of water three times per day. (Follow instructions for mixing tinctures on page 154.)

— *Slippery elm (Ulmus fulva):* The inner bark of the elm tree contains mucilage, a natural substance that can soothe a sore throat, irritated esophagus, or up-set stomach. For medicinal use, the inner bark is ground into a powder, which becomes viscous when mixed with water. The FDA has approved it as a nonprescription soothing agent that can be taken internally. It can be pur-chased online or at a health food store, in lozenge form or as powder that can be made into a tea.
Dose:

- ○ *Lozenges:* For dosage, follow the package instructions.
- ○ *Tea:* Drink one eight-ounce cup as needed, but no more than four cups per day. Mix one teaspoon of slippery elm powder with eight ounces of warm water. If you like you can add a flavoring like honey, nutmeg, cinnamon, or lemon. Do not take for more than fourteen days in a row.

Caution: If you buy slippery elm bark for gas and upset stomach, get a product that contains only slippery elm bark and is not mixed with anything else.

Notes:

1. As an experiment, you may want to try cutting out dairy (while taking a cal-cium supplement) and see if your symptoms change. Now that you're preg-nant, you may be somewhat lactose intolerant, meaning it's difficult or impossible for you to digest the sugar called lactose, found in milk. If you're lactose intolerant, you should be able to digest dairy products that don't con-tain lactose, such as hard cheeses, butter, and yogurt. Lactose-free milk and calcium-supplemented soy milk are both good alternatives to regular milk.
2. If you find that your stomach gets upset consistently within an hour or two of eating, the bacteria in your small intestine may be out of balance. In this sit-uation, take the "good" bacteria acidophilus and bifidobacter twice a day on

an empty stomach for two weeks. If your symptoms subside, continue to take "good" bacteria for the rest of your pregnancy. The problem of discomfort after a meal should clear up on its own within four to six weeks after you give birth; if you've always had this problem, it may persist, but the acidophilus should help.

You can buy acidophilus and bifidobacter in one capsule; it's sold at health food stores, some organic markets, and online. Choose a brand that guarantees between 2.5 and 5 billion live bacteria per capsule up through the expiration date.

R EAL V OICES
I had a lot of gas (in my second pregnancy). I felt like I needed to be poked with a pin, my stomach was always so bloated. In the first trimester I developed a terrible lactose intolerance. That actually went away during my second trimester, but before it did, if I had a bite of dairy I would just swell up like a balloon.

Mary, mom of two

Hair and Nail Growth

• *When it happens:* Throughout pregnancy.

• *What happens:* During pregnancy, your blood volume increases, as does circulation to the scalp (and the rest of the body), which can stimulate hair and nail growth. In fact, the cycle of hair growth and loss shifts during pregnancy so that a greater percentage of your hair is in a growth cycle, increasing its volume and thickness. In addition to hair changes, you may notice that your nails are stronger. Starting about three months after you give birth and continuing through the end of the first year postpartum, you'll shed some of that extra hair. (This is known as *telogen effluvium* or "the shedding.") When it happens, it may seem like quite a lot of hair is falling out. Your hair may or may not return to its pre-pregnancy state—it's unpredictable.

One other, less-welcome hair change you may notice during pregnancy is more hair may grow on places other than your head—often the face, and possibly the arms, legs, or back. This is known as "hirsutism" and should recede within six months after you give birth.

• *What you can do:* Electrolysis and waxing are safe during pregnancy, and plucking the occasional random hair is fine. There's no evidence that depilatory creams are harmful at all to the fetus, but I most often recommend that women avoid them because they're packed with chemicals. That said, since the creams aren't known to cause harm, if the excess hair is really bothersome or upsetting and a depilatory cream is the best solution, then go ahead and use it. (For more on beauty treatments during pregnancy, see page 311.)

Headaches

- *When it happens:* Throughout pregnancy.
- *What happens:* Triggered by a range of factors—fluctuating hormones, tension, low blood sugar, colds, stuffy rooms, or some combination thereof—headaches are common during pregnancy. If you were prone to headaches or migraines before you conceived, it's hard to predict how your body will respond during your pregnancy. You may be virtually headache-free throughout; or, unfortunately, you may have them more often.
- *What you can do:*
  - *Slow down:* Frequent headaches can be a signal that you're overdoing things. You may feel like you're just doing what you "normally" do—working, socializing, planning, taking care of what needs to be taken care of. But when you're pregnant, there's a difference between what your mind thinks is "normal" to do and what your body has the energy to do. Try to find ways to slow down, and see if that helps your headaches. If you work long hours, try to pace yourself by taking more breaks or by working for shorter periods over more days. Instead of running errands, ask your partner or a friend to help you out with getting things done while you take a nap, a walk, or a bath.
  - *Get some fresh air:* If you usually get headaches at work, the air quality of your office may be the cause. Try to go outside every two hours for a quick walk around the block—even if the weather's bad. Moving your body will feel good, and the fresh air will help clear your head. Allergens, like dust and mold, may also trigger headaches. You can improve air quality with an air ionizer, a small machine that changes the composition of the air and filters out allergens. You can get a portable unit to wear around your neck or a larger unit to treat an entire room.
  - *Avoid foods that trigger headaches:* Certain foods tend to trigger headaches. Common culprits include chocolate, aged cheeses, red wine, and foods with

processed sugar. Try not to eat them, even if you crave them, and see if your headaches improve.

— *Eat more proteins:* Proteins are the building blocks of chemicals in the brain. Since your body needs more protein during pregnancy, eating a protein-rich diet is a practical nutritional intervention for frequent headaches. Theoretically, it improves the balance of brain chemicals, decreasing the likelihood of headaches. Snack on foods like hummus, nuts, fresh peanut or almond butter, and protein bars. (For a chart of protein-rich foods, see page 229.)

— *Apply a cool compress:* This old-fashioned remedy really works for tension headaches. Place a cool compress on your forehead or neck, close your eyes, and breathe deeply.

— *Close your eyes:* With a bad headache, resting quietly in a dark room can relieve the pain.

— *If coffee helps:* If you know that a cup of coffee can nip your headache or migraine in the bud, drink one.

— *Take acetaminophen:* When nothing else helps, or when you're at work and need some relief, two extra-strength acetaminophen (Tylenol) tablets are perfectly safe to take. However, avoid over-the-counter headache medication unless you've already discussed taking it with your caregiver.

— *Massage:* Ask your partner or a friend to gently rub your temples, neck, and shoulders. An hour-long Swedish or shiatsu massage will also help reduce tension and ease pain.

— *Acupuncture:* Acupuncture treatments can relieve persistent headaches. Before you schedule an appointment, ask the practitioner if she has experience treating pregnancy-related headaches. If you decide to have a session, ask how quickly you'll feel relief and if you'll need to come in regularly.

Caution: The headache acupressure point between your thumb and index finger is commonly known to relieve headaches. While this is true, it's also a point that's used to induce labor. If you tend to have headaches, and if you used that acupressure point for relief before you became pregnant, avoid pressing it frequently during your pregnancy.

Notes:

1. If in addition to headaches you have eczema, joint pain, or feel depressed, your immune system may be overworked and inflamed. If this is your situation, talk to your caregiver about it and increase your daily dose of omega-3

essential fatty acids to 3 grams (3,000 mg) of EPA/DHA daily. *Only take a supplement that guarantees it's free of PCBs and heavy metals.* (See page 522 for sources.)

2. If you have frequent headaches and your nose is often stuffy, you may be sensitive to dairy products made from cow's milk (as opposed to goat's or sheep's milk or soy). Try cutting out cow's milk dairy products for fourteen days, being sure to maintain consumption of 1,500 mg of calcium daily. (For nondairy calcium sources, see pages 220–222.) Talk to your caregiver before taking this step, and if you decide to try it, consider meeting with a nutritionist.

If your headaches are persistent and nothing seems to give you relief, talk with your doctor or midwife about what conventional medications besides acetaminophen might help. Keep in mind that headaches have a stress component. If nothing helps, the next time you have one, try asking your headache what it's telling you. It might be a pointless exercise, and you might feel a little silly doing it, but it won't hurt you, and I've worked with women for whom this strategy has helped identify and improve situations that were triggering stress headaches. (For more on "asking" your symptom for feedback see "Back Pain," page 152.)

Caution: If you're in your third trimester and you've had fairly bad headaches for two or three days in a row, *or* if you have an unusually severe headache, *or* if you have headaches and blurry vision *together* for even one day, contact your caregiver right away. The headaches may be a symptom of high blood pressure or preeclampsia. (Preeclampsia is a syndrome consisting of high blood pressure, swelling (edema), and protein in the urine. High blood pressure alone can develop before, during, or after a pregnancy.) If you have high blood pressure, your doctor or midwife will have to determine if it's an isolated symptom or indicative of preeclampsia. If you're working with a midwife, this may be a situation in which she calls in a consulting physician. (For more on preeclampsia, see page 357.)

Heartburn (acid reflux) and Indigestion

- *When it happens:* Second and third trimesters.
- *What happens:* As your pregnancy progresses, you're more likely to experience heartburn and indigestion because: (1) progesterone relaxes the muscles in the esophagus and stomach walls, so the flap that separates the two (the pyloric valve)

doesn't close tightly, making it easier for food and gastric juices from the stomach to travel up the esophagus and cause an uncomfortable burning sensation; (2) as the baby grows, it presses against the stomach, which in turn puts pressure on the pyloric valve, pushing gastric juices up into the esophagus.

- *What you can do:*
  - *Eat small meals slowly and frequently:* Chew food slowly and thoroughly and eat small meals often. This will keep your stomach occupied (acid sloshes around an empty stomach, causing nausea and heartburn), and it'll keep you from having a too-full stomach, which would put additional pressure on the pyloric valve. As a test, try having a snack a little more than an hour before you go to sleep so you have something in your stomach most of the night. This may keep you more comfortable. If you're digesting food slowly, however, the pre-bed snack might make you uncomfortable. You might lie down and discover you're still a little full. All you can do is try it and see if it works for you.
  - *Eat simple foods:* Don't eat spicy or acidic foods. Also, peppermint and chocolate can both increase stomach acid; if you have heartburn and crave either, eat it very moderately, or see if you feel better when you don't eat it at all.
  - *Drink between meals:* Water helps both to neutralize stomach acids and to move food into the small intestine.
  - *Let gravity help:* Eat sitting up; prop yourself up when you sleep; and try to maintain good posture throughout the day. When you slump, your stomach gets even more compressed and has less room to work.
  - *Take an antacid:* These work sometimes, but not all the time—and for some women they make things worse. The only way to know for sure is to test what works for you. Try Tums, Maalox, or Mylanta.
- *Herbal remedies:*
  - *Marshmallow tea (from the plant Althaea officinalis):* Both the root and leaf of this plant contain mucilage, a substance that becomes gooey when you add water to it. It's been used for centuries to soothe sore throats and protect the lining of the esophagus, and it's rich in vitamins. Marshmallow tea is available at health food stores, natural markets, and online. (For recommendations, see page 523.)

  Dose:
    ○ Drink one eight-ounce cup as needed, up to four cups a day. You can get either tea bags or the raw herb. To make tea from raw herb, mix two to

Mind-Body Medicine: Autogenics

✦ Autogenics, also known as "self-hypnosis," is a mind-body technique that allows you to actually change your physiology simply by sitting quietly and repeating a specific phrase to yourself at least six times. It can be a powerful tool in relieving headaches. For example, if you repeat, "My arms are heavy and warm . . . I am at peace," you'll begin to notice that your arms are, in fact, heavy and warm. (To prove that your body temperature has changed, you can buy something called a BioDot at a drugstore or online. It's a small adhesive thermometer you can put on your finger. As your temperature changes, the colors go from greenish-yellow to a purple.) There are six autogenic phrases that studies have shown can change body functions. They are:

- My arms are heavy and warm.
- My legs are heavy and warm.
- My heartbeat is calm and strong.
- My forehead is pleasant and cool.
- My breathing is calm and relaxed.
- My abdomen radiates warmth.

In my own practice, I always suggest adding "I am at peace" after the first statement. For example, for pregnancy-related headaches, I would recommend repeating, "My forehead is pleasant and cool . . . I am at peace" six times, followed by six repetitions of "My breathing is calm and relaxed . . . I am at peace."

To do this, make yourself comfortable by sitting or lying down in a room where the temperature is neither too hot nor too cool. Turn off the phone, and if there's anyone home with you, ask not to be interrupted for fifteen minutes to a half hour. Begin by saying to yourself, slowly and steadily, "My forehead is pleasant and cool," pause for approximately two seconds, then say "I am at peace." Pause for a few more seconds, and then repeat the whole thing at least five more times. This should take three to five minutes, after which you should continue to lie or sit and breathe quietly for a minute or so. Begin the process again, this time using the phrase "My breathing is calm and relaxed . . . I am at peace." You can experiment by trying one, two, or as many of the phrases as you like. See how working with different phrases affects you. Or you can simply sit quietly and focus on your breathing for a couple of minutes. As you inhale, think of the word "calm," and as you exhale, think of the word "peace."

You might find it helpful to make an audiotape of yourself or a friend who has an appealing voice slowly saying the phrases at least six times, leaving enough time between each expression for you, or someone else, to repeat the phrase slowly and deliberately. The tape would go like this:

Voice: My forehead is pleasant and cool . . . I am at peace. (Pause.)
You: Repeat slowly, either silently or out loud in a quiet voice.
Voice: My forehead is pleasant and cool . . . I am at peace. (Pause.)
You: Repeat silently or out loud in a quiet voice.

Continue for a total of six repetitions.

three teaspoons of marshmallow tea in a half cup (four ounces) of cool water. Let the water sit for about an hour and a half, strain it, then warm it up over a medium flame. Follow package instructions for tea bags. Don't take for more than fourteen days in a row.

Caution: Marshmallow tea can affect blood sugar levels; don't drink it if you have gestational diabetes. Also, it may slow the absorption of prescription medication. If you're taking medication regularly, check with your doctor or midwife before trying the tea.

— *Meadowsweet (Filipendula):* Taken in tincture or tea form, this herb soothes and heals the lining of the gastrointestinal tract, and it reduces excess acidity. Meadowsweet contains salicylates, substances that are used to relieve pain and lower fevers. (Aspirin contains them as well.)

Dose:

  ○ Tincture: Take 2 to 4 ml (typically 50 to 120 drops, depending on the viscosity of the tincture; follow instructions on the bottle) three times daily. (Follow instructions for mixing tinctures on page 154.)

  ○ Tea: Up to three eight-ounce cups per day.

— *Slippery elm (Ulmus fulva):* Like marshmallow tea, the inner bark of the elm tree also contains mucilage. For medicinal purposes, slippery elm is ground into a powder, which becomes thick and gooey when water is added. It's

FDA approved and can soothe a sore throat and an irritated esophagus and belly. Slippery elm lozenges, powder, and tea are available at health food stores, natural markets, and online.

Dose:

○ Drink one eight-ounce cup as needed, up to four cups a day. Pour eight ounces of hot water over one teaspoon of slippery elm powder. Do not take for more than fourteen days in a row. Follow the package instructions for dosage if you are taking lozenges.

Caution: For an upset stomach, buy lozenges that contain only slippery elm and nothing else.

Note: Over-the-counter heartburn medications like antacids are safe to take occasionally when you're very uncomfortable. However, I wouldn't recommend taking an over-the-counter version of stronger drugs such as Zantac, unless directed by your physician.

Hemorrhoids and Varicose Veins

- *When it happens:* Third trimester.
- *What happens:* The baby creates pressure in the pelvis, slowing blood flow in leg veins, whose walls have already been relaxed by progesterone. The relaxed veins can't pump blood as effectively as usual, so blood begins to pool in them, and they swell into varicose veins. This can happen in your labia (see "Swollen Labia," page 192), legs, and rectum. Rectal varicose veins are commonly known as hemorrhoids. They feel like a soft swollen mass near your rectum that can be as small as a pea or as big as a grape. Hemorrhoids can be itchy, uncomfortable, or painful, and sometimes they bleed when you have a bowel movement.
- *Hemorrhoids—what you can do:*
  - *Use arnica gel:* Once you notice a hemorrhoid, apply arnica gel every time you go to the bathroom, even when you urinate. Arnica gel is a homeopathic cure for inflamed muscles; it also comes in a cream form, but don't use the cream for hemorrhoids. For reasons I can't explain, the experience of my patients is that the gel works much better than the cream. It's available at health food stores, natural markets, and online.
  - *Don't push and don't wait:* Try not to strain when you go to the bathroom, and don't put it off.

Herbal Medicine: Does It Work?

✦ We know that compounds in plants, as well as in fruits and vegetables, have been used for medicinal purposes for centuries. And many modern medicines are derived from plant substances. We also know that all herbs aren't benign. As with conventional medications, some can be quite dangerous, and you need to know what to take when and for how long. Doctors, midwives, homeopaths, and herbalists who use botanical medicine combine as best they can the historical knowledge developed over centuries with modern clinical use and scientific analysis in order to prescribe herbs safely and effectively.

That said, conventional doctors and scientists could say that the jury is out in terms of *scientific* proof that botanical medicine works. As a broad statement, that's true—but it misses the complexity of the situation. Herbs function differently from conventional medications. Some herbs must be tailored to individuals. Standard, therapeutic doses of many common herbal medications have yet to be determined. And, as with conventional medicine, for ethical reasons you can't always study how herbal medicine behaves in pregnancy.

Certainly there's a lot to be learned and proven about how botanical medicine can be best used. But while the scientific studies continue, the centuries of knowledge accrued by practitioners of herbal medicine can be put to use. Modern herbalists, medical professionals (like me) who use herbs regularly, and patients find that, carefully used, botanical medicine is too effective to be ignored or discarded.

- *Eat fiber:* This will help minimize constipation, which will reduce irritation from straining.
- *Invert:* Resting for a few minutes a day with your legs up against the wall (a yoga pose called *viparita karani*) is helpful for both varicose veins and hemorrhoids. (See page 278 for a description of the pose.)
- *Drink more water:* It'll help soften stool, which in turn will minimize irritation from straining when you go to the bathroom.
- *Varicose veins in the legs—what you can do:*
  - After you give birth, varicose veins may be treated through a procedure called sclerotherapy. In it, the blood vessel is injected with a solution that

More Vein Changes

✦ *Spider angiomata:* These are little spiderlike blood vessels that typically crop up on the upper body and face between the second and fifth months. They look like spiders, with a central vessel and tiny feelers coming out of it. A spider angioma may be raised or flat; larger angiomata tend to be raised. They often clear up on their own within three months of giving birth, but if they don't, a dermatologist can treat them with a laser.

• *Spider veins on the legs:* These are enlarged veins or capillaries that crop up on the legs for the same reason as varicose veins—pressure from the baby in the pelvis slows circulation and causes blood to pool in the veins. They're much more common than true, bulging varicose veins. Some people will get both spider and varicose veins; some will get just one or the other. Like varicose veins, spider veins won't clear up on their own. If you want to get rid of them, a dermatologist can treat them with a laser or sclerotherapy (see "Varicose Veins," page 170).

irritates its lining, causing it to collapse; the vessel is then absorbed into the body. If this doesn't work or isn't the right choice, a procedure called "vein stripping" performed by a vascular surgeon, may be appropriate.

Itchiness in General and Heat Rash

• *Itchiness in general—when it happens:* Throughout pregnancy.

• *What happens:* You may find that you're just itchy a lot of the time because your skin is stretching, hot, and irritated by clothing or by rubbing against itself. If you find that you're extremely itchy, let your doctor or midwife know. Extreme itchiness may be caused by an increase in bile acids and can be treated with medication.

• *Heat rash—when it happens:* Second and third trimesters.

• *What happens:* Progesterone, a hormone crucial to pregnancy, raises your body temperature and prompts your sweat glands to work harder to cool you off. As a result, your skin may be warmer and sweatier. In addition, your skin may chafe because it's rubbing more against itself or your clothing. Combine chafing with warmer, sweatier skin, and you have the ingredients for an itchy heat rash.

- *Itchiness and heat rash—what you can do:*
  - *Soothing baths:* For both heat rashes and general itchiness, take an oatmeal bath or add two parts cornstarch to one part baking soda to a tub full of warm water. (Cooler water is more soothing to itchy skin than hot water.)
  - *Cold packs:* Apply cold compresses or ice packs to the itchy area.
  - *Moisturize and hydrate:* Drink plenty of water and don't skimp on the moisturizer. Dry skin is itchy skin.
  - *Menthol creams:* Available over-the-counter, these creams can be very soothing. Ask for them at your local drugstore.
  - *Cortisone creams:* Over-the-counter cortisone ("anti-itch") creams are safe, but they should be used sparingly. If you develop a rash along with the itchiness, your caregiver may recommend a prescription-strength cortisone cream.
  - *Antihistamines:* Over-the-counter antihistamines, like Benadryl, may help very bothersome itching. Start with 25 mg every four hours as needed. (Check the box to see how many mg are in each capsule; if 25 mg doesn't help, you may increase the dose to 50 mg every four hours as needed.) You may take Benadryl (or its generic equivalent, see the chart on page 212) for up to two weeks. Benadryl may make you drowsy, and you should avoid any activity, like driving, for which you need to be wide awake. *Always talk to your caregiver before taking any medication.*

Caution: If a rash doesn't go away after fourteen days, if it's very uncomfortable, or if it covers a large amount of your body (your entire torso, for example), call your caregiver and have it evaluated to be sure it's not a more serious skin condition.

Leg Cramps

- *When it happens:* Second and third trimesters.
- *What happens:* The pressure from the baby in the pelvis reduces blood flow to the legs, causing not only varicose veins (see page 170) but also cramping. Leg

cramps, which feel like a charley horse in the calf, can happen intermittently in the second half of your pregnancy, and they usually occur at night. (Some women have them every night.) Leg cramps may be a signal that you're not getting enough potassium, magnesium, or calcium. All are nutrients that can affect how muscles contract.

REAL VOICES

At about five and a half months I started having middle-of-the-night leg cramps. I would wake up startled by the pain in my calf and begin hollering. At first my husband, Michael, didn't know what to make of it, or, for that matter, what to do, and I didn't associate the cramps with the pregnancy. In fact, I was surprised to find they're a common symptom, which we learned because Michael was reading *The Expectant Father*. We followed the book's advice to flex the foot and massage the muscle in spasm. I'd wake up yelling in pain, and Michael, who'd be equally startled, would grab my foot, flex my leg, and start massaging. The cramps would disappear in a matter of minutes, or maybe it was just seconds, but it always felt like an eternity. Since they were occurring nightly, they began to interfere with both of our sleep. In fact, Michael thought it was nature's way of preparing us for a baby crying in the middle of the night.

I tried everything people recommended: stretching during the day, rotating my ankles, increasing my water intake, taking calcium supplements, and eating bananas and oranges for the potassium. Of all these remedies, the only ones I think had any impact were rotating of the ankle and keeping hydrated. But even still my leg cramps persisted, sometimes in the back of my calf, sometimes along the shinbone.

In the end, what helped me most was a recommendation our childbirth educator made for dealing with labor contractions. She said to let your body go with the wave of a contraction instead of bracing against the contraction. With the leg cramps continuing into my eighth month, I've tried to apply this strategy. Now, when the cramp comes, I still wake up startled, but I've stopped yelling. Most of the time, I even let my husband sleep through them. I calmly massage my leg, flex and rotate my foot, and breathe with the spasm, knowing that it'll go away. I'm not sure Michael's right about the preparation for a crying baby, but I often wonder whether this is a little bit of practice for all those contractions yet to come.

Johanna, pregnant

- *What you can do:*
  - *Stretch:* When the cramp begins, straighten your leg, flex your foot, and press back on your toes. Then gently point and flex your foot. This will hurt at first, but it'll relieve the cramp fairly quickly.
  - *Eat more fruit:* If you're getting leg cramps with some regularity, try eating fresh fruit to get more potassium and magnesium. Add three to five servings to the five you're already eating. If you're not eating five servings a day, work your way up to that and see if it helps. (A serving is about the size of your palm—one medium apple is one serving of fruit.)
  - *Keep up the fluids:* Because your blood volume increases by 40 to 50 percent, as a pregnant woman you need a lot of fluid to support its circulation. If you're not drinking enough water or clear fluids, dehydration may be contributing to your cramps.
  - *Increase calcium:* Make sure you're getting 1,500 mg of calcium per day. Take a calcium citrate supplement if you're not getting enough from your diet. (For more on calcium, see page 218.) Sufficient calcium may help prevent or relieve the intensity of leg cramps.
  - *Exercise:* Moderate exercise will help improve circulation and reduce the frequency and intensity of the cramps. Walk, swim, dance, take a tai chi or prenatal yoga class as often as you can.
  - *Rotate your ankles:* From time to time throughout the day, roll your feet and ankles around to get the blood flowing.
  - *Support hose:* If you have leg cramps and varicose veins, support hose will help keep the blood from pooling in your veins, improving overall circulation and possibly relieving cramps.
- *Herbal remedies:*
  - *Red raspberry leaf tea (Rubus idaeus):* Red raspberry leaf tea is an excellent source of calcium and contains many other nutrients. Drinking it regularly may help reduce the frequency and intensity of leg cramps. (It's also thought to tone the muscles of the uterus and generally support the body during pregnancy.) Drink up to four eight-ounce cups in a day. Red raspberry leaf tea is available in most health food stores, natural markets, and online.

Nosebleeds and Stuffy Noses

• *When it happens:* Second and third trimesters.

• *What happens:* The hormones of pregnancy may irritate and inflame the membrane lining of your nose, and that irritation can trigger mucus production. In fact, some women have stuffy noses during their entire pregnancies. In addition to inflamed membranes, the blood vessels throughout your body swell while you're pregnant, and your blood volume increases. The combination of swollen blood vessels, more blood, and irritated membranes means you're more likely to get a nosebleed.

• *Nosebleed—what you can do:*

   – *Lean forward to stanch bleeding:* When a nosebleed starts, point your head forward and slightly down. Press your nostrils together gently. Don't lie down or tip your head back.

   – *Stay hydrated and moist:* Drink a lot of water, sleep with a humidifier, and try to avoid stuffy rooms. If the air in your office is very dry and stale, try saline nose drops to keep your nostrils moist. Another way to keep them moist is to gently rub a vitamin E–based salve, sold in most health food stores, or A&D ointment, just inside the nostril.

   – *If nosebleeds are very frequent:* I recommend a consultation with an ear, nose, and throat specialist to see if cautery (burning blood vessels to keep them from bleeding) is appropriate for you.

Caution: If you can't staunch a nosebleed because the bleeding is very heavy, call your doctor.

• *Stuffy nose—what you can do:*

   – *Stay hydrated:* Drink a lot of water, sleep with a humidifier, and try to avoid stuffy rooms.

   – *Use a saline nasal spray:* Medicated nasal sprays should only be used occasionally because, whether you're pregnant or not, their repeated use can irritate the nasal tissue further, which can lead to more swelling and mucus.

   – *Essential fatty acids:* Omega-3 essential fatty acids DHA and EPA will reduce inflammation. When nasal membranes are less inflamed, the nasal passages remain open and produce less mucus. Increase intake through your diet by eating foods rich in essential fatty acids. (For a list of foods high in essential fatty acids, see page 227.) Or take supplements. When you're very stuffy, take 3,000 mg daily. As a preventive measure, take 1,000 mg of DHA daily.

Only take omega-3 essential fatty acid supplements that are guaranteed free of PCBs and heavy metals. (For resources, see page 522.)

— *NAC:* N-acetylcysteine (NAC) is derived from an amino acid and thins mucus. Take 500 mg two times a day when symptoms are especially bothersome. Don't take NAC for more than two weeks; NAC is safe during pregnancy, but if after two weeks your symptoms are still very bad, you need to check with your caregiver to make sure you don't have sinusitis. (See "Sinusitis" on page 207). NAC is available in most health food stores, natural markets, and online.

Note: If you often had a runny nose before you became pregnant and it's worse now, you may be sensitive (or allergic) to dairy products made from cow's milk. This is different from being lactose intolerant, which means you're unable to digest lactose, a sugar in cow's milk, and typically shows up as gas and diarrhea. With a dairy sensitivity or allergy, the molecular structure of cow's milk triggers a low-level immune response that causes inflammation throughout the body, including the nasal passages. Nasal passages produce more mucus when they're inflamed. (There are gradations between dairy sensitivity and dairy allergy. You can be sensitive to dairy without having a full-blown allergy, so cutting out dairy could be helpful if you have a persistent runny nose but not the other symptoms of a full-blown allergy, such as headaches and eczema.)

If you suspect you may be sensitive to cow's milk dairy, I recommend cutting out all dairy products—from cow, goat, and sheep's milk—for two weeks, to see if you start producing less mucus. (You may notice you expel a large amount of mucus after a few days off dairy.) If you have other symptoms of a cow's milk dairy allergy (e.g., headaches, eczema), they may subside, too. Keep up your calcium levels (1,500 mg a day) with green leafy vegetables, calcium-fortified orange juice and soy milk, red raspberry leaf tea, and supplements. (For a chart of the calcium content of a variety of foods, see page 220.)

If you decide to try to cut out cow's milk dairy, let your caregiver know; he may have specific dietary recommendations. Alternatively, you could meet with a nutritionist who has experience working with pregnant women to develop a food plan that's appropriate for you.

Pimply Rash (PUPPP)

- *When it happens:* Third trimester.
- *What happens:* Well under *1* percent of first-time pregnant women have outbreaks of *extremely* itchy, raised, red bumps on their abdomen, buttocks, thighs, and limbs. This is called PUPPP (pruritic urticarial papules and plaques of pregnancy). Let your doctor or midwife know if you suspect this. The rash usually clears up on its own by two weeks after giving birth, and it usually doesn't recur in a second pregnancy. PUPPP is often treated with topical steroids. You may have to have a skin biopsy to rule out other, even rarer pregnancy-related rashes, which may be more serious.

REAL VOICES
By the end of my pregnancy (with twins), I'd been on bed rest since twenty weeks, I was swollen, I didn't feel great, and then I developed this thing called PUPPP. It was awful! But you know what? I was so thrilled to be pregnant and so thrilled every passing week that my pregnancy was more and more viable.

Katherine, mom of two

Pink/Red Palms

- *When it happens:* Usually between the second and fifth months.
- *What happens:* While you're pregnant, you have more blood, and the muscular walls of your veins are somewhat relaxed by the extra progesterone. As a result, veins may become more prominent (see "More Vein Changes" on page 172), and your palms, which are full of veins, may look very pink or red. Your hands should go back to their usual color within three months postpartum.

Pins and Needles in the Hands

- *When it happens:* Usually in the third trimester.
- *What happens:* You may notice a little tingling, sometimes accompanied by numbness, in your hands and feet. If your hands or feet start to tingle, twirl them

around to get the blood flowing. If the situation improves, you know that slower blood circulation is the culprit. Let your doctor or midwife know about it at your next appointment. If the sensation doesn't go away quickly when you twirl your hands around, if it happens almost daily, or if the tingling or numbness bothers you in your daily routine, call your caregiver. Recurrent tingling and numbness in the hands and feet is just one of the symptoms of MS (multiple sclerosis), an autoimmune disorder that can appear in women during their childbearing years, and your caregiver will want to rule it out.

LET YOUR BODY TAKE THE LEAD

You may experience many of these side effects or very few of them. And for some women, not having many symptoms can actually trigger some anxiety. In this situation, it's helpful to keep in mind both that every body responds differently to pregnancy and that the range and intensity of symptoms don't correlate to your health or the baby's. You can have a perfectly healthy pregnancy and experience relatively little discomfort. If you're concerned about the nature of your symptoms, talk over the specifics of your situation with your caregiver.

Pins and Needles: Carpal Tunnel Syndrome

- *When it happens:* Third trimester.
- *What happens:* If you notice tingling, numbness, and weakness in your palm, thumb, second and third finger, and the lower half of your ring finger, especially if these symptoms happen in the middle of the night, you may have carpal tunnel syndrome. During pregnancy, the median nerve, which runs through the carpal tunnel in your wrist, can swell and press up against the tunnel wall, causing carpal tunnel syndrome. Besides tingling, other symptoms include pain in your forearm and wrist, feeling like your hand is falling asleep, and pain running up to your shoulder. Sometimes, carpal tunnel syndrome can weaken the hand enough to make it difficult to do simple tasks like gripping or opening a jar. Luckily, carpal tunnel syndrome from pregnancy almost always goes away after you give birth.
- *What you can do:*
  - *Reduce swelling:* Cut out salty foods and snacks from your diet because they might contribute to swelling.

– *Ice your wrist:* Apply cold compresses to the affected wrist for fifteen minutes a day.

– *Wear a splint:* For more serious cases, a splint can reduce the pressure on the nerve and thereby relieve the symptoms.

– *Eat cucumbers:* Cucumbers are a gentle, natural diuretic. Eat one or two servings a day. You can chop cucumbers in a salad with tomatoes and red pepper, slice them on a sandwich, or toss them in a green salad. (Usually diuretics aren't given to pregnant women because they need the extra fluid their bodies produce. But cucumbers and other natural diuretics—see below—are mild enough to be used safely during pregnancy.)

– *Increase omega-3 essential fatty acids:* Take a supplement to get 3,000 mg a day of EPA and DHA, which will reduce inflammation around the nerve. *Only buy a supplement that guarantees it does not contain PCBs or heavy metals.*

• *Herbal remedies*

– *Nettle (stinging nettle, Urtica dioica):* This herb is a very mild, natural diuretic that balances the body's fluids, which will relieve some of the pressure on the nerves in the wrist. Typically, pregnant women should avoid diuretics, but the natural action of this herb is gentle enough to be safe in pregnancy.

Nettles, in tea and tablet form, are often available at health food stores, natural markets, and online. Raw nettles, nutritious leafy greens, may be available at health food stores and specialty markets.

Dose:

  ○ *Tablets:* Take two 250-mg nettle tablets twice a day on an empty stomach.

  ○ *Tea:* Drink one eight-ounce cup of nettle tea (made from nettle root) per day.

  ○ *Raw:* Eat one serving daily of nettles. Fresh nettles are a green leafy vegetable that you can sauté with garlic in olive oil.

– *Dandelion greens (Taraxacum officinale):* This is another herb that gently balances body fluids. You can have dandelion greens fresh or drink a tea. Both may be available at health food stores and specialty markets. (For recommendations, see page 523.)

Dose:

  ○ *Tea:* Drink no more than two eight-ounce cups of tea a day.

  ○ *Raw:* Eat one serving daily of dandelion greens sautéed with garlic in olive oil or raw in a salad. (If you eat them raw, consider yourself forewarned—they are very bitter.)

Note: Physical therapy can help relieve carpal tunnel syndrome, as can yoga therapy. With the latter, look for an Iyengar yoga teacher who has experience working with carpal tunnel syndrome.

REAL VOICES

I was very swollen—no high blood pressure, but I was all puffy like a beach ball—which was rough. And I had such bad carpal tunnel syndrome at the end of my pregnancy that I still get it now if I'm not careful. At the end I slept with my Rollerblading wrist guards on for the carpal tunnel.

Jennifer, mom of one

Rib Pain and/or Pain in the Middle Back

• *When it happens:* Usually from the second trimester forward.

• *What happens:* This is a somewhat unusual—but not unheard-of—pregnancy symptom. Some women experience a sharp, persistent pain, most often under their right ribs and on the right side of their middle to upper backs, but it can also occur on the left side. If it happens on the right side, particularly if the pain is worse after meals, it may be related to the gallbladder. During pregnancy, the extra estrogen pregnant women produce can lead to a gallbladder problem.

Alternatively, the pain could be caused by pressure on the ribs from the baby or the ribs stretching. Tell your caregiver about the pain. Depending on your symptoms, she may ask you to have an ultrasound to evaluate the liver, gallbladder, kidneys, and pancreas. Whatever the cause, the pain should clear up after giving birth.

• *What you can do:*

— *Cut out greasy and fried foods:* If the pain is on your right side, creating the possibility that it's gallbladder-related, greasy, fried foods will aggravate the pain.

— *Maintain your posture:* Try doing exercises and stretches that stretch your spine (as in prenatal yoga, see chapter 14) and try to maintain good posture. Both will create more space in the abdomen.

— *Acupuncture:* Depending on your situation, acupuncture may help relieve the pain.

Sciatica

- *When it happens:* Third trimester.
- *What happens:* Your growing baby may be lying in a way that puts pressure on the sciatic nerve, which runs through your low back. If this happens, you may feel a sharp pain from the back of your hip down the back of your leg. The pain, which can occur in either leg, can make it difficult to find a comfortable position to sit, lie down, or even walk. The pain from sciatica can be frustrating because even though you can take steps to relieve it, it can last through the end of a pregnancy. The good news is that the sciatica should clear up after you give birth.
- *What you can do:*
  - *Find a comfortable position:* To relieve the pressure on your sciatic nerve, find the position that is most comfortable for you, rest there for about ninety seconds or as long as you want, and then come out of it. Repeat this several times each day.
  - *Apply heat:* Every evening, put a heating pad set on medium on the spot where the pain seems to originate for fifteen minutes.
  - *Take acetaminophen:* Take two extra-strength acetaminophen (Tylenol) tablets every four to six hours as needed. Applying heat along with taking acetaminophen may help.
  - *Acupuncture:* As with low back pain, acupuncture can be effective in managing sciatica in pregnancy.
  - *Chiropractic:* An experienced chiropractor can help relieve the pressure and pain from sciatica.
  - *Massage:* Deep-tissue massage can help relieve the pressure on the sciatic nerve.
  - *Osteopathy:* An osteopath, who is trained in musculoskeletal issues, can do some hands-on therapy, such as trigger-point therapy, and possibly recommend certain exercises to help with your particular situation.

Note: If you choose a complementary approach to easing sciatica, be sure to find a practitioner or doctor who's experienced working with pregnant women and sciatica.

REAL VOICES

Sciatica was one of the worst symptoms I had. I got an air mattress and slept on it. It really helped until the cat punctured it!

Stephanie, mom of one

Sharp Pain or Dull Ache in Lower Abdomen or Groin
(round ligament pain)

- *When it happens:* Typically between weeks 10 and 18.
- *What happens:* The uterus is anchored by two big bands—the round ligaments. As it grows, the uterus stretches the round ligaments, which can cause either a dull ache or sharp, stabbing pain, especially if you've had an active day. You may notice round ligament pain as early as ten to twelve weeks. Usually it lets up after about eighteen weeks.
- *What you can do:*
  - *Apply heat:* Set a heating pad to medium (not high) and let the heat do its soothing work.
  - *Take acetaminophen:* For intermittent aches and pains like this, acetaminophen may help.

Ovarian Cysts

✦ During the first ten to twelve weeks of pregnancy, the corpus luteum (the shell of the ovarian follicle that once contained the egg that became your baby) produces the hormones (like progesterone) that you need to maintain a healthy pregnancy. Sometimes, while it's producing these hormones, the corpus luteum becomes a fluid-filled cavity, or a cyst. Ovarian cysts can grow to several centimeters in diameter, but they're usually harmless and often painless. They're frequently discovered during first-trimester ultrasounds, and patients have no idea they have one. Occasionally, an ultrasound is ordered especially to investigate first-trimester pain, and a cyst is discovered as the cause.

The corpus luteum, whether or not it's become a cyst, disintegrates between the tenth and twelfth week, when the placenta takes over hormone production. Rarely, a cyst will rupture instead of disintegrate. This may or may not be painful (some women find it very painful, others don't know it happened), but knowing that you had a cyst will help your caregiver diagnose any pain from a rupture, should one occur.

Sharp Pain Low and On One Side
Later in Pregnancy? It May Be a Fibroid

✦ If you had fibroids before you became pregnant, the estrogen that your body produces to support your pregnancy may make them grow relatively quickly from early in your pregnancy. Then, by the second or third trimester, a fibroid, which needs both estrogen and blood to stay "alive," may not be getting the blood it needs—either because it's too big or because the position of the uterus cuts off blood flow to it. Either way, without a steady blood supply, a condition called "necrosis" might set in; in other words, the fibroid begins to die. This usually isn't dangerous to you or the baby, but you may experience fairly intense pain, which will subside in anywhere from a few days to a couple of weeks. Some women, however, don't have any pain from their fibroids during pregnancy. It's unpredictable.

• *What you can do:*
  – *Apply heat and take acetaminophen:* Take two extra-strength Tylenol every four to six hours, as needed, and put a warm compress on the area.
  – *Call your doctor or midwife:* She will probably ask you to come in for a sonogram that can confirm that it is, in fact, the fibroid causing the pain.

Caution: In *very* rare cases, a large fibroid can trigger preterm labor. (Defined as labor that begins before thirty-seven weeks; for more on preterm labor, see page 363.) There are two ways this can happen: (1) the fibroid's decay triggers the production of inflammatory chemicals that in turn cause the uterus to contract, prompting preterm labor; (2) the fibroid becomes so big that there's no room left for both it and the growing baby. If you have a large fibroid and are at risk for preterm labor, chances are your caregiver will keep a close watch for symptoms of preterm labor.

REAL VOICES
Around twenty-eight weeks or so in my first pregnancy, I got this really awful pain one weekend when I was visiting family. We'd gone for a walk in the

woods, and I couldn't walk at all. Up until then, I'd been walking at least an hour a day with my dog in addition to working out in the gym for an hour. So you can see the pain was really bad. But it was also finite—it definitely had a beginning and an end. Once we went in for the sonogram, just knowing that it was a fibroid and not anything more serious allowed me to work through the pain.

Ami, mom of one, stepmom to two, pregnant

Caution: Round ligament pain most typically feels like an occasional stitch. If you're very uncomfortable over an extended period of time, say a day or two, call your doctor or midwife. You may have fibroid-related pain (see page 184) or an ovarian cyst (see box, page 183).

Skin Tags

- *When it happens:* Anytime, more common in the third trimester.
- *What happens:* Wherever skin rubs against skin—under your bra, under your arms, on the neck, sometimes in the folds of the groin—little flaps of skin, known as skin tags, can form. They usually don't go away after delivery, and a dermatologist can remove them in a very simple procedure done in the office.

Sleep Problems

- *When it happens:* Third trimester.
- *What happens:* As your belly grows and your due date nears, you may find it hard to sleep through the night. Physically, it may be difficult to find a comfortable position, and because the baby may be pressing against your bladder, you may have to get up to urinate throughout the night. Emotionally, you may find that as your baby's birth gets a little closer, your mind is buzzing—with excitement, anxiety, anticipation, all of the above. As the big day approaches, it can be hard to quiet all the chatter and relax into sleep.
- *What you can do:*
  - *Spend time outside:* Walking in a nature preserve or along an easy trail can remind us of our connection to the natural world. Many of the women I work with find that tapping into this connection helps them manage the anxiety that develops as their due date approaches.

– *Don't go to bed hungry:* Have a light snack a little more than an hour before you plan to go to sleep. That way, your blood sugar will stay elevated and you won't wake up hungry in the middle of the night. Try not to eat within an hour of going to sleep, though. The digestive activity may keep you up.

– *Take calcium supplements:* Calcium supplements can help with sleep because they're filling and somewhat soothing for nerves. About an hour before you go to bed, take 1,000 mg of calcium (preferably calcium citrate, see pages 218–220) with 500 mg of magnesium. If you prefer, you could start with a smaller dose to see if that works.

– *Avoid sugar and caffeine:* Avoid caffeinated drinks after 1 P.M. Cut back on sweets after 6 P.M. You may get a sugar rush followed by a crash, leading to hunger in the middle of the night.

– *Create a bedtime routine:* If you're having trouble falling asleep, try to establish a routine that helps calm your body and mind. For example, write in your journal for at least fifteen minutes. Then draw a nice, warm bath (not too hot) and put in about twenty drops of lavender oil. Finally, as you settle into bed, spend a few minutes talking to your baby, telling him or her about your day and getting ready for sleep.

– *Use extra pillows:* Use a body pillow to support your whole body or put a pillow between your knees. Finding a comfortable position will help you sleep better and longer.

– *Aromatherapy:* The smell of lavender will help you relax. To take advantage of this effect, place a lavender pillow, sachet, or cotton ball soaked with lavender oil by your head while you go to sleep. Lavender oil is available in health food stores and aromatherapy stores. Other lavender products may be available in bath stores and specialty shops.

• *Herbal remedies:*

– *Chamomile tea:* Have one eight-ounce cup of tea about an hour before you plan to go to bed. Chamomile gently relaxes the nervous system. Drink up to four eight-ounce cups of chamomile tea in a day. It's available in health food stores and supermarkets.

– *Passionflower (Passiflora incarnata):* Late in pregnancy, if you find that you're restless at night because of anxiety, this herb may help. It's available in health food stores, natural markets, and online. Passionflower won't cause grogginess the morning after you take it. Don't use it for more than one week straight. If you think you need it for longer, consult with your care provider to rule out medical concerns such as a bladder infection that causes frequent urination.

Dose:

- ○ *Tea:* Drink one eight-ounce cup.

- ○ *Tincture:* Drop 1–2 ml of tincture (typically 25–50 drops, depending on the viscosity of the tincture; follow instructions on the bottle) into eight ounces of hot water just before going to bed. (Follow tincture instructions on page 154.)

— *Valerian root (Valeriana officinalis):* A natural sedative that's been shown to improve the quality and duration of nighttime sleep, valerian root is a good choice when you're truly exhausted but still can't sleep.

Dose:

- ○ *Tincture:* Take 30–60 drops mixed in hot water (follow tincture instructions on page 154) thirty minutes to an hour before going to sleep. It's available in health food stores, natural markets, and online. It won't cause grogginess the morning after you take it.

Notes:

1. While valerian is generally considered safe in pregnancy, a small percentage of people find it works as a stimulant. If you're trying it for the first time at night, take a smaller dose—about half the normal dose—as a trial.

DIY: SLEEP TONIC

In my practice, we have developed a sleep tonic especially for pregnancy. For simplicity's sake I would recommend trying the valerian alone before buying three different tinctures to make the tonic yourself or working with a trained herbalist. But if you'd like to mix it, simply combine equal parts of the following herbal tinctures into a small, clean glass jar, and then put about 30 drops of the mixture into eight ounces of hot water (following instructions for mixing tinctures on page 154) or about four ounces of juice:

- Valerian
- Hops
- California poppy

Caution: Don't use tinctures if you're a recovering alcoholic.

Mind-Body Medicine for Sleep

✦ Mind-body medicine techniques, which slow down the mind and release anxiety, can help ease insomnia throughout your pregnancy. One technique that I often recommend for anxiety-related insomnia in the third trimester is to combine belly breathing with self-hypnosis, an affirmation, and/or visualization.

A simple exercise would be to combine belly breathing with a self-hypnotizing phrase. (For instructions see "Mind-Body Medicine: Autogenics" on page 168.) Begin by practicing belly breathing (see page 63 for a description) and then slowly repeat the phrase "I am calm and relaxed . . . I am at peace" to yourself at two-second intervals, between six and ten times.

If you know you're worried about a particular issue, you can try to combine belly breathing with a visualization of the situation that's weighing on you. Then, complete the exercise with an affirmation. For example, if thinking about labor is keeping you up, after getting ready for bed, lie down and do belly breathing for about five minutes. Then slowly call to mind an image of your labor and your baby's birth. Imagine it exactly how you want it to go—it can be a fantasy version or a medically accurate version, whichever feels best for you. Stay with the scene as it unfolds. Let your imagination go wherever it takes you. When you feel complete with the visualization, begin to repeat a phrase such as "My labor and birth will unfold in the way that's best for me and my baby (use a name if you've selected one) . . . I am at peace" six times at two-second intervals. You can use this combined visualization/affirmation exercise with anything that's making you anxious—a prenatal test, connecting with your baby, even a baby shower! Alternatively, you can simply relax with belly breathing and repeat an affirmation designed around whatever's weighing on you.

Other exercises: If you've found that a mind-body exercise previously described helps you clear your mind, then try using it or adapting it to help you sleep. To review basic mind-body exercises, see page 62.

2. There's extensive historical use of valerian root used in tincture or tea form as a sleep aid, and its effectiveness has been studied and proven. While its long-term safety and its safety during pregnancy haven't been scientifically assessed, I consider it safe for my patients to use occasionally (around once

or twice a week throughout the second and third trimesters or continuously for up to one week, depending on the situation). Unfortunately, it smells like stinky feet, but it works.

Sore Tailbone

- *When it happens:* Typically the third trimester.
- *What happens:* The nub at the end of the spine, the tailbone, becomes quite sore and it can be uncomfortable to sit. This is a relatively rare side effect, but not unheard-of. It's not clear why this happens—pregnant women tend to get sore in odd places. It most likely happens because of changes in posture.
- *What you can do:*
  - *Work on your posture:* Make an effort to keep your spine long, while keeping your shoulders back and maintaining a gentle curve in your low back. It might not help right away, but it may help over time.
  - *Sit on an inflatable donut:* An inflatable donut is relatively easy to carry around and provides a little extra cushion.
  - *Take acetaminophen:* If you're very uncomfortable, two extra-strength acetaminophen tablets every six hours can help.

Soreness at the Top of the Belly (diastasis)

- *When it happens:* Second and third trimesters.
- *What happens:* You may notice a funny, tingling soreness or "hot spot" at the very top of your uterus where the ribs come together. This phenomenon is known as diastasis. It happens because the abdominal muscles run vertically, starting at the bottom of your rib cage, just below the sternum (the bone in the middle of your chest), and continuing to your pubic bone. They come together in the middle of the top of your abdomen, but there isn't any muscle right there. As your uterus grows, it can push the muscles away from each other, creating a space that becomes tender. There isn't much that can be done about it; just let your doctor or midwife know if you experience any discomfort, especially if it's very uncomfortable. (Sometimes women feel like this sensation is a "small" thing and don't bring it up with their providers—but your doctor or midwife is there to help you, so even if you're experiencing something that seems minor, it's helpful for your provider to know if you're

uncomfortable.) Tylenol or a heating pad may help with the discomfort, which should go away after you give birth because the muscles are no longer being forced apart by your uterus. In extreme cases, a stitch can be put in surgically during a C-section or in a special procedure after the birth.

Stretch Marks (*striae gravidarum*)

- *When it happens:* Starting around twenty-four weeks.
- *What happens:* Many pregnant women get stretch marks (estimates range from 50 to 90 percent). As your baby and body grow, your skin stretches, and the collagen, which supports and strengthens the skin, breaks up, making lines that are anywhere from faint pink to, in extreme cases, purple. Stretch marks appear most often on the abdomen, but they also may show up on the breasts, thighs, and buttocks. Skin type, genes, weight gain, and hormonal fluctuations all contribute to the extent of the stretch marks. After delivery, they generally fade to a pale color, but they may never disappear completely. Unfortunately, there's no way to prevent stretch marks altogether; after you give birth their appearance may be improved with laser treatment.
- *What you can do:*
  - *Eat well and drink water:* Hydrated skin fed by a daily zinc supplement of 30 mg and a diet rich in protein, vitamins E and C, and bioflavonoids (found in colorful fruits like apricots, mangoes, etc., and vegetables like squash, tomatoes, carrots, and sweet potatoes) can better tolerate stretching.
  - *Keep skin moist:* Gently rub calendula ointment with vitamin E or any basic moisturizer into your skin twice a day to keep it moist and supple, which may help minimize stretching.

Note: Ointments, oils, and rubs that claim to prevent or get rid of stretch marks don't work.

Swelling (edema)

- *When it happens:* Typically in the third trimester, may begin in the second trimester.
- *What happens:* You may notice that your hands and face are a little puffy and that your feet and ankles are swollen—especially at the end of the day. While you're

pregnant, the balance of body fluids shifts, you retain more fluids, and your blood volume increases. Taken together, the extra fluid and blood can lead to swelling. Another reason your feet and ankles may swell is that as your growing uterus puts pressure on the veins in your pelvis, blood flow to your feet and legs slows. When that happens, blood can pool in veins, pushing non-blood fluids out of your veins and into your feet and ankles.

- *What you can do:*
  - *Wear loose clothing:* Clothes that are tight around the ankles and feet can exacerbate swelling.
  - *Sit when you can:* Don't stand for extended periods of time if you can avoid it. If you must stand for a long time, use a footstool and put one foot or the other up on it throughout the day.
  - *Don't cross your legs:* Sitting with legs crossed can slow blood flow in your legs even more.
  - *Drink water:* Even though it's counterintuitive, staying well hydrated will help your kidneys flush excess fluids out of your body.
  - *Eat protein:* Without enough protein, your body may retain even more fluids. (For protein-rich foods, see page 229.)
  - *Eat cucumbers:* They're a natural, gentle diuretic. Try one or two servings of cucumber salad a day.
- *Herbal remedies:*
  - *Nettles (stinging nettles, Urtica dioica):* This leafy green provides a gentle, natural diuretic that helps balance the body's fluids.
    Dose:
    - *Fresh nettles:* Eat the equivalent of a large portion of spinach once a day. You can buy nettle greens and sauté them with olive oil and garlic as you would spinach.
    - *Tablets:* Take two 250-mg tablets twice a day.
  - *Dandelion greens (Taraxacum officinale):* Dandelion greens help the kidneys get rid of excess fluids, and they're an excellent source of potassium and calcium.
    Dose:
    - *Fresh greens:* Eat a large portion tossed raw into a salad or sautéed with a little garlic and olive oil.
    - *Tea:* Drink three eight-ounce cups daily. The tea is available in health food stores, and the greens may be available in health food stores and specialty markets.

Caution: If your feet, hands, or face *suddenly* get very swollen, or if you experience swelling along with a headache or blurry vision (or all three together), call your doctor or midwife *right away,* no matter the time of day. If you notice you're just a little puffier than usual, call your doctor or midwife sometime during office hours that day. Swelling is an important symptom of preeclampsia, which is a serious complication that may need immediate attention. (For a discussion of preeclampsia, see page 357.)

REAL VOICES
I guess one thing that surprised me was how much my hands hurt. They got really swollen, and it literally hurt to bend them. I'd wake up in the morning, and I couldn't really bend my fingers. I think it was just a circulation thing and it wasn't incapacitating, but it wasn't comfortable. I knew my hands and feet would swell, but I was surprised by the stiffness and how much they hurt.

Laura, mom of one, pregnant

My feet have gotten so swollen that I can only wear flip-flops. It helps a little to keep them elevated—and for a while swimming helped reduce the swelling. Its funny, because they don't really hurt, but everyone who sees them comments on them.

Rebecca, pregnant

Swollen Labia

• *When it happens:* Beginning in the second trimester.
• *What happens:* Many times pregnant women will come into my office and say, "Something is wrong with my vagina. It looks funny!" What they're seeing is congestion in the veins of the labia, essentially varicose veins in the labia. This usually occurs in the outer labia, but in severe cases, the inner labia may also swell. This happens if the baby is resting on the veins coming into the vagina from the pelvis, slowing blood flow and causing it to pool in the veins of the labia. This is the same process that causes varicose veins in the legs and hemorrhoids in the rectum. (See "Hemorrhoids," page 170.) There's not much you can do about varicose veins of the labia, but they will go away within six weeks of giving birth.

The Rhythm Connection

✦ I'm a strong believer in the medicinal power of music in many situations, but especially during pregnancy. My belief is based on the principle of *entrainment,* where the rhythm of the body's major organs eventually merges with the rhythm of the music. (Entrainment appears in a range of disciplines including chemistry, biology, and psychology. The classic example of it shows two individual heart muscle cells, each pulsing at its own rate, that begin to pulse in unison when brought together.)

Through entrainment with music, your heartbeat becomes more regular and less variable and the nervous system is soothed, creating a more deeply relaxed state and helping you sleep. The application of entrainment to pregnancy is less scientifically documented but, in my view, no less important. Preliminary data show that the first sense a baby develops in utero, around twenty weeks, is hearing. When you play soothing music, it can synchronize your heartbeat with your baby's in a two-to-one rhythmic ratio. (The fetal heart rate is much faster than the maternal.) And the soothing effect of music on the nervous system can reduce the release of stress hormones, relax the uterus, and increase blood flow to the baby.

Taking quiet time for you and your baby to listen to music together as your bodily rhythms merge—what a wonderful way for you to connect with your baby! (To experience entrainment, you can simply listen to music or use pregnancy-specific entrainment CDs and devices, which help the music reach the baby.

Tightening of the Abdomen (Braxton Hicks contractions)

• *When it happens:* Second and third trimesters, typically beginning between weeks 20 and 22.

• *What happens:* When you feel your uterus hardening or tightening, you're having Braxton Hicks contractions. By definition, these contractions, which were named for John Braxton Hicks, a nineteenth-century English doctor who first identified and named them, don't lead to labor or delivery. Rather, they're the uterus's way to prepare for labor, and they'll become more frequent as your due date gets closer.

Women most often describe Braxton Hicks contractions as uncomfortable (although they can be *quite* uncomfortable and some women describe them as painful), and they may come at regular intervals. Unlike labor contractions, however, they don't grow more intense or start coming more closely together. If you're carrying multiples or have a (large) fibroid, you may have Braxton Hicks contractions more frequently. You don't have to call your caregiver every time you have them, but after you first notice them, let your doctor or midwife know at your next appointment.

- *What you can do:*
  - *Drink water:* Dehydration can bring on Braxton Hicks contractions.
  - *Breathe slowly:* Sit quietly for five minutes and take slow, deep breaths. Focus on the inhale, then on the exhale. This is a good way to soothe the parasympathetic nervous system. (See "belly breathing" on page 63.)
  - *Rest:* Activity can increase contractions, so if you can rest, do so.
  - *Stay calm:* Try to relax and go with it.

Cautions:

1. If you're *ever* unsure if contractions are "real" or Braxton Hicks, particularly before thirty-seven weeks, call your doctor or midwife that day.
2. Call your caregiver immediately if you have more than six contractions per hour for more than two hours and they don't stop after you rest and drink water.
3. Call your caregiver immediately if you have Braxton Hicks contractions for more than two hours and if you notice any mucus or bloody or liquid discharge.

REAL VOICES

In both pregnancies I started having Braxton Hicks at around five months. At one point in my first pregnancy I had them so much that I went to the hospital. It turned out I had gotten dehydrated for some reason, so they pumped me with fluids and the contractions stopped. In fact, I had so many contractions in both pregnancies that it affected my sex life. When I'd have an orgasm, it was kind of scary because I would have a lot of contractions. I knew it wouldn't put me into labor, but with all the Braxton Hicks toward the end of both pregnancies, I definitely shied away from sex.

Mary, mom of two

Umbilical Hernia

- *When it happens:* Third trimester.
- *What happens:* This is another very rare side effect. A space may open up at the bottom of your belly button (umbilicus), causing abdominal discomfort and possibly nausea, which you can try to manage as you would morning sickness (see page 120). If you suspect an umbilical hernia, gently place the tip of your finger in your belly button (if your nails aren't too long). If you feel a small opening at the bottom, about the size of a Life Saver hole but that you can put your finger through, you may have an umbilical hernia. Tell your caregiver if you find this. If it's not bothering you that much, it can be evaluated at your six-week postpartum appointment, when the pressure from the uterus is no longer there to aggravate it. If it's more than a little bothersome while you're pregnant, you may find that wearing a "belly bra" that supports the uterus is helpful, and you may want to consult with a general surgeon about repairing it. (In my experience surgery for this condition is rare.) Finally, it may be repaired during a scheduled C-section.

Urinary Frequency

- *When it happens:* Mostly in the first and third trimesters.
- *What happens:* There's no avoiding it: When you're pregnant, you're going to urinate a lot. There are many reasons for this. Your blood volume is increased, so the kidneys do more filtering, which creates more urine. Your uterus may be pressing into your bladder: Early in pregnancy this happens because progesterone relaxes your muscles, including the muscles of the uterus, which slump into the bladder; later in pregnancy it happens because the growing baby takes up more room. Finally, as a pregnant woman, you need to drink a lot of fluids, which always means going to the bathroom more. There's nothing much you can do about it; just go when you feel you need to. Even if only a little urine comes out, it's still important to expel it, because stagnant urine is a breeding ground for infection.

Vaginal Discharge

- *When it happens:* Throughout pregnancy.
- *What happens:* Once you're pregnant, you can expect vaginal discharge throughout the entire nine months. Pregnancy hormones trigger the discharge, known as leukorrhea, which is thin and milky white with a mild smell. You may find the discharge gets heavier as you get closer to your due date. Sometimes the discharge is heavy enough to warrant using pads or panty liners, but do not use tampons or douche. Contact your caregiver if you notice that your discharge becomes cheesy, green, yellow, or pungent, because you may have an infection. (See "Yeast Infections and Vaginitis" on page 210.)

Vaginal Pain (symphysis pubis separation)

- *When it happens:* Starting in the second trimester.
- *What happens:* This is quite rare. The pubis is made up of two bones that are connected by a strong piece of cartilage. The relaxing effect of progesterone can cause the two bones to gradually spread. Then, stress on the pubis from a wrong move, or even a structural predisposition, creates a symphisis pubis separation. You'll know if this happens because you'll experience sudden sharp pain and, if your case is severe, difficulty walking. Typically, the pain goes away after you give birth. If your situation is serious and doesn't get better after you give birth, you may need surgery. Again, this is very rare.
- *What you can do:*
  - *Sit down when you need to:* Relieving the pressure on your pubis will ease the pain.
  - *Let your caregiver know:* This is painful, and your caregiver can help manage the pain. There are devices that can help keep the baby off the pubic bone.

Herbs for Pregnancy Aches and Pains

Note: These are the herbs that I recommend and that I typically use in my practice. There are other safe and effective herbal remedies that you can use under the care of a trained herbalist, physician, and/or midwife. Follow the instructions for teas and tinctures on page 154.

Ache and Pain	Herb	Dose	Available*
Back pain	Tiger Balm, White Flower Analgesic Balm	Follow instructions	Health food stores; Tiger Balm is often available at hardware stores, online
Back pain causing insomnia	Valerian (*Valeriana officinalis*)—tincture or tea	*Tincture:* 30–60 drops in 8 oz. of hot water 1 hour before bed *Tea:* 1 8-oz. cup 1 hour before bed	Health food stores, natural markets, online
Carpal tunnel syndrome	Nettles (stinging nettles, *Urtica dioica*)—tablets, tea, or fresh greens (to reduce swelling) Dandelion greens (*Taraxacum officinale*)	*Tablets:* 2 250-mg tablets twice a day (preferably on an empty stomach) *Tea:* 1 8-oz. cup every 4 hours or as needed *Fresh greens:* 2 servings per day, sautéed in olive oil	Health food stores, natural markets, online
Gas and bloating	Fennel seeds (*Foeniculum vulgare*)	*Tea:* 3 8-oz. cups of tea per day *Tincture:* 2–4 ml (50–120 drops) in 8 oz. of water 3 times per day	Health food stores, natural markets, online
Gas and bloating	Slippery elm (*Ulmus fulva*)— lozenge or tea	*Lozenge:* as directed on package. *Tea:* 1 8-oz. cup of tea as needed (do not exceed 4 cups per day)	Health food stores, natural markets, online

Continued

Ache and Pain	Herb	Dose	Available*
Gas and bloating	Meadowsweet (*Filipendula*)	*Tincture:* 2–4 ml (50–120 drops) 3 times daily *Tea:* up to 3 8-oz. cups of tea per day	Health food stores, natural markets, online
Heartburn and Indigestion	Slippery elm— lozenge or tea	*Lozenge:* as directed on package *Tea:* 1 8-oz. cup of tea as needed (do not exceed 4 cups per day)	Health food stores, natural markets, online
Heartburn and Indigestion	Marshmallow tea (*Althaea officinalis*) Chamomile tea	*Tea:* 1 8-oz. cup of either tea as needed (up to 4 cups per day) (Do not drink marshmallow tea if you have gestational diabetes.)	Health food stores, natural markets, online
Hemorrhoids	Arnica gel	Once hemorrhoid appears, apply *every* time you go to the bathroom, or at least each time you move your bowels	Drugstores, health food stores, online
Leg cramps	Red raspberry leaf tea (*Rubus idaeus*)	One 8-oz. cup as often as you like	Health food stores, natural markets, online
Sleep problems	Lavender oil	*Bath:* add 20 drops oil *Scent:* saturate cotton ball and place next to pillow	Health food stores, natural markets, aromatherapy stores, bath stores, online
Sleep problems	Chamomile tea	One 8-oz. cup 1 hour before bed	Supermarkets, health food stores, natural markets, drugstores, online
Sleep problems (accompanied by anxiety)	Passionflower (*Passiflora incarnata*)	*Tea:* 1 8-oz. cup *Tincture:* 1–2 ml of tincture (25–50 drops) in 8-oz. of hot water just before bed	Health food stores, natural markets, online

Continued

Ache and Pain	Herb	Dose	Available*
Sleep problems	Valerian (*Valeriana officinalis*)—tincture or tea	*Tincture:* 30–60 drops in 8 oz. of hot water 1 hour before bed. *Tea:* 1 8-oz. cup 1 hour before bed	Health food stores, natural markets, online
Swelling	Nettles (stinging nettles, *Urtica dioica*)—tablets, tea, or fresh greens Dandelion greens or tea	*Tablets (nettles only):* 2 250-mg tablets twice a day (preferably on an empty stomach) *Nettle and dandelion tea:* 1 8-oz. cup no more than 2 times a day. *Fresh greens:* 2 servings per day, sautéed in olive oil	Health food stores, natural markets, online
Stretch marks	Calendula ointment Cocoa butter	Follow instructions	Drugstores, health food stores, online

*When buying herbal medications, look for products sold by reputable companies. Recommendations that I give in my practice are listed in appendix 1 on page 521, or ask a trained herbalist, acupuncturist, or integrative physician or midwife for recommendations.

12

How to Treat Everyday Illnesses

Unfortunately, being pregnant doesn't mean you won't catch common illnesses like stomach bugs and colds, and you don't even get a pass on seasonal allergies. When you get sick while you're pregnant, you may not want to take any medication at all, but there are safe ways to relieve uncomfortable symptoms. Here are some strategies for feeling better when you're under the weather.

◆　◆　◆

In this chapter you'll find:

- Allergies
  - Hay fever
  - Sinus pain
- Bug Bites
- Colds
- Fever

- Lice
- Muscle Strains/Sprains
- Sinusitis
- Stomach Bugs
- Urinary Tract Infection
- Yeast Infections and Vaginitis

A Holistic and Realistic Approach

✦ As a general philosophy, I try to gently support the body's natural ability to heal itself. I believe the best choice whenever you have a cold, flu, or some other *minor but uncomfortable* illness or allergy is to give your body the chance to heal itself, primarily by resting and drinking fluids. Much of the work of the body's infinite number of cells, systems, and chemicals is to restore health, and as long as nothing damaging is occurring, I feel it's best not to interfere. This is especially true when you're pregnant, and particularly during the first trimester. That said, there are times when intervention is necessary and important, either because there's the potential for something more harmful to develop or because you're in unnecessary pain. When it comes to choosing an intervention, I typically try to use a natural intervention first and then a conventional option. But this isn't a hard-and-fast rule. If it's clear to me that a patient needs conventional medication, or if a patient prefers conventional medication, we'll follow that route. Finally, when you're pregnant, use both herbal and conventional medications sparingly.

Note: I won't address more serious non-pregnancy–related illnesses here, since a situation calling for antibiotics or other medications requires direct attention from your doctor or midwife.

Allergies

Hay fever

Hay fever, like other allergic reactions, is the result of the immune system responding to an irritant, such as pollen or mold, and like many immune reactions, it behaves unpredictably during pregnancy. Some women find their allergies ease up, while others have a terrible time.

- *What you can do for hay fever:*
  - *Increase omega-3 essential fatty acids (EFAs):* Because they reduce inflammation, EFAs ease allergic symptoms. During a hay fever attack, take 3,000 mg a day (or 3 gm) of EPA and DHA combined. Brands vary in their dosing,

so read the label to insure you get the dose you wish. When symptoms sub-side, take 1,000 mg a day (or 1 gm; I recommend this daily dose to all the pregnant women I work with). *Only take an omega-3 essential fatty acid supplement that is guaranteed free of PCBs and heavy metals.* (For resources, see page 522.)

— *Acupuncture:* Regular sessions can relieve hay fever and seasonal allergy symptoms. Talk with your practitioner about the number of sessions you should have before feeling a difference.

• *Over-the-counter allergy medications:*

— *Sudafed (pseudoephedrine):* In my practice, I feel comfortable with pregnant women taking plain Sudafed in the second and third trimesters (not the first) if their allergies are causing real discomfort. There has been some con-flicting evidence about its safety, but the data are inconclusive. I suggest its use within the dose recommended on the package. Don't take pseu-doephedrine for longer than seven to ten days straight. If your symptoms persist for more than seven to ten days, check in with your caregiver to be sure you don't have a sinus infection.

— *Benadryl (diphenhydramine hydrochloride):* Follow dose recommendations on the package. If your symptoms persist for more than seven to ten days, let your caregiver know. Keep in mind that Benadryl or its generic equivalent may cause drowsiness.

Note: Check with your doctor or midwife before taking any over-the-counter medication.

• *What you can do for mucus from allergies:*

If your allergies trigger the production of thick mucus try the following:

— *NAC:* Derived from an amino acid, NAC (N-acetylcysteine) thins mucus. (See "Colds," page 204.) Take 500 mg twice daily while symptoms are bad. It's safe to take NAC continually for seven to ten days, but notify your care-giver if you need it longer. It's available in most health food stores.

— *Cut out dairy:* If you constantly have a stuffy nose, you may be sensitive to cow's milk dairy products. Try eliminating all cow's milk dairy products for two weeks, and see if your symptoms improve. When you cut out cow's milk dairy, be sure you still consume 1,500 mg of calcium per day by eating calcium-rich foods like green leafy vegetables, broccoli, and calcium-supplemented soy milk and orange juice, and take calcium supplements if necessary. (For calcium content in a variety of foods, see page 220.) Talk to your caregiver about cut-ting out dairy; he or she may have specific diet recommendations for you.

Sinus pain

If you tend to have allergy-related sinus pain, it may be better now that you're pregnant, but it may get worse.

- *What you can do for allergy-related sinus pain:*
  - *Acupuncture:* There are acupuncture treatments specific to allergy-related sinus pain. Talk with an acupuncturist about whether or not she's worked on sinus pain, and approximately how many sessions you're likely to need to feel relief.
  - *Saline nose spray:* Simple saline sprays clean out nasal passages without irritating membranes. Medicated nasal sprays may be effective in the short term, but continued use can cause irritation. I recommend limiting their use to a few days when symptoms are at their worst.
  - *Reduce inflammation:* Reducing inflammation will reduce pressure on the sinuses, which will relieve pain. To do so, try NAC: 500 mg twice daily while symptoms are bad. It's available in most health food stores. Or increase omega-3 essential fatty acid intake to 3,000 mg (3 gm) a day of DHA and EPA when pain is acute, or 1,000 mg (1 mg) a day of DHA and EPA as a preventive measure. *Only take an omega-3 essential fatty acid supplement that is guaranteed free of PCBs and heavy metals.* (For resources, see page 522.)
- *Over-the-counter sinus medication:*

  For sinus pain, I recommend Benadryl (diphenhydramine hydrochloride), plain Sudafed (pseudoephedrine), or plain Tylenol (acetaminophen), following the instructions given on page 201 for allergy use. *Always contact your caregiver before taking any medication.*

Note: If sinus pain is accompanied by green, yellow, or brown mucus, or if it persists for more than seven days, call your caregiver. You may have sinusitis (see page 207).

Bug Bites

If you live in an area where Lyme disease or West Nile virus is a problem, wear long sleeves and pants when you're walking in the woods or gardening and only use bug repellant that's marked safe for children (DEET is a good option). If you simply want to avoid mosquito bites, but there's no threat of Lyme disease or West Nile virus in your area, I recommend skipping the bug repellant, but still wearing long sleeves and long pants.

- *Over-the-counter cortisone (anti-itch) creams:* They're safe and effective in relieving itchiness from bug bites. Avoid calamine lotion and Caladryl unless you know they work for you. In my clinical experience, both sometimes cause itching and swelling to worsen.

Colds

When you feel a cold coming on, rest and drink as much water and clear fluids (simple soups, herb teas, etc.) as you can—up to twelve eight-ounce glasses per day. Continue to treat a cold with fluid and rest until your symptoms subside. You can supplement rest and fluids with vitamins and herbs. Let your caregiver know if your cold continues for more than two weeks.

- *Vitamin and herbal treatments:*
  - *Vitamin C:* 500 mg four times a day (2,000 mg total). Don't take all 2,000 mg at once or you could get diarrhea. If you don't get loose stools on 2,000 mg a day, you can increase your dose to 3,000 mg a day.
  - *Zinc:* 15 mg twice a day (30 mg total).
  - *NAC:* 500 mg twice a day (1,000 mg total). Derived from an amino acid (L-cysteine), NAC (N-acetylcysteine), thins mucus. It's available in health food stores, natural markets, and online.
  - *Echinacea:* In the second and third trimesters, take about 30 drops of tincture in warm water or juice three or four times a day. Echinacea tastes bad, so you can "chase" the dose with any drink you like. It's available at health food stores, natural markets, and online.

Note: Lozenges that contain vitamin C and zinc are widely available. Some contain vitamin C, zinc, and echinacea, some also contain elderberry (see "Fever," page 205). These are all safe to take in the second and third trimesters. Those with echinacea should be avoided in the first trimester.

Cautions:
1. Do *not* take echinacea in the first trimester; if you're at risk for preterm labor (see page 363); or if you have an autoimmune disease such as MS or lupus.

2. Do not take *goldenseal* at any time while you're pregnant; it may bring on contractions or preterm labor. Goldenseal is often combined with echinacea in tablets and tinctures, so double check any echinacea you have to be sure there is no goldenseal in it. (If you take echinacea with goldenseal once, don't worry about it, just be sure not to take it again.)

3. Read the label of zinc/vitamin C lozenges carefully. They should *not* contain goldenseal or additional vitamin A. (Your prenatal vitamin already meets your daily vitamin A requirement.)

- *Over-the-counter (OTC) cold medications:*
  - *Plain Robitussin:* Plain Robitussin (or its generic equivalent) can soothe a cough. If plain Robitussin doesn't help your symptoms, talk to your caregiver about other options. Take as directed on the package.
  - *Tylenol (acetaminophen):* Take two extra-strength acetaminophen tablets every four to six hours (or as directed) for cold-related body aches and headaches.
  - *Mentholated rubs:* Mentholated rubs (like Vicks) are safe to use as needed and per package instructions.

Note: Check with your doctor or midwife before taking any OTC medication.

Q: Can I take NyQuil? It really helps me sleep when I have a cold, but it has alcohol.
Dr. Evans: The *occasional* use of a cold medication like NyQuil (during a bout with a cold), which contains a fair amount of alcohol, is *probably* safe in the second and third trimesters. I wouldn't recommend taking it for more than ten nights in a row, and I would avoid it entirely in the first trimester.

REAL VOICES
I got a terrible cold recently when I was about twenty-five weeks. Honestly, since I'd had a stuffy nose for much of my pregnancy so far, I didn't realize I was sick right away. I thought I was just extra tired and my nose was a little runnier. But as things got worse, I figured it out.

Beth, pregnant

Fever

A high fever (above 100.4 degrees Fahrenheit) that lasts more than seven days can be dangerous to a fetus. (The nervous system of a developing fetus or very young baby is extremely sensitive to heat.) If you have a fever, your number-one priority is to get it down below 100.4 degrees Fahrenheit.

Every caregiver will have her own guidelines for when to call with a fever. Mine are as follows: If you have a fever that is between 100.4 and 102 degrees Fahrenheit, and it's the middle of the night, call the next morning; if you have a fever that is 102 degrees or higher, call anytime day or night. Ask your caregiver for her fever guidelines and follow them.

- *To lower a fever:*
  - *Acetaminophen (Tylenol):* Take two extra-strength tablets every four to six hours as needed. These may lower your fever and relieve body aches.
  - *Sleep:* As much as you can.
  - *Take a lukewarm sponge bath, bath, or shower:* The water temperature shouldn't make you shiver; it should simply feel cooling. Do not rub your body vigorously with a towel when you're done. (It can raise your body temperature.) Gently pat yourself down instead.
- *Herbal treatments:*
  - *Elderberry juice syrup or lozenges (Elder, Sambucus nigra L):* Elderberry has been shown to be safe and effective in fighting fever from a flu virus. Elderberry syrup and lozenges are available in most health food stores.

  Dose:
    ○ *Syrup:* Four tablespoons of syrup three times a day, or as directed by the package.
    ○ *Lozenges:* Take lozenges as directed on the package.

Note: If your symptoms persist for more than two days, put a call in to your caregiver to make sure there's no underlying problem that needs to be evaluated.

Lice

If you're around school-age kids, there's always a chance you could get lice. If you do, use RID, *not* Kwell; RID's ingredients are safer. As always, check with your doctor or midwife before using anything.

Muscle Strains/Sprains

It's a little easier to trip and sprain something when you're pregnant because your growing belly shifts your center of gravity, meaning you can lose your balance more easily. Plus, your tendons are relaxed and more prone to injury. If you regularly play tennis, take aerobics, or participate in other activities that require quick, shifting movements, be extra careful now that you're pregnant. And if you've never played tennis or taken an aerobics class, now's not the time to start. Likewise, pay close attention when you're biking or Rollerblading, since you may lose your balance more easily than usual.

- *What you can do:*
  - *Ice:* Apply ice for fifteen minutes immediately after an injury to reduce swelling. After the initial impact of an injury has passed, apply a heating pad (set to medium) for fifteen minutes. This will enhance blood flow to the injured area.
  - *Tiger Balm or White Flower Analgesic Balm:* Ask your partner to rub either balm into the affected area—as long as the rubbing doesn't aggravate the strain. Both are available at health food stores.
  - *Acetaminophen (Tylenol):* Acetaminophen can relieve some of the pain from muscle strains and sprains. If pain persists for more than five days, and its intensity doesn't lessen, put a call in to your caregiver.

Notes:
1. If you absolutely need an X-ray, tell the technician that you're pregnant and be sure your belly is *completely* covered by a lead apron.
2. Do not take pain relief medication with ibuprofen, such as Advil or Motrin, when you're pregnant.

Sinusitis

Call your doctor or midwife if you suspect you have sinusitis, a bacterial infection in your sinuses; you may need an antibiotic. Symptoms include profuse mucus that's green, yellow, or brownish, and pain over the sinuses—on either side of the nose, under the eyes, or in your forehead. Before taking an antibiotic, see if you can weather the worst of it. Steam your sinuses with a face steamer (available at most drugstores) or by simply boiling a pan of water and leaning over the steam with a towel over your head. Don't take a hot steaming shower, and stay out of steam rooms, especially; you don't want your body temperature to rise.

Note: If you take an antibiotic at any point during pregnancy or while you're breastfeeding, I strongly recommend taking a probiotic as well, such as acidophilus, to maintain the good bacteria in your gut. While on antibiotics, take two acidophilus (lactobacillus) tablets per day.

- *Over-the-counter sinus medications:*
  - *Benadryl (diphenhydramine hydrochloride):* Take as directed for sinus pain. Keep in mind that it causes drowsiness.
  - *Tylenol (acetaminophen):* Extra-strength acetaminophen tablets can relieve some of the pain associated with sinusitis.
  Note: Check with your doctor or midwife before taking any OTC medication.

Stomach Bugs

Rest and fluids are the keys to recovery from a stomach bug. Unfortunately, if you have something that's causing diarrhea or vomiting, it's usually best to let the bug simply work its way through your system, which usually takes twenty-four to forty-eight hours. If you have diarrhea and/or vomiting, you must replace lost fluids and electrolytes. To do so, drink as much as you can. Sports drinks like Gatorade will help replace electrolytes; they contain a lot of sugar, which can irritate your stomach, so drink them in moderation—for example, one glass of Gatorade once or twice a day—unless you know that they don't bother you. Alternatively, electrolyte drinks like Pedialyte have less sugar, and you can drink those more often if you wish.

Caution: Rarely, between twenty-four and thirty-five weeks, diarrhea can be the first sign of preterm labor, particularly if it's accompanied by back pain and a change in your vaginal discharge. Ask your provider for guidelines about when to call if you develop diarrhea during that time period.

If you know you have a higher risk for preterm labor, your provider will probably recommend that if you start to have diarrhea, you call right away, even if it's the middle of the night. If you're not at risk for preterm labor, your provider may suggest that you simply drink a lot of fluids and electrolytes and call him in the morning.

Urinary Tract Infection (UTI)

The urethra, the tube that urine comes out of, relaxes along with everything else during pregnancy. As a result, urine can stagnate in both the bladder and urethra, creating a breeding ground for infection. Because a UTI can bring on uterine contractions, it's important to let your caregiver know if you experience any burning when you go to the bathroom. If a pregnant patient has a UTI, I always prescribe an antibiotic since a UTI can progress into a kidney infection, which is very serious, or it can trigger preterm labor.

- *What you can do:*
  - *Contact your caregiver:* If you have a UTI, you'll probably need an antibiotic. In addition to the antibiotic:
    - *Drink a lot of fluids:* At least eight eight-ounce glasses of water daily.
    - *Drink four ounces of unsweetened cranberry juice four times a day:* It's available in health food stores, organic markets, and some supermarkets. You can dilute it with water or seltzer. This fluid counts toward your daily water intake. Don't drink sweetened cranberry juice; the sugar will aggravate the infection.
    - *Eat a palmful of dried cranberries twice a day.*
    - *Wear cotton underwear.*
    - *Wipe from front to back:* So you don't introduce more bacteria into the area.
    - *Don't hold urine in:* Go whenever you need to.
- *Herbal medication:*
  - *Echinacea:* Thirty drops in warm water four times a day for seven days.

Note: I don't recommend echinacea alone for a UTI. It can be used *in addition to* an antibiotic if the infection takes an especially long time to clear up (more than seven days) or is recurrent.

  Cautions:
  1. Do *not* take echinacea in the first trimester, if you're at risk for preterm labor (see page 363), or if you have an autoimmune disease such as MS or lupus.
  2. Do not take goldenseal at any time while you're pregnant; it may bring on contractions or preterm labor. If you're taking echinacea, double-check that the preparation contains no goldenseal.

Yeast Infections and Vaginitis

The combination of pressure from the baby, extra blood flow, and increased hormones makes vaginal infections much more common during pregnancy. If your discharge becomes yellowish or thick and cheesy, let your doctor or midwife know because you may have an infection known as vaginitis, which your caregiver can treat. Likewise, if your vagina looks red, it's very itchy, and your discharge smells yeasty (as opposed to mild), let your caregiver know because you may have a yeast infection.

• *Treating yeast infections:* In the first trimester, I try not to treat vaginitis or a yeast infection with medication. Instead, I ask the women I work with to follow the interventions listed below. In the second and third trimesters, if the infection is persistent, I may prescribe a suppository or recommend using an over-the-counter yeast infection medication. That said, if you have a yeast infection, you can:

— *Drink more water:* It might seem impossible, but try. When you want to clean your system, nothing does it like water.

— *Dress comfortably:* Avoid tight clothes, choose loose skirts over jeans, and wear cotton underpants.

— *Wipe from front to back.*

— *Cut out refined sugar:* Sugar is a breeding ground for yeast. Avoid it as much as possible because its presence only strengthens the yeast.

— *Cut down on wheat:* Like sugar, yeast, which is live bacteria, thrives on wheat. If your infection is very bad or persistent, cut wheat out entirely.

— *Acidophilus:* Take two tablets of acidophilus every day. Or, have one eight-ounce container of yogurt with *live* lactobacillus/acidophilus cultures daily. Daily acidophilus can help prevent a yeast infection from developing.

Note: As I've mentioned before, I like to limit cow's milk dairy products when it's both possible and practical, just in case someone has an undiagnosed sensitivity to them. However, if eating yogurt with live acidophilus culture daily is the most practical way to get the acidophilus you need, and especially if you don't have any of the symptoms of a sensitivity to dairy (e.g., excess mucus, eczema, frequent headaches), then there's absolutely no problem with yogurt.

• *Medication for yeast infections:* I prefer to prescribe Terazol 7 vaginal cream for bad or recurrent yeast infections in the second and third trimesters. A natural alternative is boric acid vaginal suppositories, 600 mg in size zero gel capsules, used twice daily for seven days. Many pharmacists can make this up, and it may require a prescription in some states. My own OTC choice is Monistat vaginal cream or suppositories.

Medication in Pregnancy: How the FDA Rates Drug Safety in Pregnancy

✦ The Food and Drug Administration (FDA) assigns all over-the-counter and prescription drugs a rating to reflect their relative safety during pregnancy. Because of the complex ethical and practical issues involved with evaluating drug safety during pregnancy, these categories are broad and somewhat vague, but they can still be useful if you and your caregiver are trying to figure out the risks and benefits of taking a certain medication.

Category A: These drugs have been evaluated in controlled human studies and have been shown to pose no risk to a fetus.

Category B: Based on studies in humans and animals, these drugs are believed to pose no significant risks to a fetus. Some category B drugs have been evaluated in animals with no adverse effects, but no studies in humans have been done. Other drugs in this category have shown a risk in animal studies but not in human studies.

Category C: The data on these drugs are inconclusive because either there haven't been studies done in humans or animals, or animal studies have shown a risk but there have been no studies in humans.

Category D: These medications have been shown to pose a risk to a fetus, but they may be used in pregnancy when the benefit to the mother outweighs the risk to the baby. Certain prescription drugs for chronic conditions (like epilepsy) fall into this category.

Category X: These drugs should not be taken. They pose a risk to a fetus that is not outweighed by their benefit to the mother.

Note: Many OTC drugs fall into "Category C," which is why it's important to refer to the list of medications your caregiver considers safe, to ask about any medication you're unsure of before taking it, and to be moderate when taking any medication.

Over-the-Counter (OTC) Medications for Everyday Illnesses

The following OTC medications are considered safe to take while you're pregnant:

Illness	Brand-name OTC medicine*	Active Ingredient	Dose
Allergies/Hay fever	Sudafed, Benadryl	Pseudoephedrine, diphenhydramine hydrochloride	Follow package instructions. Do not exceed 14 days' continuous use.
Bug bites	Cortaid, etc.	Hydrocortisone	Follow package instructions.
Constipation	Metamucil	Psyllium (a natural fiber)	Follow package instructions. Can be used throughout pregnancy.
Cold—stuffy nose, mucus	Sudafed, Benadryl	Pseudoephedrine, diphenhydramine hydrochloride	Follow package instructions. Do not exceed 14 days' continuous use.
Coughs	Robitussin (plain)	Guaifenesin USP, dextromethorphan hydrobromide	Follow package instructions. Do not exceed 14 days' continuous use.
Cuts	Neosporin (antibiotic ointment)	Bacitracin, zinc	Follow package instructions. Use as needed.
Fever, headaches, body aches, sprains	Extra Strength Tylenol**	Acetaminophen	Follow package instructions.
Sinus pain/allergies	Saline nasal spray, Extra Strength Tylenol	Acetaminophen	2 tablets every 4 hours, per package instructions.
Sinusitis (See your doctor or midwife if you suspect a sinus infection.)	Benadryl, Extra Strength Tylenol	Diphenhydramine hydrochloride, acetaminophen	Follow package instructions. Do not use for more than 14 days.
Yeast infections— 2nd and 3rd trimesters only	Monistat	Clotrimazole	Follow package instructions.

*Other brand-name or generic medications that are the equivalent of these drugs are considered safe as well.

**Tylenol may be taken daily for an indefinite period of time. However, if you need it for a fever or headache for more than 2 days, contact your caregiver to make sure there's no underlying condition that needs to be treated. Similarly, if pain from a muscle strain persists for more than 5 days without lessening in intensity, put a call in to your caregiver.

Note: Many OTC medications are available in compound formulas that treat a range of symptoms. Some ingredients of those medications may be safe during pregnancy, while others should be avoided. Therefore, I recommend sticking with the plain formulation of these brand-name medications.

Caution: Do *not* take ibuprofren (Advil, Motrin, etc.) at any point in pregnancy or when you're trying to conceive. It used to be considered safe in the first and second trimesters, but recent studies show a link between ibuprofren and miscarriage.

Remember: To call your doctor or midwife before taking *any* medication.

Herbs, Supplements, and Vitamins for Common Illnesses

Illness	Herb,* Supplement, and Vitamin	Dose	Where to Find It
Allergies/Hay fever	Omega-3 essential fatty acids, especially DHA**	3,000 mg a day during attack, 1,000 mg a day preventive	Health food stores, organic markets, online
Allergies/Hay fever with thick mucus (with thick mucus, consider sensitivity to cow's milk dairy)	NAC (N-Acetylcysteine)	500 mg twice a day for 14 days	Health food stores, organic markets, online
Allergies/Sinus pain	NAC (N-Acetylcysteine)	500 mg twice a day for 14 days	Health food stores, organic markets, online
Colds	1. Vitamin C 2. Zinc 3. NAC 4. Echinacea***	1. 500 mg 4 times a day (2,000 mg) 2. 15 mg twice a day (30 mg) 3. 500 mg twice a day 4. 30 drops 3 to 4 times a day, do not exceed 14 days	Health food stores, organic markets, online
Flu/Fever (Keep fever below 100.4 degrees F.)	Elderberry juice syrup or lozenges	*Syrup:* 4 tbsp 3 times a day or as package instructs *Lozenge:* as per package; do not exceed 14 days	Health food stores, organic markets, online

Continued

Illness	Herb,* Supplement, and Vitamin	Dose	Where to Find It
Urinary tract infections	1. Sugar-free cranberry juice 2. Dried cranberries 3. Echinacea***	1. 4 oz. 4 times a day 2. 1 palmful twice a day 3. 30 drops 4 times a day. (In addition to antibiotics for difficult infection; do not exceed 7 days.)	Health food stores, organic markets, online
Yeast infections	Acidophilus (PCB8)	2 tablets twice a day (It's safe to take daily throughout pregnancy.)	Health food stores, organic markets, online

*The active ingredients in most herbs are not fully understood. Therefore, we cannot claim to know the exact active agents in all of these herbs.

**Only take an omega-3 essential fatty acid supplement that guarantees it does not contain PCBs or other heavy metals. See appendix 1 for recommendations.

***Do not take echinacea in the first trimester, if you're at risk for preterm labor, or if you have an autoimmune disease. Do not take goldenseal at any time while you're pregnant; it may bring on contractions or preterm labor.

Remember: Call your doctor or midwife before taking any OTC medication or herbal remedy.

• Pregnancy Weight Gain and Where It Goes
• Foods to Avoid

Building a Balanced Diet

Even if you typically eat a healthy diet with a variety of foods, pregnancy often requires dietary adjustments—some minor, some

Prenatal Nutrition

While you're pregnant, there are many good reasons to eat a healthy, balanced diet: For one, you need about twice as many nutrients daily to keep up with the demands of your changing body and growing baby. Proteins, carbs, and fats are now building blocks to good health instead of code words for weight loss. This doesn't mean you have to follow a stringent food regimen or deny yourself your favorite foods, but it does mean giving a little extra thought to your food choices to figure out how you can both live your life and meet the nutritional demands of pregnancy without driving yourself up the wall. Doing that means moving beyond the myths about diet in pregnancy (for example, you don't have to give up coffee) and embracing what you know in your heart to be true (an apple a day is a good and tasty thing, and sometimes you need a cookie). When you understand what nutrients your body needs and your own eating habits, you can make informed decisions about your food and, hopefully, enjoy the act of nourishing your body and baby.

◆ ◆ ◆

In this chapter you'll find:

- Building a Balanced Diet
- The Big 5 Nutrients
- Food Preparation and Planning
  - Clean Foods

- Pregnancy Weight Gain and Where It Goes
- Foods to Avoid

Building a Balanced Diet

Even if you typically eat a healthy diet with a variety of foods, pregnancy often requires dietary adjustments—some minor, some more substantial. Making these changes, however, can be challenging. Food, besides tasting good and satisfying cravings, is full of emotional meaning. It can offer solace during stressful times, represent love and family, and signal community ties. Beyond its emotional weight, sometimes you have to eat on the run (which usually means eating less healthy food), and sometimes it's hard to carve out the time to shop for and prepare healthy meals. Given everything that's wrapped up in what we eat and the time food preparation takes, if you're trying to modify your eating habits it's helpful to keep a few key concepts in mind:

- *Understand what you eat and why:* We ask our pregnant patients to keep a food journal for one week. (See "How to Keep a Food Journal," page 217.) The journal allows you to keep track of not only what you eat, but also how you feel before, during, and after eating. After a week of tracking your meals, it'll be easy to see how certain foods affect you both physically and emotionally.

- *Identify trends:* With the help of a food journal, you can identify the major trends in your diet. Most often we find women eat too much processed sugar or not enough protein. These trends provide an obvious starting point for dietary adjustments.

- *Start slow and set realistic goals:* When you know the trends, you can start by simply changing one thing in your diet instead of trying to change everything at once. For example, if you always have a large cookie as an afternoon snack and as dessert after dinner, swap a piece of fruit for either the afternoon snack or dessert. Then, after a week or two, begin modifying another big trend.

- *Don't give up everything:* Eating a healthy diet means finding the right balance; there's room for your favorite foods—fried chicken, mac and cheese, ice cream, etc. But enjoy what you love in moderation. For example, have a smaller portion of ice cream once a week instead of a larger portion three times a week. And when you eat something you love, do so mindfully, letting yourself experience *all* the satisfaction of a particular food. (See "Mindful Eating," page 225.)

• *Ask for help:* If you think it'll help, ask your partner or a friend to join you in the big changes to your diet, to share chores like shopping, cooking, and cleaning up.

• *Be compassionate with yourself:* This is a process. There's no right or wrong, good or bad. Some changes will be easy to make, others harder. Don't worry if you feel you've taken two steps forward and one step back—you're still one step ahead!

Note: Food aversions and nausea can dictate what you eat throughout your pregnancy. Sometimes, you simply have to do your best and eat what you can. For strategies to cope with nausea and vomiting, see page 120.

How to Keep a Food Journal

✦ *In general:* At the eight-week visit (the first OB visit), we give each pregnant woman a form on which she'll list everything she eats as well as the feelings that accompany each meal and snack. After a week, the nurse practitioner I work with, Monique Class, does an in-depth review of the journal, evaluating the strengths and weaknesses of each woman's eating habits. We most often find that the women we work with don't eat enough protein or calcium, and they eat too many carbohydrates and processed sugars.

Since we do this exercise in the middle of the first trimester, we don't ask women who are grappling with daily nausea or vomiting to do it. They need to focus on eating what they can when they can until the nausea has passed, usually between weeks 12 and 16. If this is your situation, by all means eat whatever you can keep down, and once the nausea lifts you can begin to keep a journal. Some women choose to keep a journal intermittently throughout their pregnancies just to see what kind of new habits they've developed and adjustments they'd like to make.

• *What to do:* To keep a food journal for a week at any point in your pregnancy, get a small notebook or copy the form printed in appendix 4. *Every* time you eat, simply note the time, place, what you're having, and how you feel (emotionally as well as physically) before, during, and after eating a specific food. At the end of a week, either review the journal on your own for major food trends (see the following pages for daily nutrient requirements and foods to meet them) or share the journal with your caregiver. If your caregiver doesn't usually review food journals, let her know you're planning to keep one for a week and that you'd like to discuss it with her or someone she recommends, such as a nurse practitioner or nutritionist who regularly works with pregnant women.

• *What to watch for:* Noting your emotions that accompany eating can mean tapping into powerful feelings. The journal may become a starting point for understanding the complex emotional forces that can drive eating habits. When I'm working with someone for whom a food journal triggers very powerful feelings, I often recommend she meet at least once with a therapist who specializes in food-related issues. That way she can start to develop a more nuanced understanding of how food affects her. If this seems like an appropriate route for you, talk with your doctor, midwife, pastor, or a mental health care professional you already know about finding a counselor who specializes in food-related concerns.

For a sample food journal, see appendix 4.

The Big 5 Nutrients

Every day, you should eat calcium, complex carbohydrates, fat, iron, and protein. Here's a rundown of how much of each you need and why.

• *Calcium:* As you probably know, you and your baby both need calcium for strong teeth and bones. But calcium does more than build healthy bones—among other things, it helps the body maintain regular circulation, muscle action, and nerve function. Since the baby will take the calcium he needs from you no matter what, you need to replenish your own stores of the nutrient. While you're pregnant and nursing, I recommend a total of about 1,500 mg of calcium a day (official guidelines recommend 1,250 mg a day), close to a third more than the requirements for a nonpregnant woman of childbearing age. (But there is a limit to how much calcium you should have. Don't consume more than 2,500 mg a day.)

Dairy products are famous for calcium, but a wide variety of foods besides dairy are calcium-rich, for example: green leafy vegetables, legumes, nuts, soy products, and certain fish. (See chart, pages 220–222.)

If you can't get enough calcium through your food, take a daily calcium supplement. Two kinds of supplements are widely available: calcium citrate and calcium

Can You Eat Too Much Dairy?

✦ It would be relatively easy to meet all of your calcium needs through cow's milk dairy products. I think, however, that it's wise to try to get your calcium through a wide variety of foods and consume a moderate amount of dairy.

Why? Both the conventional and holistic medical communities agree that the molecular structure of cow's milk can activate some people's immune system, resulting in physical symptoms ranging from mild to severe. A mild response could be defined as a sensitivity to dairy, which typically shows up as excess mucus production (a constantly running or stuffed nose, whether pregnant or not). Or it could be a full-blown dairy allergy with symptoms such as eczema, headaches, and joint pain.

Broadly speaking, the conventional medical community believes a fairly limited number of people suffer from a sensitivity or allergy to dairy. In contrast, the holistic community believes that many people unknowingly have some kind of immune reaction to cow's milk dairy products. This belief is based on our experiences observing patients who improve substantially once they stop eating dairy, not from data collected through long-term clinical studies.

As an obstetrician, I like to limit anything that could potentially cause an immune reaction in a pregnant woman, because *theoretically* a maternal immune reaction could influence a fetus's developing immune system, making the fetus more allergic (or sensitive) to a range of foods, and stimulation of the fetal immune system could *possibly* contribute to autoimmune disease later in life.

I want to be clear: This is my own theory based on my understanding of nutritional medicine and biochemistry. Strong scientific evidence doesn't (yet) exist to support the idea that cow's milk dairy can affect a developing fetus's immune system.

Putting aside the theoretical issues of fetal health—in practical terms, I've seen a real difference in maternal health when pregnant patients have eliminated or reduced their dairy intake. They have more energy and feel stronger, plus they have fewer colds, and less abdominal pain, gas, and bloating. Their experiences are significant enough for me to recommend that all my pregnant patients look for calcium in a variety of foods, using dairy as just one of many.

Of course, if you moderate dairy, you must do so in a way that's practical and reasonable. (If you eliminate it altogether, you must take calcium supplements as well as eat calcium-rich nondairy foods.) For example, if you have yogurt or cottage cheese every day, try cutting back to two or three times a week. If you drink a glass of milk daily, try substituting eight ounces of calcium-fortified soy milk instead (but don't drink more than 8 ounces of soy milk per day, because too many isoflavones can affect your hormonal balance). And if you have ice cream or frozen yogurt every night, cut back to once a week.

Finally, when you buy dairy products, look for those that are from cows that haven't been given antibiotics and growth hormones and, ideally, are fed pesticide-free grass.

carbonate. Calcium carbonate is less expensive and easier to find, but it can be difficult to digest and it must be taken with food. Calcium citrate, which I typically recommend, is easier to digest, can be taken at any time of day, and is more easily absorbed by the body. Whether you choose calcium citrate or carbonate, make sure the supplement also has magnesium (about half of the amount of calcium per dose), which helps the body absorb calcium.

Calcium-rich Foods

Cow's Milk Dairy	Serving Size	Calcium Content
Cheddar cheese	1 oz.	200 mg*
Cottage cheese	½ cup	115 mg
Ice cream	1 cup (8 oz.)	300 mg
Milk (whole)	1 cup	300 mg
Milk (1% and 2%)	1 cup	321 mg
Yogurt (low-fat)	1 cup	415 mg

Fish	Serving Size	Calcium Content
Salmon (canned with bones)	1 cup (8 oz.)	431 mg
Salmon (fresh)	about ⅓ cup (3 oz.)	10 mg
Sardines (with bones)	1 cup	300 mg
Trout	3 oz.	57 mg

Continued

Calcium-rich Foods (continued)

Fruits and Nuts	Serving Size	Calcium Content
Almonds	24 whole	70 mg
Figs	3	80 mg
Peanuts (roasted)	25 whole	13 mg
Raisins	1 cup	81 mg

Legumes	Serving Size	Calcium Content
Baked beans	1 cup (8 oz.)	142 mg
Black beans	1 cup	46 mg
Chickpeas (garbanzos)	1 cup	77 mg
Soybeans, boiled	1 cup	175 mg
Soybeans, cooked	1 cup	261 mg
Soybeans, roasted	1 cup	237 mg

Soy and Tofu	Serving Size	Calcium Content
Soy milk (calcium fortified)	1 cup (8 oz.)	300 mg
Tofu (regular with calcium sulfate)	½ cup (4 oz.)	434 mg
Tofu (firm with calcium sulfate)	½ cup	860 mg

Vegetables	Serving Size	Calcium Content
Bok choy	½ cup (4 oz.) cooked	80 mg
Broccoli	½ cup cooked	40 mg
Collard greens	½ cup cooked	75 mg
Dandelion greens	1 cup (8 oz) cooked	147 mg
Kale	1 cup cooked	90 mg
Mustard greens	1 cup cooked	104 mg
Rhubarb	½ cup	174 mg
Turnip greens	1 cup cooked	148

Continued

Sundries	Serving Size	Calcium Content
Blackstrap molasses	2 tablespoons	275 mg
Orange juice (calcium fortified)	1 cup	250 mg
Total cereal	½ cup	258 mg

*Calcium content in grams is an estimate. Sources vary in how they calculate the nutritional content of all foods.

Note: There's some evidence to support consuming 1,500 to 2,000 mg of calcium daily to help reduce the likelihood of preeclampsia, a serious complication of pregnancy. (For more on preeclampsia, see page 357.)

REAL VOICES
For me, my diet during pregnancy means just getting by. I have to eat what appeals to me, and that's not always what's necessarily the best for me.

Stephanie, mom of one, pregnant

• *Complex carbohydrates:* Along with proteins and fats, complex carbohydrates are a basic source of energy; during pregnancy you should eat between six and eight servings daily.

Carbohydrates can be divided into two (very) broad categories: simple and complex. (Note: The way we understand how the body processes carbohydrates is rapidly becoming much more sophisticated. Foods once labeled as either a simple or complex carb are now given a "glycemic index" that reflects how efficiently the body metabolizes them. For the purpose of pregnancy nutrition, however, the old-fashioned terms are still useful.)

Complex carbohydrates contain sugar, fiber, and starch. During digestion, they're slowly converted into sugar, entering the bloodstream at a moderate pace and creating a steady source of energy that the body can use over several hours.

Simple carbohydrates are primarily sugar with no fiber or starch. The body converts these foods very rapidly, and they flood the blood with sugar, which creates a burst of energy (a "sugar buzz"). The body then releases the hormone insulin, which lowers blood sugar levels. This means simple carbs only provide energy for a short period of time, leaving you hungrier sooner than you would be after eating a complex carbohydrate. In addition, once insulin lowers your blood sugar, you may experience a "sugar crash," or a sudden drop in energy and mood followed by intense cravings for more sugar. If you eat more sugar, the cycle of buzz-and-crash will continue. Some women who have had this roller-coaster response to sugar before pregnancy find it's worse now, and some pregnant women who've never had sugar highs and lows before may find they're experiencing them for the first time.

Complex carbs are typically found in whole grains—multigrain, rye, and pumpernickel breads, enriched semolina pasta, couscous, and brown rice. Fruits and vegetables are also good sources of carbohydrates (but they don't fall neatly into the complex/simple groups).

Simple carbohydrates include foods made from grains that have

THE BENEFITS OF INDULGENCE

There really might be benefits to eating chocolate in pregnancy. A Finnish study asked 305 new mothers to rate their six-month-old babies' temperaments. Those who ate chocolate daily or weekly gave their babies better ratings than those who didn't. The mothers who gave their babies the lowest temperament ratings were those who reported stress during their pregnancies and didn't eat chocolate regularly. The bottom line? Don't feel guilty if you love chocolate, and eat it in reasonable amounts throughout your pregnancy. It can make you feel good about everything—including your baby!

been stripped (e.g., white rice and anything made with white flour, like white bread and most baked goods), white potatoes, and processed foods that contain the ingredients dextrose, sucrose, and fructose.

Finally, a low-carb diet is unhealthy for pregnant women *and* their babies. If you eat fewer complex carbohydrates and more protein—which most low-carb diets require—your proteins and carbohydrates won't be balanced, which can lead to ketosis, a condition where your body creates substances called ketone bodies to make energy. Ketosis (the condition in which ketone bodies are being produced) may be a good buzzword for weight loss, but in pregnancy, ketones are toxic to fetal brain development.

If you're concerned about moderating your weight gain while you're pregnant, work with your health care provider or an experienced nutritionist to develop a reasonable plan that balances all the nutrients you need.

It's *never* a good idea to try to diet or lose weight during pregnancy.

Tip: Complex carbohydrates can satisfy hunger for longer periods when they're paired with protein. For example, excellent protein-carb snacks include a piece of multigrain bread with peanut butter or a salad of couscous, chickpeas, cucumber, tomato, and parsley.

Complex Carbohydrates	Serving Size
Rice: brown or wild	½ cup (4 oz.)
Bulgar, millet, kasha, barley	½ cup
Whole wheat bagel, English muffin	½
Whole grain cereals	1 oz
Whole wheat, multigrain breads, rye, pumpernickel	1 slice
Wheat germ	2 tablespoons
Rice or whole wheat crackers	2
Enriched pasta	½ cup

Q: How big is a serving size?
Dr. Evans: A serving size is an amount that's equivalent to the size of your palm or your clenched fist. For example, a large apple would be approximately two servings of fruit, and six ounces of chicken would equal one serving of protein.

• *Fats:* Fats are important building blocks in a balanced pregnancy diet. They keep maternal and fetal cells soft and pliable, and make it easier for cells to transmit and receive information. But, as with carbohydrates, there are "good" fats and "bad" fats.

• *Good fats:* Primarily monounsaturated fats and omega-3 essential fatty acids, good fats are found in salmon, nuts, seeds, flaxseed, avocados, olive oil, and other vegetable oils

• *Bad fats:* "Hydrogenated," "partially hydrogenated," or "trans fats" are found in fried foods and processed foods (like snack chips). Foods with bad fats tend to be high in calories, with little nutritional value, and they contribute to heart disease.

• *Protein:* While you're pregnant, you need two to three servings of protein each day or the equivalent of 60 to 80 grams (about 15 percent more than when you're not pregnant). Proteins are the building blocks of everything from DNA to neurotransmitters to muscle mass. They're made of smaller units, called amino acids. The body needs twenty amino acids in all; it produces eleven, which are called "non-essential amino acids." (Because the body makes them, it isn't essential that we eat them.) The other nine amino acids, known as "essential amino acids," must come from food.

Mindful Eating

✦ *In general:* Like walking, sitting, or chopping vegetables, eating is something we can do either without a second thought or mindfully, by slowing down and turning our attention solely to the experience of feeling, smelling, tasting, chewing, and swallowing each piece of food. So often we'll sit in front of the TV with a snack, say a bowl of popcorn, and before we know it, it's gone and we've barely tasted a thing. One goal of eating mindfully is to tap into feelings that we're not fully aware of that may lurk behind our eating habits. A second is to experience the pleasure from our food more completely.

• *The exercises:* To start, sit down with three grapes. Look carefully at one of the grapes. What color and shape is it? Is there water on its skin? Does it look appealing? Pick it up, feel it between your fingers. Is it a little heavier than you expected? Is it cold or wet to the touch? Bring the grape into your mouth—how does it feel? Start to eat it, chewing slowly, noticing if the sensation of the grape in your mouth changes as you eat it. Continue to chew until the grape is completely dissolved and you've swallowed it. Move on to the next grape, and go through each stage of the exercise again. Notice if you want to rush, or if you don't even want to continue. Repeat with the third and final grape and see if your feelings might have shifted. Are you bored? Can you bring as much attention to the third grape as to the first? Do you want more grapes? There is no right answer to any of these questions; there's only your own evolving experience of eating three grapes. You may want to jot down a description of your experience doing this exercise—what surprised you, how you felt, and what you learned.

Another day, you might want to repeat the exercise slightly differently. Start with a plate that has three grapes and three chocolate kisses. Pay attention to the different thoughts that go through your mind as you decide whether you'll choose the grapes or the chocolate. Have you had a difficult day and feel you "deserve" the chocolate? Do you want the grape because you think it's better for you? Did you feel guilty once the chocolate was in your mouth or shortly thereafter? Did you feel proud of yourself for choosing the grape? Whatever your thoughts or feelings, try to write them down as a way of gaining insight into how you choose food. If you feel "stuck," uneasy, or unable to free yourself from troubling thoughts about food, please get a referral to a therapist who is knowledgeable about food issues.

• *In practice:* The next time after doing these exercises that you eat something you know has more calories than nutrients, bring some of your experience from the awareness meditation to the table with you. If, for example, you decide to have a bowl of ice cream, really focus your attention on it and eat it slowly and mindfully. Notice the creamy consistency, the cold in your mouth, the intensity of the flavor. Also pay attention to how you feel physically—do you feel satisfied or maybe a bit bloated or nauseated?

• *The benefits:* What are the benefits of mindful eating? In general, I believe in eating with delight as opposed to guilt, and enjoying every aspect of food—whether you're eating an apple or a piece of fried chicken. And when you eat mindfully, you more fully experience—and appreciate—the act of eating, as well as your food. I would go so far as to say that when you really enjoy your food, you get more out of it. After all, a bowl of ice cream is not only sensual and tasty, but it's also full of calcium. I think by focusing on what's good in food and embracing the pleasure it gives you—as opposed to feeling guilty for eating what you "shouldn't" have, feelings that can trigger the release of the stress hormones cortisol, epinephrine, and norepinephrine, which can interfere with digestion—your body gets more of the nutritional value of the foods you eat.

Examples of Foods with Good and Bad Fats

Foods with Good Fats	Foods with Bad Fats
Avocado	Chips (potato, tortilla, corn, etc.)
Mayonnaise	Fried foods (fried chicken, french fries, fritters, etc.)
Nuts (almond, peanut, cashew, etc.) and seeds (pumpkin, sunflower)	Bacon
Nut butters (peanut, almond, etc.)	Butter*
Plant oils (olive, canola, flaxseed)	Half-and-half, heavy cream, sour cream
Tahini	Coconut*

*Butter, particularly organic butter, and coconut, while high in fat, are both acceptable in moderation.

Foods that contain all nine essential amino acids are considered "complete proteins." These include: poultry, soy, eggs, dairy products, fish, shellfish, and red meat. Foods with some of the essential amino acids—"incomplete proteins"—include: plant products like grains, nuts, legumes, fruits, and vegeta-

The New Prenatal Nutrients:
Omega-3 Essential Fatty Acids and Choline

✦ *Omega-3 essential fatty acids (EFAs):* These are especially important during the second half of pregnancy—some people go so far as to call them "the new folic acid." For the baby, omega-3 EFAs promote brain and eye development. Recent studies show they encourage fetal weight gain, particularly at the end of pregnancy. Another recent study showed that when women with asthma increased their intake of omega-3s, their children were 71 percent less likely to develop childhood asthma. To take advantage of these benefits I would recommend eating twenty-four ounces (three eight-ounce servings) per week of foods rich in omega-3 EFAs.

Other studies have shown that omega-3 EFAs may prevent preterm labor, and they can increase the nutritional value of breast milk. They reduce inflammation throughout the body, easing the effect of seasonal allergies and colds in pregnancy, without drugs. EFAs have also been shown to stabilize mood and prevent depression during pregnancy, and they may help alleviate the baby blues after delivery.

In addition to eating foods rich in omega-3 essential fatty acids, I typically recommend a baseline supplement of 800 mg daily. Omega-3 essential fatty acids are alpha-linolenic acid (ALA), eicosapentaenoic acid (EPA), and docosahexaenoic acid (DHA).

Foods rich in omega-3 EFAs include: salmon, halibut, flaxseed, flaxseed oil, canola oil, soybeans, soybean oil, pumpkin seeds, pumpkin seed oil, purslane, perilla seed oil, walnuts, and walnut oil. (For directions for grinding fresh flaxseed, an excellent daily source of omega-3 EFAs, see page 115.)

Notes:
1. Only take an omega-3 essential fatty acid supplement that's guaranteed free of PCBs and heavy metals. See page 522 for resources.
2. Organic eggs fortified with omega-3 essential fatty acids are always a good choice, but alone they cannot provide enough of the nutrient except when eaten in large numbers. Also, the amount of omega-3 EFAs in eggs varies from brand to brand; look for the brand with the highest omega-3 EFA content.

Caution—Omega-6 EFAs: If you have or are at risk for preeclampsia or preterm labor, don't eat red meat or seafood, including scallops, shrimp, lobster, clams, oysters, and crab. They contain arachidonic acid, an inflammatory omega-6 EFA that can aggravate either condition. Also the study of fish and asthma mentioned above found that mothers eating fried fish sticks, which contain omega-6 EFAs, may increase the incidence of asthma in their children, whether or not the mothers have asthma.

✦ *Choline:* Recent studies have shown that a nutrient called choline plays an important role in fetal memory development. In fact, studies of rats whose mothers were given choline supplements during pregnancy showed signs of improved memory into old age. The FDA currently recommends pregnant women eat 450 mg of choline daily, but leading experts in the field of choline research and prenatal nutrition recommend closer to 750 to 1,000 mg daily. The good news is choline tends to be found in many common foods. Good sources of choline include: eggs, wheat germ, beef and chicken liver, spinach, whole wheat bread, peanuts, peanut butter, fava beans, dandelion greens, cauliflower, and oranges. If you eat these foods frequently throughout your pregnancy, you'll get sufficient choline.

bles. Incomplete proteins can be paired to create a complete protein—for example, rice and beans. You don't have to eat two incomplete proteins together at the same meal; you can eat them in the same day and still get the benefit of a complete protein.

Finally, protein, while important throughout pregnancy, is especially important in the second and third trimesters. If in the first trimester you're too queasy to eat protein-rich foods, try your best to maintain your protein intake, but don't worry if you can't. If you choose to breastfeed, you'll need to continue to eat 60 to 80 grams of protein daily.

Note: If you're carrying multiples, specialists recommend a diet that's *very* high in protein—130 to

COMPLETE PROTEIN FOOD PAIRS

Peanut, almond, or cashew butter on whole wheat bread
Rice and beans
Lentil soup with rice
Split pea soup and rye bread
Hummus and whole wheat pita

150 grams daily, even early in pregnancy. A protein-rich diet will help you maintain the pregnancy to as near to term as possible, and it promotes fetal growth.

REAL VOICES

I ate so much protein when I was pregnant with my twin girls, it was coming out of my ears . . . I still know how much protein is in a glass of milk and an egg because I kept a journal every day.

Rochelle, mom of three

Protein-rich Foods

Beans (incomplete)	Serving Size	Protein Content
Black beans	1 cup (8 oz.)	15 grams*
Chickpeas (garbanzos)	1 cup	13 grams
Lentils	1 cup	16 grams
Lima	1 cup	8 grams
Navy	1 cup	15 grams
Peas	1 cup	16 grams
Pinto	1 cup	22 grams

Dairy and Eggs (complete)	Serving Size	Protein Content
Cheddar cheese	1 oz.	9 grams
Cottage cheese	1 cup (8 oz.)	26 grams
Egg	1 (preferably organic, DHA/EPA fortified)	6 grams
Milk (low-fat, regular)	1 cup	9 grams
Parmesan cheese	1 oz.	9 grams
Yogurt (any type)	1 cup	8 grams

Continued

Protein-rich Foods (continued)

Fish (complete)**	Serving Size	Protein Content
Cod	4 oz. (½ cup)	22 grams
Flounder	4 oz.	22 grams
Lobster	4 oz.	20 grams
Salmon	4 oz.	22 grams
Shrimp	4 pieces	20 grams
Trout	4 oz.	22 grams

Meat and Poultry (complete)	Serving Size	Protein Content
Chicken	4 oz. (½ cup)	20 grams
Beef	4 oz.	22 grams
Ham	4 oz.	16 grams
Lamb	4 oz.	20 grams
Liver	4 oz.	20 grams
Turkey	4 oz.	20 grams
Veal	4 oz.	23 grams

Vegetarians and Vegans

◆ Vegetarian diets come in many forms, and for the most part, they're all safe in pregnancy. If you follow a vegetarian diet, you have to be sure you get enough protein daily. If you don't eat fish, you may have trouble getting enough omega-3 essential fatty acids. For non–fish-eating vegetarians, I recommend adding two tablespoons of ground organic flaxseed to your daily diet as a vegetarian source of omega-3 EFAs. (If you decide to take an omega-3 EFA supplement, take one that's guaranteed free of PCBs and heavy metals.)

If you're a vegan and don't eat any dairy or egg products, it will be challenging to get enough protein, iron, and omega-3 essential fatty acids. But, with careful planning, it can be done. If you're a vegan, I strongly recommend consulting with a nutritionist who has experience working with pregnant women.

Protein-rich Foods (continued)

Nuts (incomplete)***	Serving Size	Protein Content
Almonds	1 cup (8 oz.)	21 grams
Cashews	1 cup	19 grams
Peanut butter	⅓ cup (just under 3 oz.)	13 grams
Peanuts	1 cup	30 grams
Pignoli (pine nuts)	1 cup	35 grams
Sunflower seeds	1 cup	26 grams
Walnuts	1 cup	17 grams

Soy & Tempeh (complete)	Serving Size	Protein Content
Soy milk	1 cup (8 oz.)	6 grams
Soybeans (cooked)	1 cup	30 grams
Tempeh	1 cup	38 grams
Tofu (firm)	½ cup	8–15 grams

*Protein content in grams is an estimate. Sources vary in how they calculate the nutritional content of all foods.

**Because of concern over mercury content in fish, current federal guidelines state that pregnant women should not eat more than twelve ounces of fish per week. For more information, see "Fish: Is It Safe?" below.

***If nut allergies run in your family, talk with your care provider about whether or not you should eat them while you're pregnant.

Fish: Is It Safe?

✦ Whether it's safe for pregnant or nursing women and young children to eat fish is a hotly debated and confusing issue, and there's little agreement. The major concern with fish is its methylmercury content. Methylmercury is a contaminant from coal-fired power plants and other industrial sources. The power plants spew out smoke with polluting particles, which land in the water and get into the food fish eat. Over time, methylmercury levels in fish go up, particularly in large, predatory fish like swordfish and shark (which eat smaller fish, adding the methylmercury load of their prey to their own). In large doses, methylmercury can seriously damage the neurological system of a fetus, and in smaller amounts it *may* cause more subtle developmental problems in a baby.

Because of concern over mercury content in fish, current FDA guidelines state that pregnant and nursing women should not eat more than twelve ounces of fish a week. Pregnant and nursing women should not eat swordfish, shark, king mackerel, and tilefish, and if they need to eat white (albacore) tuna, they should eat no more than six ounces per week (light tuna is a better choice; see lists below). New federal guidelines for fish caught by friends or family members state that pregnant and nursing women should eat no more than six ounces of home-caught fish per week. Check your state department of health for local guidelines. (These should be available online.)

In addition, there are growing concerns over PCB levels (polychlorinated biphenyls, a cancer-causing agent) in farmed salmon, and environmental issues with overfishing and fish farming in general.

Even with all of that, a well-chosen piece of fish is still an excellent source of protein and omega-3 essential fatty acids. In my own risk-benefit analysis and in my recommendations to patients, I suggest:

1. Follow the FDA's twelve-ounces-weekly rule. (An average serving size of fish is six to eight ounces.)
2. Take off the skin and broil or roast fish to cook off fat, where methylmercury is stored. (Grilling is also a good option, but avoid char.)
3. Choose fish with the following lists* in mind:

• *Fish with low levels of methylmercury:* Salmon, preferably wild Atlantic or wild Pacific (if you can, limit farmed salmon to once a month), sardines, tilapia, ocean perch, red snapper, sole, flatfish, cod, haddock, white crappie, black crappie, yellow perch, line-caught sea bass (Chilean sea bass is safe, but extremely overfished; some restaurants won't even serve it anymore), canned "light" tuna (light comes from smaller fish than white albacore tuna, and has lower methylmercury levels).

• *Fish with medium levels of methylmercury:* canned white (albacore) tuna, halibut, smallmouth bass, catfish, largemouth bass, carp

• *Fish with high levels of methylmercury:* swordfish, shark, king mackerel, tilefish, northern pike, walleye

• *Two additional points:*

1. I recommend avoiding scavengers like catfish and flounder, but that's a personal preference not supported by scientific literature. Flounders do have low levels of methylmercury and are considered safe on that front.
2. I personally recommend that my patients avoid tuna altogether in pregnancy, but if you can't, choose light tuna as opposed to white albacore.

*Sources: the Center for Women's Health; "FDA Prepares Warning on Tuna," John J. Fialka, *The Wall Street Journal,* 12/10/03; the Wisconsin Department of Health and Family Services.

Q: I try to limit my cholesterol and fat in general. Does pregnancy change that?

Dr. Evans: Cholesterol is the precursor for all the steroid hormones, which include estrogen and progesterone. Since your body is now producing high levels of these hormones, it needs cholesterol. Just as with carbohydrates and fats, there's "good" (HDL) and "bad" (LDL) cholesterol, but generally speaking you don't have to worry about cholesterol levels during pregnancy, unless you have a specific pre-existing medical condition for which you follow a low-cholesterol diet.

• *Iron:* Iron, a mineral, allows the blood to carry oxygen throughout the body. During pregnancy, you need twice as much iron (about 30 mg daily) for several reasons. First, by the end of pregnancy, the average increase in blood volume is 40 to 50 percent—since you have more blood, you need more iron. Second, your baby needs iron to produce her own red blood cells. Finally, as childbirth nears, it's important to maintain healthy iron levels because whether you give birth vaginally or by Cesarean, childbirth involves blood loss. When you lose blood, you lose iron, and if your iron levels are low before delivery, even if they're not low enough to be called anemic, you could become anemic postpartum, when fatigue from anemia is

---

POWER FOODS (FOODS WITH SOME COMBINATION OF HIGH LEVELS OF PROTEIN, CALCIUM, AND IRON)

Almonds
Broccoli
Chickpeas/Hummus
Dark, leafy greens
Figs
Peanuts/Peanut butter
Raisins
Salmon
Tofu

CHECKLIST: WHAT TO EAT EVERY DAY

Meeting the body's nutritional needs may seem overwhelming, but it doesn't have to be. Simply do what you can to follow these guidelines:

- Eat a serving of whole grains with most meals or as a snack (e.g., brown rice, whole grain breads and cereals, whole wheat pasta, for a total of about six servings a day).
- Use plant oils such as olive or canola.
- Eat as many vegetables* as you like. Green leafy and orange-red vegetables (e.g., carrots, yams, squash, tomatoes, peppers) are especially rich in nutrients.
- Eat two to three servings of fruit* a day.
- Eat a handful of nuts one to three times a day.
- Eat two servings of protein from (organic) chicken, fish, (EPA/DHA-fortified) eggs, or legumes daily
- Be sure to get 1,500 mg of calcium a day.
- Minimize how much white rice, white flour products, potatoes, and sweets you eat in any given day.

*Choose fresh, organic fruits and vegetables. If they're not available or affordable, choose fresh conventionally grown produce, followed by frozen organic vegetables, and then frozen conventional vegetables. Avoid canned vegetables, which tend to be very salty. Finally, microwaved vegetables lose many of their nutrients in the cooking water. If you can, steam vegetables or use less water when you microwave.

Note: One serving equals the size of your palm or a small fist.

the *last* thing you need. Maintaining a healthy iron level throughout your pregnancy is a simple way to prepare for good health postpartum. As with calcium, if you don't get enough iron to meet your baby's iron demands, he'll take all the iron he needs from your blood.

Your doctor or midwife will test your iron levels first early in pregnancy, then again between weeks 24 and 28, and once again at thirty-four weeks to make sure that you haven't developed anemia (a red blood cell deficiency). This happens if you're not able to produce enough red blood cells to keep up with the demands of the growing baby and your own increasing blood supply. (Technically this is known as *physiologic anemia,* because the anemia is the result of a natural process, not an illness, injury, or medication.)

Symptoms of anemia include fatigue, irritability, and achy muscles, and while these are common pregnancy symptoms, let your caregiver know if you've been experiencing them or suspect there's a problem. (For more information, see page 339.)

It's most important to eat iron-rich foods in the second and third trimesters. If you're nauseated in the first trimester, simply eat what you can. As your pregnancy progresses, if you're not getting enough iron, try taking an iron supplement that's nonconstipating. If you do develop anemia while you're pregnant, your caregiver will watch your iron levels until they return to normal, which they usually do by the six-week postpartum checkup.

Note: Vitamin C helps the body absorb iron, while dairy products, bran, coffee, tea, and antacids slow iron absorption. Therefore, pair iron-rich foods with vitamin-C foods, like citrus and tomatoes.

REAL VOICES

In the middle of my first pregnancy, I was taking a nonconstipating form of iron, I think it's like 25 mg. Then my doctor called and said I needed to take 325 mg a day—that would have been like seventeen tablets. I tried a stronger kind of iron, but it was really hard on my stomach. So I decided to eat liver and steak a couple of times a week—even though I'm mostly vegetarian. I bought free-range meat, and it was easier on my stomach than the pills.

Glenda, mom of two, stepmom to one

Iron-rich Foods	Serving Size	Iron Content
Almonds	½ cup	3.3 mg*
Apricots (dried)	5	1.7 mg
Artichokes	1 cup	5 mg
Barley	1 cup	5 mg
Blackstrap molasses	2 tablespoons	7 mg
Broccoli	1 cup	1.1 mg
Chicken	4 oz.	92 mg
Chickpeas (garbanzos) (cooked)	1 cup	7 mg
Eggs	2	8 mg
Figs (dried)	5	2 mg
Kidney beans (cooked)	1 cup	5.2 mg
Liver	4 oz.	8 mg
Oysters	6	5.6 mg
Peaches (dried)	5	5.3 mg
Pears (dried)	5	3.7 mg

Continued

Iron-rich Foods	Serving Size	Iron Content
Potato with skin	1	2.7 mg
Quinoa (cooked)	1 cup	6.3 mg
Raisins	½ cup	2.2 mg
Squash/pumpkin	1 cup	3.4 mg

*Iron content in grams is an estimate. Sources vary in how they calculate the nutritional content of all foods.

Q: I'm on bed rest. Do I just eat like I normally would?

Dr. Evans: When you're on bed rest, you need the same nutrients as any pregnant woman. But since your activity is so restricted, you'll need fewer calories, so I typically recommend focusing on nutritionally rich foods and limiting as much as possible "empty" calories from foods without nutritional value. (For more on coping with bed rest, see page 353.)

> REAL VOICES
> I went on bed rest with my twins at around twenty weeks, when I started to have preterm labor. I was trying to eat a lot of protein, so every morning my husband would leave a huge jar of peanut butter, apple slices, nuts, you know, stuff that could be by me all day—it was so boring.
>
> Katherine, mom of two

Food Preparation and Planning

There's no way around the fact that maintaining a healthy diet means doing some planning and preparation. Weekly shopping trips, cooking enough for leftovers, packing a lunch—these are all useful steps toward making the most of what we eat. Shopping, cooking, and cleaning up take time, but you don't have to do all the work on your own. Ask your partner or a friend to share the work a healthy diet requires; that way you can divide the tasks involved. By sharing the work and committing to a healthier diet, you're agreeing to take care of each other and your baby.

Q: Is it safe to cook with wine or other kinds of alcohol while I'm pregnant?

Dr. Evans: Generally there's not enough wine per serving for me to be really concerned about the wine content in cooked food. Plus, when wine, sherry, or other alcoholic beverages are heated to boiling, their alcohol content cooks off. So as long as the dish or sauce reaches boiling, it's safe to cook with alcohol.

REAL VOICES

The first time, I was all about pasta with meat sauce or meatballs (this isn't something I eat ordinarily). I also craved chocolate and lemonade. This second pregnancy, I have a crazy thing for super-spicy food—I've been eating pizza (another thing I don't eat a lot of normally) loaded with extra-hot, pickled jalapeños (it's really very delicious). And I have to have an apple every day, as well as a ton of chocolate.

Kate, mom of one, pregnant

I craved very random things at different times in the pregnancy: bagels with cream cheese, chicken-fried rice, orange juice, chocolate, guacamole. Toward the end of my pregnancy, I just had to have cheesesteaks and would get very cranky when one wasn't forthcoming (thank god I live in Philadelphia).

Suzanne, mom of two

In my first pregnancy, I ate a lot of potato salad. I always had a big bowl of it in the house.

Andrea, mom of three

In my first pregnancy, it was meat and avocados. I was a raging carnivore. As for the avocados, I'd have them on pepperoni pizza, or I'd put a whole avocado on a bagel. My stepdaughters thought I was nuts, but I just had to have it. Now, I'm craving fish and fruit. Go figure.

Ami, stepmom to two, mom of one, pregnant

The first time, the only thing I ate for about three months was cottage cheese and Ruffles potato chips. I would dip the Ruffles potato chips in the cottage cheese. Now in my second pregnancy, I'm finding myself dipping things in cottage cheese again. I. Love. Cottage. Cheese.

Asha, mom of one, pregnant

Dried apricots and mint chip ice cream.

Allison, mom of two

With my first pregnancy, it was cheese omelets, apples, and always chocolate. In my second pregnancy, I ate a lot of pomegranates and other fruit, and I *had* to have a chocolate bar every afternoon.

Glenda, mom of two, stepmom to one

Grapefruit! I always wanted grapefruit. I'd even have it for dessert at the end of the day.

Martha, mom of two

Sample Daily Menus

A NON-VEGETARIAN MENU
Drink eight eight-ounce glasses of water throughout the day.

Breakfast: Calcium-fortified orange juice; oatmeal with berries, banana, and one tablespoon ground flaxseed sprinkled on top; coffee or tea (decaf optional)

Snack: Apple; one slice of whole grain toast with peanut butter; a cup of herbal or red raspberry leaf tea.

Lunch: Egg salad on rye or whole grain bread with lettuce and tomato; salad with greens, carrots, red pepper, tomatoes, cucumbers, and raisins, with oil and vinegar dressing.

Snack: Handful of almonds; three (dried) figs; a cup of herbal or red raspberry leaf tea

Dinner: Grilled salmon* fillet; mango salsa (mango, garlic, cilantro, lime juice, a little bit of olive oil, salt); brown rice; bok choy sautéed in olive oil with garlic.

Snack: One peanut butter cookie with a glass of calcium-enriched soy milk.

*If you can, choose wild salmon over farmed salmon, which can be high in PCBs.

A VEGETARIAN MENU
Drink eight eight-ounce glasses of water throughout the day.

Breakfast: Smoothie with banana, blueberries, yogurt, one tablespoon ground flaxseed, and soy milk.

Caffeine: How Much Is Too Much?

✦ While you're pregnant, it's safe to have up to 300 mg of caffeine each day. An eight-ounce cup of coffee has about 150 mg of caffeine. Keep in mind, though, that in the age of super-sizing, coffee servings are often larger than eight ounces. For example, a Starbucks tall coffee is twelve ounces, a grande is sixteen ounces, and a venti is a whopping twenty ounces. (Note: Starbucks doesn't give estimates of the caffeine content of its drinks.) But caffeine can be found in a variety of foods and drinks beyond coffee, so here's a chart of the caffeine content in common foods.

Food/Drink*	Serving Size	Caffeine Content
Brewed coffee	1 cup (8 oz.)	135 mg
Decaffeinated coffee	1 cup	5 mg
Arizona Iced Tea (assorted varieties)	16-oz. bottle	15–30 mg
Diet Coke	12 oz.	46.5 mg
Coca-Cola, classic	12 oz.	34.5 mg
Sunkist Orange Soda	12 oz.	42 mg
Minute Maid Orange Soda	12 oz.	0 mg
Häagen-Dazs coffee ice cream	1 cup	58 mg
Häagen-Dazs coffee frozen yogurt, fat-free	1 cup	40 mg
Dannon coffee yogurt	1 cup	45 mg
Stonyfield Farm cappuccino yogurt	1 cup	0 mg
Hershey milk chocolate bar	1 bar (1.5 oz.)	10 mg
Cocoa or hot chocolate	1 cup	5 mg

*Source: Center for Science in the Public Interest.

Continued

Caffeine in Tea*

Tea (assumes 1 tea bag per 8 oz. water)	Average Caffeine per Serving	Range	Per Ounce
Black	40 mg	25–110 mg	5 mg
Oolong	30 mg	12–55 mg	3.75 mg
Green	20 mg	8–30 mg	2.5 mg
White	15 mg	6–25 mg	2 mg
Decaf	2 mg	1–4 mg	2 mg
Herbal	0 mg	0 mg	0 mg

* Source: *www.stashtea.com/caffeine.htm.*

Snack: Two slices of toasted whole grain bread with peanut butter and raisins; a cup of herbal or red raspberry leaf tea

Lunch: Lentil soup with rice; green salad with red pepper, avocado, and one tablespoon slivered almonds

Snack: Carrots with hummus; a cup of herbal or red raspberry leaf tea

Dinner: Whole wheat pasta with broccoli, pine nuts, and sun-dried tomatoes

Snack: Pear; one peanut butter cookie; chamomile tea

Note: If you're constipated, avoid bananas.

Q: I've heard that there are certain teas you shouldn't drink while pregnant. Which herbal teas are safe?

Dr. Evans: Generally speaking, herbal teas that you buy in the grocery store—for example, peppermint, ginger, chamomile, Red Zinger, etc.—are safe. You may have heard that peppermint and chamomile should be avoided, and that's true when you're talking about medicinal doses of these herbs. But packaged teas are not strong enough to cause harm. (That said, I still recommend drinking no more than four eight-ounce cups of peppermint or chamomile tea in a day.) Some caution against drinking red raspberry leaf tea because they fear it could cause uterine contractions, but as I've discussed elsewhere, one to four eight-ounce cups a day of red raspberry leaf tea is very good for pregnant women because it tones the uterus and provides many nutrients.

The teas you have to watch out for are those that make health claims. As with any herbal supplement, you need to treat these teas like you would an over-the-counter drug, which means proceed with caution and call your caregiver before taking any. Avoid any teas with goldenseal, black or blue cohosh, ephedra, dong quai, feverfew, juniper, pennyroyal, St. John's wort, rosemary, and thuja.

Note: If you're keeping track of calories, the latest research shows that the number of calories you need depends on both your pre-pregnancy weight and your trimester. A woman with an average body mass index (BMI; for more on BMI, see appendix 4) who's moderately active needs:

In the first trimester: about the same number of calories a day as she did before pregnancy (about 2,200, on average).

In the second trimester: about 350 extra calories daily.

In the third trimester: about 500 extra calories daily.

The change from trimester to trimester reflects the growing demands on the body that pregnancy

---

SAMPLE WEEKLY SHOPPING LIST AND PANTRY STAPLES

Weekly Shopping List
- Calcium-enriched soy milk
- Calcium-enriched orange juice
- 1 large container low-fat cottage cheese
- Parmesan cheese
- 1 dozen eggs (preferably EPA/DHA fortified)
- 1 loaf multigrain bread
- 1 package enriched semolina pasta
- 1 box multigrain cereal
- 1 bag almonds or peanuts (unsalted)
- Soup (or ingredients for it): green pea, lentil, or mushroom barley (Canned soups are high in sodium. Choose a low-sodium option or dried packaged bean soups.)
- Broccoli
- Mustard greens
- Romaine lettuce
- Cucumbers
- Red peppers
- Tomatoes
- Sprouts
- Carrots
- Sweet potatoes
- Avocado
- Fresh herbs: e.g., parsley, rosemary, cilantro
- Lemons/limes
- Fresh fruit: e.g., apples, bananas, pears
- Mango
- 1 package firm tofu (preferably organic)

makes. In other words, calories supply energy, and when you're pregnant, your body needs more and more energy to simply maintain itself in a resting state.

If your BMI is above or below normal, you would adjust your caloric intake according to your own needs. If you're concerned about caloric intake, talk with your caregiver about how to manage your diet, and how your diet should change, throughout your pregnancy.

Clean Foods

While you're pregnant, it's worthwhile to think about how "clean" your food is, along with how nutritious it is. By "clean" food, I mean food that doesn't have (too many) chemical additives and preservatives. This is part and parcel of a holistic approach to diet, because by choosing foods with fewer chemicals, you get closer to a diet that promotes optimal health and well-being (whether you're pregnant or not). For example, diet soda and sugar-free yogurt contain artificial sweeteners. According to the FDA, they're safe to eat while you're pregnant, but because they contain many chemicals, from a holistic perspective you'd want to have them only occasionally.

The unfortunate truth is we live in a world where much of our food supply has some level of contamination. I do what I can to avoid eating foods contaminated with pesticides or toxins, as well as preservatives and other artificial ingredients. I know from personal experience that you could drive yourself crazy trying to avoid contaminants altogether—it's an almost impossible task. So when I'm eating foods that I know are not as "clean" as I'd like, I choose to focus on the positive and express gratitude for what's good in them. A conventionally grown tomato may have some pesticide residue on it, but it's also filled with important nutrients like vitamin C and lycopene. We need those nutrients. I believe we get more of their benefits if we don't worry so much about the pesticides, but instead focus on the pleasure and goodness the foods bring, expressing gratitude toward nature for providing us with sustenance. The bottom line is: Do what you can to eat a cleaner diet, and celebrate the virtues—sensual and nutritional—of whatever you eat.

SIMPLE STEPS TOWARD A CLEANER DIET

- Drink spring or filtered water.
- Eat organic fruits and vegetables when you can.
- Wash conventional produce vigorously (soak in water mixed with one drop of soap for fifteen minutes, rinse thoroughly).
- Choose meat, poultry, and dairy products that are free of antibiotics and growth hormones.
- Avoid foods made with chemical preservatives and artificial flavors and sweeteners.

For more information on a clean diet, see page 28.

Pregnancy Weight Gain and Where It Goes

• *The pace of pregnancy weight gain:* Official guidelines on pregnancy weight gain state that a woman shouldn't gain any weight in her first trimester, then gain about a pound a week after that. Some women I work with naturally follow that, others don't. To be honest, I keep track of weight gain, but I don't pay much attention to it as long as a pregnant woman is eating well, her baby is growing at a healthy rate, and there's no sudden spike or loss of weight, which might be a warning sign of a complication. (For example, a sudden gain of several pounds accompanied by obvious swelling could be a warning sign of preeclampsia.) Fundamentally, there are so many different ways that the body responds to pregnancy that it's much more important to focus on eating habits than on weight gain.

In other words, if you're eating well and gaining more or less weight than the guidelines say, don't worry about it. As long as the baby's growing, you're fine. Generally speaking, moderate pregnancy weight gain is recommended for three reasons:

1. To lower the risk of gestational diabetes (see page 340).
2. To lower the chances that a baby will be lighter than 6 pounds or heavier than 8.5 pounds, the latter of which *may* lead to a complicated childbirth. Many small babies are perfectly healthy, but babies who weigh less than five pounds face the *risk* of more serious complications. Larger babies may have low blood sugar immediately after birth, a situation that's absolutely manageable. In fact, many hospitals check blood sugar levels of all babies above a certain weight automatically after birth.
3. To ease many of the common aches and pains of pregnancy, for example swelling, low back pain, carpal tunnel syndrome, fatigue.

If you're concerned about weight loss postpartum, keep in mind that what you eat during pregnancy is more important than how much weight you've gained. If you eat a relatively healthy diet, the weight will come off fairly easily, regardless of how much you want to lose.

REAL VOICES
Your body changes in unbelievable ways, and you just have to let it go—however you can. For example, I turn around so I don't see my weight gain. Otherwise I'm like, "I gained eleven pounds this month? How do you gain eleven pounds in a month?" So I don't look, and it's really helpful.

Asha, mom of one, pregnant

• *Weight gain guidelines:* Guidelines exist to give you an idea of about how much weight you're expected to gain based on your pre-pregnancy body mass index (BMI)*:
    – A BMI in the normal range: gain between twenty-five and thirty-five pounds
    – A BMI in the underweight range: gain between twenty-eight and forty pounds
    – A BMI in the overweight range: gain between fifteen and twenty-five pounds

*To calculate your BMI, see appendix 4.

– A BMI in the obese range: gain at least fifteen pounds
For twins, add five to fifteen extra pounds.

• *Where the weight goes:* By the end of your pregnancy, weight typically distributes as follows*:

6–8 pounds: Baby

7 pounds: Your own stores of protein, fat, and other nutrients

3–4 pounds: Blood (blood volume increases by 40–50 percent during pregnancy)

4 pounds: Body fluids

2 pounds: Uterus

1–2 pounds: Breasts

1–2 pounds: Amniotic fluid

1.5 pounds: Placenta and umbilical cord

Total: 25.5–30.5 pounds

REAL VOICES

I only gained twenty-two pounds—I couldn't eat that much because I was so nauseous for most of my pregnancy. At different points in my pregnancy, people would say, "You're too small," which was upsetting. My doctor was wonderful about it. She said, "It's absolutely not a problem. And if I say it's not a problem, then don't worry about what people say to you or tell you. Block it out of your mind." And I did.

Silu, mom of one

I gained forty-five pounds. It's definitely more than you're supposed to. But no one said anything to me about it. I was really skinny when I started, so I think the midwives probably thought it was good.

Maia, mom of one

In each pregnancy, I gained exactly the same amount of weight—almost to the pound. I delivered my daughter three weeks early, and she weighed 5.1. My son was born a week early, and he weighed 8.5 pounds.

Mary, mom of two

---

*Source: American College of Obstetricians and Gynecologists.

I hate to say it, but I got just about as big with the singleton as I did with the twins. My midwife questioned me on it and said, "If you're comfortable with it, you're fine." And I'd say, "I'm fine. I'll lose it later." And she'd say, "Okay, you're fine."

Rochelle, mom of three

Foods to Avoid

Building a healthy pregnancy diet means getting the right balance of nutrients, eating a cleaner diet, and avoiding certain foods altogether because they're more likely to carry food-borne bacteria like E. coli and salmonella. While most of these bacteria won't necessarily threaten the baby, they can be very difficult to treat during pregnancy and extremely uncomfortable. Listeria is the food-borne bacteria you need to be most careful of. While it's relatively rare, it's extremely dangerous. It can infect both the placenta and fetus, and can cause miscarriage, preterm labor, even death. Therefore, foods that could carry listeria warrant extra precautions.

- *Foods you should avoid while pregnant:*
  - *Meat pâtés, blue cheeses (e.g., Maytag, Roquefort, Stilton), unpasteurized (raw) dairy products, and soft cheeses:* Raw milk and raw milk hard cheeses can be found in gourmet shops. Avoid them and any other raw milk dairy product you come across. Unpasteurized soft cheese is illegal in the U.S. Whether or not pasteurization is sufficient to kill dangerous listeria bacteria in soft cheeses is a subject of some debate. Recent studies suggest that it isn't, and to be completely safe, avoid all soft cheeses, even those made with pasteurized milk.

    Why? They may be contaminated with listeria.
  - *Hot dogs, cured meats (salami, pepperoni, bacon, sausage, ham, etc.), and cold cuts:* Unless you are 100 percent confident that they've been consistently refrigerated or they're cooked.

    Why? They may be contaminated with listeria. Also, there's some evidence linking chemicals in cured meats eaten during pregnancy with a higher incidence of childhood brain tumors. The risk of a neurological cancer seems to rise if two or more servings of cured meats are consumed daily. If you have a reliable source for cold cuts and cured meats, consider eating them very moderately during pregnancy. Cooking deli meats will kill the listeria.

— *Unpasteurized juices:*

Why? They may be contaminated with E. Coli. It *is* safe to make your own juice at home, if you wash your fruits and vegetables thoroughly and keep your juicer clean.

— *Raw fish and shellfish (including "seared" fish that's cooked on the outside and raw on the inside):*

Why? Raw fish may contain parasites. Avoid raw oysters and clams because they, too, may be contaminated with dangerous bacteria as well as parasites. Raw shellfish in general (including shrimp) puts you at risk for contracting hepatitis.

— *Raw and undercooked meat:* According to the USDA, ground beef should be cooked to 160 degrees Fahrenheit on a meat thermometer (medium). Muscle meat (roasts) can be cooked to a minimum of 145 degrees Fahrenheit (medium rare).

Why? It may be contaminated with E. coli, which is killed at high temperatures. Bacteria are generally found on the surface of whole meats, meaning if the outside is cooked, the meat should be safe. With ground meat, there's no surface, which is why you have to cook it so it's no longer pink. (See "Handling Raw Meat" below.)

— *Runny yolks and raw eggs:* Some Caesar salad dressings are made with raw eggs, as is fresh mayonnaise. Egg yolks should be hard cooked.

Why? They may be contaminated with salmonella.

— *Swordfish, shark, tilefish, and king mackerel:*

Why? They're known to contain high levels of methylmercury, a contaminant that can cause neurological damage to a developing fetus. (See "Fish: Is It Safe?" on page 231.)

Note: Wash all vegetables and herbs from your garden or a friend's thoroughly. Because neighborhood cats may go to the bathroom on or near them, they're a potential source of toxoplasmosis. (See page 321.)

• *Handling Raw Meat and Poultry:* When you want to take extra precautions against food-borne bacteria, follow these steps when cooking raw meat and poultry:

1. Wash your hands before and after handling raw meat and poultry.
2. Don't put cooked meat or poultry back on a plate or surface that was used for raw meat.

3. Meat and poultry should be refrigerated at 40 degrees Fahrenheit, in shallow, sealed containers for no more than three days.

4. From a contamination perspective, there's no limit on how long meat or poultry may be frozen. However, make sure meat or poultry is thawed completely before cooking, so it will cook evenly and completely.

5. Don't reuse a cutting board where raw meat or poultry has been for anything else before washing it with hot, soapy water.

6. If barbecuing, cook all meat or poultry thoroughly until it's hot and cooked through. Avoid char from charcoal grilling. It contains toxic compounds called herocyclic amines.

7. Poultry is done when the juices run clear and the meat isn't at all pink.

14

Exercise and Pregnancy

Being physically active is an important component of a healthy lifestyle. For some people, that means working out at the gym three times a week; for others, it means walking to work and taking the stairs instead of the elevator. Whatever it means for you, now that you're pregnant, being physically active offers both physical and emotional benefits.

✦ ✦ ✦

In this chapter you'll find:

- Getting Started
- Exercise Guidelines
- Prenatal Yoga
- The Basics
  - Yoga *asanas* (poses)
  - Two prenatal yoga sequences

Getting Started

- *Overview:* During pregnancy, regular physical activity in general, and moderate exercise in particular, has many benefits. Emotionally, it can help you manage stress and anxiety. If you're having mood swings, it can help you feel more in control, and it can even relieve mild depression. Physically, exercise improves sleep, circulation, and digestion. Regular, moderate exercise will keep your muscles strong and help prepare you for childbirth. Labor is physically demanding; maintaining strength in your leg, back, and abdominal muscles won't necessarily make your labor progress any faster, but it will give you stamina for the experience.

Having said all that, being pregnant makes enormous demands on your body. It affects everyone differently, and how you feel will change from day to day. Honor what your body tells you each day. If you've planned to take a long walk and wake up feeling tired, take a short walk instead. If you're used to working out intensively, try not to be disappointed if you can't continue to work out with the same intensity and regularity now that you're pregnant. (You may be able to some days, but others you may not feel like it.) On the flip side, if you don't usually make time for physical activity, you may find you're more motivated to exercise now.

• *Starting out:* If you exercised regularly before you became pregnant, try to continue, adjusting your activities as appropriate. If you didn't exercise regularly before you became pregnant, keep in mind that pregnancy isn't the time to start an intensive exercise regime. Start slowly, and see how you feel at each stage. For example, if you want to start exercising, begin with an easy-paced fifteen-minute daily walk. As you feel more comfortable walking for fifteen minutes, start adding five minutes to your walk each day, until you're walking for a half hour. You can also mix your walks with swimming or riding a stationary bike for fifteen minutes and slowly increase the time you spend in each activity. You can even simply dance around your living room for fifteen minutes whenever the mood strikes. Finally, look into a prenatal exercise class of any type—for example, yoga, Pilates, general exercise, or tai chi class. If you attend a "regular" (non-prenatal) class, let the instructor know in advance that you're pregnant and ask about any adjustments you might need to make. (For more on prenatal yoga, see page 255.)

It's best to do some form of moderate exercise (dancing, walking, yoga, whatever is accessible and appealing) every day, but do what you can as often as you can. If you can't exercise, take steps to add more activity to your daily routine. Park your car at the far end of the parking lot or a block from your destination—even a few extra minutes of walking can be beneficial. What's important is to start thinking about physical activity as a regular part of your lifestyle.

REAL VOICES
I didn't exercise at all the first time; I'm not normally much for working out. But this time I've continued the brisk two-mile walk to work that I started

after my last maternity leave. I think it's made a big difference so far. I feel better and sleep better.

Kate, mom of one, pregnant

Exercise Guidelines

- *General guidelines:*
  - *Listen to your body:* Don't push it. If you feel tired, dizzy, or short of breath, or if something you're doing is uncomfortable, causes pain, or even just feels "funny," stop immediately.
  - *Keep your heart rate under 140:* You can check this by taking your pulse—find your pulse in your wrist or on the side of your neck, count the beats for six seconds, and multiply by ten. If you can talk while you're exercising, your heart rate is probably within an acceptable range.
  - *Pay attention to your center of gravity:* Throughout your pregnancy, it'll shift, making it easier to stumble and fall. You want to be cautious because even a soft fall the wrong way can trigger labor.
  - *Drink plenty of fluids before, during, and after exercising:* Your body needs more fluids during pregnancy, so it's easy to become dehydrated when you're working out.
  - *Don't get overheated or exercise in very hot weather:* Stay cool by drinking fluids; some women even keep a small, handheld fan nearby.
  - *Warm up, stretch out, and cool down each time you exercise.*
  - *Don't lie flat on your back:* After week 20, don't do exercises that require you to lie flat on your back, even for a short period. The pressure from your uterus against the major blood vessel in the pelvis (vena cava) can limit the amount of blood, oxygen, and nutrients that get to the baby.
  - *Be careful of your back, especially your low back:* Don't do exercises that take the curve out of your low back, increase the curve, or strain your back in any way.
  - *Don't overstretch:* With the hormone relaxin loosening ligaments, it's easy to feel extra flexible and push too deeply into a stretch. Resist the temptation and listen to your body for its natural limits.
  - *Maintain good eating habits:* And eat an extra serving of carbohydrates on days you exercise.
  - *Never try to lose weight while pregnant.*

REAL VOICES

Exercising definitely helped me feel good about myself. I didn't do stomach crunches or anything like that, but I would go to the gym and jog on the treadmill or ride the bike, and later on I would do fast walks. It was just good to feel that I was doing a positive thing for both me and my daughter.

Suzanne, mom of two

- *Do not exercise if:*
  1. You have any pain, anywhere.
  2. You have bleeding in the second or third trimester.
  3. You're having frequent Braxton Hicks contractions.
  4. You're at risk for or have been in preterm labor. (See page 363.)
  5. You have placenta previa past twenty-six weeks. (See page 350.)
  6. You have a weak (aka "incompetent") cervix or cerclage. (See page 343.)
  7. You have preeclampsia. (See page 357.)
  8. You have intrauterine growth retardation (IUGR). (See page 345.)
  9. You have heart disease.

- *Check with your caregiver before exercising if:*
  1. You have anemia.
  2. You're pregnant with twins. If you're pregnant with triplets, don't exercise.
  3. You've never exercised before.

REAL VOICES

I ran until six months, and then I just walked . . . a lot, especially toward the end. It made me feel physically more comfortable. Until the very end, I never had that cumbersome feeling like I can no longer be comfortable in any position. Plus I slept pretty well all the way through. And I think exercise must have helped with my labor, or maybe it was just that I had a general sense that I was strong, so I went into labor feeling confident.

Maia, mom of one

- *Stop exercising if:*
  1. You feel pain.
  2. You have shortness of breath or dizziness.
  3. You feel any vaginal fluid leaking.
  4. You feel physically weak.

Activities with Equipment: Are They Safe?

✦ *Biking and Rollerblading:* Technically, both are safe during pregnancy. If you did either regularly before you become pregnant, you may continue to do so. Keep in mind, however, that your shifting center of gravity can have a strong effect on your sense of balance. You don't want to fall because (1) it can trigger labor and (2) you don't want to have to have an X-ray while you're pregnant. If you feel at all unsteady, stop what you're doing. And as your pregnancy progresses into the third trimester, you may want to stay off the bike and blades altogether.

• *Downhill skiing:* The danger from downhill skiing is twofold: (1) you may fall and (2) you may be hit by another skier. Besides the risk of going into labor after a fall, a broken bone may be hard to diagnose because, again, you don't want to be X-rayed and expose the baby to radiation. Only you can decide what you're comfortable with, but be careful, whatever you do.

• *Horseback riding:* Don't ride horseback until your pregnancy is over. It's too jarring.

• *Racket sports:* Tennis and other racket sports typically demand quick shifts from one side to the other, which can be hard when you're pregnant. Also, as your center of gravity shifts, something that would normally be easy for you to do on the court could throw you off balance, leading to a fall. Proceed with caution.

• *Waterskiing:* Do not water-ski. When you fall, you fall hard, and it's too risky.

5. You have a headache.
6. You have vaginal bleeding or have been bleeding in the last two days.
7. You notice decreased fetal movement. (For how to track fetal movement, see page 347.)

REAL VOICES
I did a lot of the pregnancy exercises. I definitely think it helped me maintain a positive outlook, and it helped keep me flexible, especially with the second pregnancy. I was doing a lot with twins—they were two when their brother was born—so even though I was carrying a lot of extra weight, working out was really important to keep my body from breaking down.

Rochelle, mom of three

Q: Is it safe to lift weights while I'm pregnant?

Dr. Evans: If you did so before you were pregnant, working with three- or five-pound free weights should be safe. Don't lift weights heavier than ten pounds, which can strain your abdominal muscles, and don't lift weights above your head, which can increase the pressure in your abdomen and therefore on the uterus. (If you've worked with heavy weights for at least a year before conceiving, consider working with a trainer with pregnancy-related experience to develop a safe workout regimen.) Finally, if you didn't lift weights before you were pregnant, don't start now unless you're working with a trainer with pregnancy-related experience.

Q: Is it okay to take an aerobics class while I'm pregnant?

Dr. Evans: Aerobics isn't necessarily dangerous, but it may not be comfortable and it's not an ideal form of exercise during pregnancy. The bouncing may become painful, and you may lose your balance shifting from side to side, so be careful when you take an aerobics class. Wear clothing that supports your belly and your breasts, and wear shoes that support your ankles and arches. Drink water throughout the class, and stop if your breathing becomes too labored or your heart rate goes above 140. (Check to see if you can talk; if you can, you're probably fine.) Many gyms and community centers offer special prenatal fitness classes. I would recommend exploring those, because they are designed specifically for pregnant women.

Q: Is Pilates safe during pregnancy?

Dr. Evans: I'm a big fan of prenatal Pilates classes. You have to be more careful in regular (non-prenatal) Pilates classes because the exercises can create pressure on the abdominal cavity. If you're taking a regular Pilates class, let the instructor know you're pregnant so you can modify the exercises.

Q: What activities do you recommend during pregnancy?

Dr. Evans: I think you should do what you enjoy, within reason. For example, if you're a runner and running feels good, do so. Talk with your caregiver about your exercise habits and any special precautions that might be appropriate given your own life and medical history. Dancing, walking, swimming, prenatal yoga classes, prenatal Pilates, tai chi, and qi gong are all excellent forms of exercise.

Prenatal Yoga

This prenatal yoga material, unless otherwise noted, was prepared by Joan White, certified Advanced Jr. Iyengar Yoga Teacher, in collaboration with Dr. Geeta Iyengar, author of *Yoga: A Gem for Women*.* Joan, who's taught yoga for over thirty-two years, is among the most experienced Iyengar yoga teachers in the U.S. (For "Iyengar yoga," see glossary, page 525.)

- *What are the benefits of prenatal yoga?*
  - A regular prenatal yoga practice builds strength and improves balance, making it easier to manage the extra weight and shifting center of gravity that comes with the second half of pregnancy.
  - Yoga postures (*asanas*) stretch and strengthen the spine and open the chest. This improves circulation and mood—chest openers in particular can help lift the spirits when you're feeling depressed. The spine work improves your posture, which in turn can relieve any strain on your lower back.
  - Breathing exercises (*pranayama*) can give you energy and quiet the nervous system. Yoga breathing is especially helpful during labor, when long, soft exhalations should help you push more easily. Learning to hold your breath at the end of the exhale can help you manage pain better. (In fact, many of the breathing techniques developed by Dr. Fernand Lamaze are based on yoga breathing techniques.) These are best taught in a class setting.
  - Throughout your pregnancy, you can adapt most yoga poses to suit your particular body, needs, and mood. Also, since it brings your attention to how you feel in a particular pose at a particular moment in time, a regular yoga practice can help you stay connected to the range of physical and emotional changes you're experiencing.

REAL VOICES
I know that in pregnancy you're more flexible, your body's literally opening, but there are certain things you just forget to do. Your posture devolves, it's really hard to maintain, and for me it's important to open my back because

---

*Geeta Iyengar's knowledge and generosity deserve special mention and thanks. Joan also thanks B. K. S. Iyengar for his pioneering work in this area.

General Prenatal Yoga Guidelines

1. *Focus on your spine:* While you're in a particular posture, think about strengthening and lengthening your spine while keeping your abdomen soft.

2. *Make adjustments:* As your pregnant body changes, how you do postures—the props you use, the placement of your limbs—will change, and the postures will feel different, too. Go with the changes. Get out of poses that feel bad, seem to put pressure on the baby, or make your heart race.

3. *Let postures be easy and soft:* Don't jerk or jump into or out of a pose, and don't strain or push once you're in one.

4. *Notice your breathing:* Throughout your practice your breathing should be smooth and regular. If you find that you're panting or breathless, or your breathing feels labored in any way, stop what you're doing.

5. *Notice your strength:* Some days you'll feel stronger than others. You must pay attention to what feels right on this particular day and act accordingly—without comparing it to how a pose felt at any other time.

6. *Breathe and relax:* Breathing exercises (*pranayama*) and relaxation (*savasana*, or corpse pose) are energizing for both you and the baby.

7. *After practicing yoga:* Ideally, you should feel calm and good after a yoga practice. If you feel exhausted, either the sequence isn't right for you or you're working too hard.

that's where I hold it all. So yoga helped me open up my body in certain ways, it helped me stay grounded and get into a good mind-set, and really I feel like it helped me have a great birth experience.

Ami, stepmom to two, mom of one, pregnant,

The Basics

You can practice yoga anytime, from before you conceive, through your pregnancy, and into the postpartum period. If you're new to yoga and interested in trying it now that you're pregnant, the sooner you begin the better. Look for an experienced, certified prenatal yoga teacher. (See box, page 259.) Whenever you practice, pay attention to the messages your body sends you. You don't want to push or strain when you practice yoga during pregnancy.

As you become acquainted with different postures and how they make you feel, you can tinker with your practice, choosing more relaxing poses when you're feeling tired or stressed, for example, or spending a longer time in poses that feel especially good.

REAL VOICES

I thought the yoga was great, and physically it just felt so good. I felt that yoga and the breathing exercises I learned prepared me for labor more than anything. I took a Lamaze class but I didn't really think of any of that while I was in labor. I thought more about the pelvic tilt and the things I learned in yoga to keep your body feeling good.

Mary, mom of two

Yoga *asanas* (poses)

Yoga poses fall into six groups: standing, sitting, forward bends, backward bends, reclining poses, and inversions.

Standing poses

- In the first trimester, don't do standing poses if you've miscarried even once, because they're very strenuous and, if done incorrectly, can put a lot of pressure on the uterus. If, however, you were able to get a diagnosis for the miscarriage—for example, if there was a chromosomal abnormality or an infection—you should be able to do them.
- If your abdomen feels tight when doing a standing pose, use a prop—a block, stool, or chair. It will make the pose easier and more beneficial. For example, in triangle pose (see page 271), use a block for the arm that reaches toward the ground. This will create space in your torso and keep your abdomen from compressing.
- As your pregnancy progresses, do standing poses against a wall, kitchen counter, or the back of a couch. The extra support will help you maintain balance and proper alignment.
- If you're tired, support your head on blocks, pillows, or blankets when you're in downward facing dog, even in the first trimester. Later in your pregnancy, you may want to use a head support no matter what.

Sitting poses

- As you get further along in your pregnancy, sit up on blankets, towels, or pillows. It will relieve the pressure your growing abdomen puts on your pelvis and groin.
- Sit against a wall. It will help you maintain a long spine when your abdomen feels heavy.

Forward bends (both standing and sitting)

- Work on creating a concave spine by stretching from your tailbone through the top of your head, and stretch your collarbones away from each other to open up your chest. Don't worry about reaching your feet with your hands. (It will become increasingly difficult as your pregnancy progresses anyway.)
- Use a belt, towel, or old tie to reach your feet, keep your spine concave, and your chest open.
- When you bend forward, rest your head on a chair.

Backward bends

- Give up back bends at the end of the first trimester unless you're practicing with a certified teacher.
- Advanced practitioners *may* be able to continue a limited backward bending practice, but still only with the guidance (and in the presence) of a certified teacher.

Reclining poses

- After the first trimester, prop yourself up in all reclining poses, including *savasana*. Use blankets, pillows, and/or a bolster to prop yourself up to at least a fifteen-degree angle, or wherever you can rest comfortably.

Inversions

- Don't do handstand after the first trimester. You could injure yourself either by twisting when you come up or by losing your balance and falling.
- Only do headstand if you did so regularly before you became pregnant. When you practice headstand during pregnancy, keep your legs open. You may also press your feet together and open your knees, as in bound angle pose (*baddha konasana*).
- If you practice headstand at the wall, ask a friend to help you lift your legs so you don't strain your abdomen coming up. If it feels like you're straining once

Notes from a Prenatal Yoga Teacher

✦ Alma Largey teaches prenatal yoga at in New York City. (For *"vinyasa* yoga," see glossary, page 529.) Here she talks about her classes and what to look for in a teacher.

Q: What's the difference between a prenatal yoga class and a "regular" yoga class?

Alma Largey: A "regular" yoga class focuses on breathing exercises and *asanas* (poses) done in a certain sequence based on the goals of that particular class (for example, opening shoulders, preparing for back bends, etc.).

In prenatal yoga classes, we tailor the sequences to the specific needs of pregnant women. My classes have mostly newcomers to yoga. We don't do any poses that would tax the abdomen or the baby, such as inversions (like headstand), wheels (back bends), or vigorous breathing exercises. Instead, we do breathing exercises specifically for pregnancy that tone the abdomen. We do Kegels for the pelvic floor, and we chant to tone the voice to prepare for labor and connect with the baby. We also do a lot of poses with partners; they help the moms meet each other and develop a sense of community. Plus, after working with a partner in class, moms know how to do the poses with their partners at home.

On the emotional/spiritual side, one idea I emphasize in my own prenatal classes is impermanence. Pregnancy can be a complicated journey and sometimes women feel stuck and unhappy. Yoga class can be a time for women to check in with how their bodies are changing and how they feel about themselves. The really beautiful thing is that they're able to give birth—it's not every woman who can. So some days and some moments might be difficult, but I think yoga can help show how there's beauty in every moment, even the challenging ones.

Q: So you recommend women practice at home between classes?

Alma Largey: If possible, yes (see sequences below). One video I like for home practice is *Shiva Rae's Prenatal Yoga.*

Q: What should someone look for in a prenatal yoga class?

Alma Largey: Look for an experienced, mindful teacher. By mindful, I mean a teacher who's attentive and focused. She should teach a well-paced and gentle class that has a consistent atmosphere every time you attend. It's hard to put a finger on this, but the environment should be one that helps you connect with your child and yourself physically, emotionally, and spiritually.

you're up, come out of the pose. Also come down if you feel blood rush to your head, pressure on your eyes or ears, or any pain in your neck.

- If you're new to yoga, only do shoulderstands (*salambas sarvangasana*) with instruction from a certified yoga teacher.
- Only do "legs-up-the-wall" pose (*viparita karani*) if you have someone there to help you get into it. The pose looks very simple, but lifting your legs against the wall and lying with your pelvis propped up may strain your abdomen.

REAL VOICES

Yoga is too mellow for me. I like to jump up and down if I'm exercising. I usually run, and I stopped running right away with both pregnancies; it just seemed counterintuitive. So I swam, I kept lifting weights, and I did the elliptical.

Glenda, mom of two, stepmom to one

I like just going (to prenatal yoga class) and being in a room full of pregnant women and sharing that experience. I also like the strengthening and the stretching and feeling like it's going to help my body in labor. I feel like I'm connecting with certain muscles that I wouldn't necessarily take the time or think to connect with.

Michele, mom of one, pregnant

Two prenatal yoga sequences

The first trimester

Generally speaking, a first trimester yoga practice should be simple and easy. You can do most poses, but don't push yourself in any of them. Don't hold poses for too long, try to keep your body temperature cool, and adjust your practice to how *you're* feeling—whether in a class or at home. If you get tired, rest in *adho mukha virasana*, which is sometimes called extended child's pose. You do the pose by sitting on your heels with your knees apart, feet facing back and touching. Bring your torso forward, resting your abdomen on pillows or a bolster and your head on a blanket or your folded hands. Extended child's pose is very restful and creates less pressure on the groin than regular child's pose.

Caution: Talk with your doctor or midwife before starting to practice yoga or continuing a vigorous practice. Don't practice vigorously if you have high blood pressure, if you're bloated, putting on weight quickly, or if you've recently learned that you have protein in your urine. (For a first trimester sequence, if you have some yoga experience and you're feeling energetic, please turn to page 533.)

A restorative sequence

You can do this series of poses at any point in your pregnancy when you're feeling tired. The actions of these poses are extremely gentle, but they improve circulation, lengthen the spine, and help the body stay aligned, even when you're exhausted. Restorative poses typically use props like bolsters and blankets, whether you're pregnant or not. When you're in your second and third trimesters, *always* do reclining poses on a bolster or blankets, so you're lying at an angle (see drawings).

Cross bolsters:

1. Take two yoga bolsters or two sets of rolled-up blankets.
2. Put one bolster down horizontally and the other vertically over the center of the first bolster.
3. Lie back with your pelvis on the center of the top bolster and your shoulders

---

CHECKLIST: WHAT YOU'LL NEED

- 1 sticky yoga mat
- 2 belts (you can use old men's ties or towels)
- 2 to 3 blankets (wool or cotton; if you don't have blankets, you can use towels)
- 2 yoga blocks or large books like phone books
- 2 yoga bolsters or 2 more blankets rolled up
- 1 chair (like a folding or kitchen chair)
- Wall, the back edge of a couch, or a kitchen counter to act as a support

Note: Try not to be overwhelmed by setting up props like books and blankets. Used well, props can help you get and stay comfortable in poses that are extremely beneficial.

IN THE FIRST TRIMESTER AVOID

- Jumping into poses
- Deep twists (like revolved triangle pose)
- Poses that create pressure in the abdomen (like boat pose, *paripuna navasana*, and leg lifts)
- Inversions if your breathing becomes heavy or labored

(comfortably) on the ground. If your shoulders don't reach the ground, put a blanket underneath them.

4. Keep your legs slightly apart. If your back hurts, put your feet up on blocks or books.

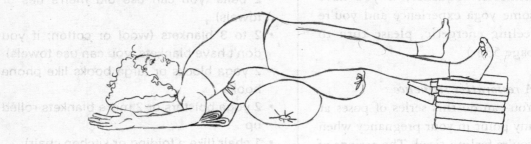

Reclined crossed leg pose *(supta sukasana):* Have a bolster or folded-up blankets lined up vertically behind you, with a small pillow for your head.

1. Sit in front of the bolster, and simply cross your legs in front of you, with the sides of your feet on the ground.

2. With the bolster touching your low back, gently lie back, resting your whole spine on the bolster. If your low back hurts, fold up a towel or blanket and put it under your buttocks. Rest here for a few minutes, then repeat, changing the cross of your legs so the other leg is in front. As you get further along in your

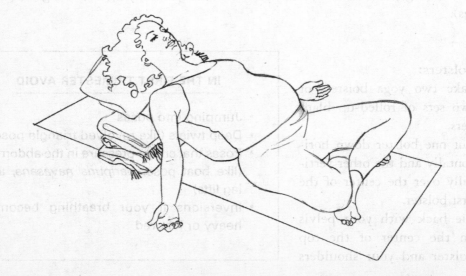

pregnancy, you can add height by putting a blanket or two under the far end of the bolster where your head rests.

3. If you feel any strain in your shoulders, or if your hands start to tingle, place a book or block under each hand.

4. Uncross your legs, gently roll onto your left side, place your hands on the floor, and slowly push yourself up.

Reclined bound angle pose *(supta baddha konasana):*

1. Have a bolster or rolled-up blanket lined up vertically behind you. If you have a strap, press your feet together, knees out to the side, and loop the strap around low on your back (below your pelvis), over your inner thighs, and around the outside of your feet (see drawing, page 264).

2. Press the soles of your feet together, bringing them in close to your groin. The strap helps you maintain this position. Think about your thighs releasing away from each other. If this is hard on your knees, or if you're not using a belt, put a rolled-up towel under each thigh as support (see drawing below).

3. *In the third trimester,* place a block or book between your feet, which will help widen the pelvis.

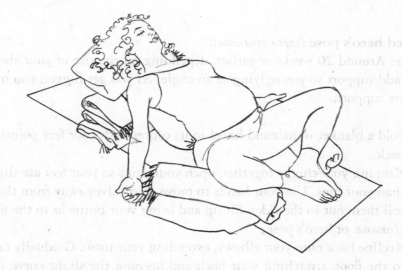

4. With the bolster against the back of your waist, gently lie back, resting your spine on the bolster. If your low back hurts, the bolster may be too high. If this is the case, fold a blanket and put it underneath your buttocks. If your neck hurts, fold up a towel or blanket as a pillow for your head.

5. If you feel any strain in your shoulders, or if your hands start to tingle, place a book or block under each hand.
6. Rest here for a few minutes.
7. If you're using a strap, release it. Straighten your legs, gently roll onto your left side, place your hands on the floor, and slowly push yourself up.

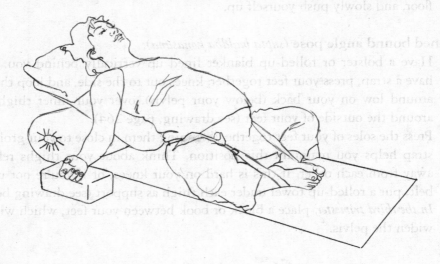

Reclined hero's pose (*supta virasana*):

Note: Around 20 weeks or earlier, depending on the size of your abdomen, you should add support so you're lying at an angle. As you get bigger, you may want to add more support.

1. Fold a blanket in half and kneel in its center with your feet pointing straight back.
2. Keeping your thighs together, open your shins so your feet are slightly wider than your hips. Use your hands to move your calves away from the knees and roll them out to the sides. Sit up and bring your buttocks to the floor. This is *virasana,* or hero's pose.
3. Recline back onto your elbows, extending your torso. Gradually take yourself to the floor, stretching your back and keeping the slight curve in your low back.
4. If you don't reach the floor, use a bolster or roll several blankets together. After twenty weeks, always use a bolster and a little pillow for your head so you're propped on an angle. Toward the end of your pregnancy, your support

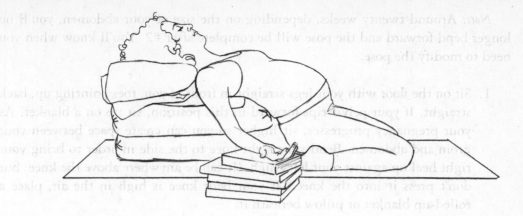

should be higher. (See drawing; this shows highest support. You can use less padding if it's more comfortable for you.)

5. If you feel any strain in your shoulders, or if your hands start to tingle, place a book or block under each hand.

6. Breathe here for as long as is comfortable (up to five minutes).

7. Using your elbows, slowly come back up to a sitting hero's pose. If you feel pain or like you're suspended from the ligaments in your knees, put a block, book, or folded blanket underneath your buttocks.

Head to knee pose *(janu sirsasana):*

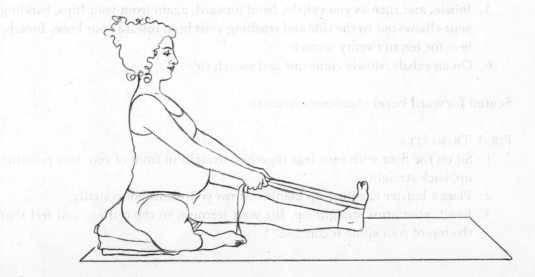

Note: Around twenty weeks, depending on the size of your abdomen, you'll no longer bend forward and the pose will be complete after #2. You'll know when you need to modify the pose.

1. Sit on the floor with your legs straight in front of you, toes pointing up, back straight. If your pelvis tips forward in this position, sit up on a blanket. As your pregnancy progresses, sit higher so you can create space between your groin and abdomen. Bend your right knee to the side in order to bring your right heel up against your left thigh. (It can be anywhere above the knee, but don't press it into the knee.) If your bent knee is high in the air, place a rolled-up blanket or pillow beneath it.
2. Adjust your torso so it's in line with your left leg (this is a slight twist), which is still straight, left toes still pointing up to the ceiling. As you become bigger, move your left leg out to the left. Loop a belt around the ball of your left foot and make your spine concave, holding onto both ends of the belt and looking up. From around twenty weeks forward (depending on the size of your abdomen), this will be the final pose.
3. On an exhale, bend forward. Think about bending from your hips, not your upper back; extend the low back so you don't come down with a dome shape in your upper back.
4. Grab hold of your left foot with both hands. If reaching your foot means bending your left leg, loop a belt or a towel around the ball of your left foot and hold onto the ends.
5. Inhale, and then as you exhale, bend forward, again from your hips, bending your elbows out to the side and reaching your head toward your knee. Breathe here for ten to twenty seconds.
6. On an exhale, slowly come out and switch sides.

Seated forward bend *(paschimottanasana):*

FIRST TRIMESTER
1. Sit on the floor with your legs together, straight in front of you, toes pointing up, back straight.
2. Place a bolster or rolled-up blanket across your shins horizontally.
3. Reach your arms straight up, lift your sternum to the ceiling, and feel that the top of your spine is concave.

4. Slowly reach forward toward your feet, bending from the hips and keeping the spine concave. Rest your head on the blanket or bolster for twenty to thirty seconds or as long as you're comfortable.
5. On an inhale, slowly lift up out of the pose.

SECOND AND THIRD TRIMESTERS

1. Have a kitchen chair in front of you or use a belt. Place one or two folded blankets under your buttocks.
2. Sit with your legs slightly apart, wrap a strap around the balls of your feet or place your legs beneath the seat of the chair. Make sure that your padding is high enough under your buttocks that you have room for your stomach and to elongate your spine.
3. Reach your arms straight up, lifting your sternum to the ceiling and feeling that the top of your spine is concave.
4. Slowly reach forward, bending from the hips and keeping the spine concave. Grab hold of the strap or fold your arms onto the seat of the chair, and rest your head on your arms, relax your arms, neck, and head. Rest here for a minute, or as long as you're comfortable (see drawings). *Make sure your abdomen doesn't feel compressed in any way. If it does, come out of the pose.*
5. On an inhale, slowly lift up out of the pose.

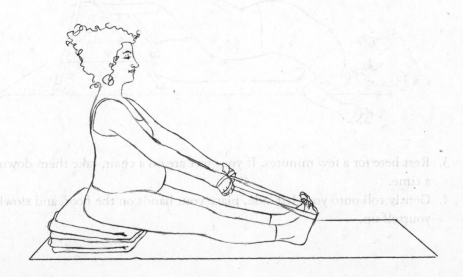

Shoulder stand *(sarvangasana):* If you know the pose or are in a prenatal yoga class with a certified teacher.

Supported plow pose *(halasana):* If you know the pose; put your legs on a chair and keep them apart.

Supported bridge pose *(setu bandha sarvangasana):* As your pregnancy progresses, add height to the support and, if the pose becomes uncomfortable, support your legs by placing them on a chair with bent knees.

1. Lay a bolster or rolled-up blanket down vertically behind you. Place a chair, a book, or a second bolster or blanket on the floor perpendicular to the first, about a leg's length away. (You may want to set the book up against a wall.)
2. Lie down on the first bolster. Slide back over the bolster's top edge until your shoulders and head are resting on the floor. Your chest should be open. Place your feet on the book or second bolster. Separate your feet a few inches. Or you may feel more comfortable with your knees bent and resting on a chair.

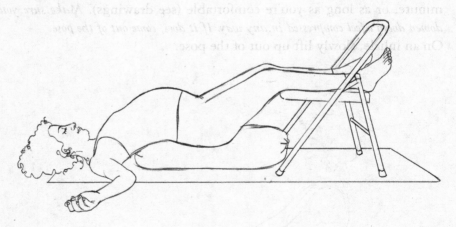

3. Rest here for a few minutes. If your feet are on a chair, take them down one at a time.
4. Gently roll onto your left side, place your hands on the floor, and slowly push yourself up.

Corpse pose (*savasana*):

Note: Use modifications around twenty weeks or earlier, depending on the size of your abdomen. You'll know when you need to modify the pose.

1. Lie on your back, with your feet apart and arms out to the side (so they're not touching your body).
2. Close your eyes, stretch your arms and legs, and then let everything relax.
3. Lie here for as long as you can comfortably.
4. When you're done, slowly start to deepen your breath and roll onto your left side. Then gently return to a comfortable seated position.
5. *Modification:* From around the twentieth week forward, lie on your left side with a bolster or rolled-up blanket between your knees. You may want to put a pillow behind your head and another rolled up behind your back.

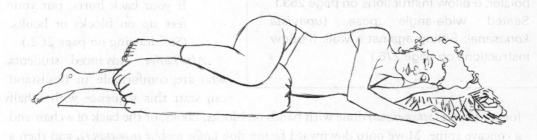

An active sequence for the second and third trimesters

As you get further along in your pregnancy, keep in mind the idea that through practicing yoga, you're creating more space for the baby while becoming stronger. Continue to modify your practice to meet your own needs on any given day.

This series can be done as often as you like, and you can adapt it to your mood. If you add poses, do so according to their group. For example, insert standing poses between triangle pose and intense wide-legged stretch. (If you have some yoga experience and would like to try a longer sequence for the second and third trimesters, turn to appendix 3.)

3 POSES FOR EVERY DAY

These three poses gently open the hips. Practice them as often as you can—daily is ideal. Even if you don't have the time or energy for a full practice, you'll benefit from spending a little time doing these.

- Bound angle pose (*baddha konasana*): Sitting against a wall. (Follow instructions on page 276.)
- Reclined bound angle pose (*supta baddha konasana*): In the second and third trimesters; always do reclining poses on a bolster. (Follow instructions on page 263.)
- Seated wide-angle pose (*upavista konasana*): Sitting against a wall. (Follow instructions on page 276.)

Cross Bolsters:
1. Take two yoga bolsters or rolled-up blankets.
2. Put one bolster down horizontally and the other vertically over the center of the first bolster.
3. Lie back with your pelvis on the center of the top bolster and your shoulders (comfortably) on the ground. If your shoulders don't reach the ground, put a blanket underneath them.
4. Keep your legs slightly apart. If your back hurts, put your feet up on blocks or books. (See drawing on page 262.)

Alternative: Advanced students who are comfortable in headstand can start this sequence with a half forward bend (*uttanasana*) done with hands on blocks, books, or the back of a chair and a concave spine. Move onto downward facing dog (*adho mukha svanasana*), and then a headstand (*sirsasana*). Headstand should be done with feet resting on the wall and legs apart (you can ask someone to put a roll of paper towels between the tops of the thighs in order to maintain the proper width) or in bound angle pose. Stay up for as long as you're used to, one to five minutes, then continue with the rest of the sequence.

Triangle pose (*utthita trikonasana*):
1. Start with your feet hip-width apart and stand against a wall.
2. Use the wall for support throughout the entire pose.
3. Step your feet about four feet apart; keep them parallel to each other. Turn your right foot out to the side and your left foot slightly in—your right heel should line up with the center of your left arch.
4. Stretch your arms out to the side, lifting up your abdomen, chest, and leg muscles.

Chest and Shoulder Openers

✦ You can do chest and shoulder stretches any time of day (at your desk, when you're watching TV), not just during a yoga practice. By regularly opening your chest and shoulders, which carry a lot of tension, you'll improve circulation and help the body's energy move freely.

- With a straight spine (maintaining the curve in your low back), lift your arms up overhead, palms facing forward. Keep your elbows straight and don't let your shoulders get too close to your ears.
- *Gomukhasana* ("cow face" pose) arms: With a straight spine (maintaining the curve in your low back), lift your right arm straight up overhead and bend it at the elbow so your hand is touching your back. Take your left arm out to the side, turn the palm to face the wall behind you, bend your left arm so the back of your hand is touching your back, and clasp both hands. If your hands don't reach (or if they only reach on one side) hold onto a strap or a belt. Repeat on the other side.
- Standing with legs a little wider than hip distance apart, bring both arms behind your back, keep them straight, and clasp your hands together. Slowly bend forward, bringing your clasped hands overhead. As you get further along, you can rest your head on a chair or countertop.

5. As you exhale, extend your right arm out to the right and bring it down onto your leg—at whatever point you reach easily—or a block.
6. As you press your right hand down, stretch up with your left arm, gently turning your chest and head toward the ceiling, keeping the abdomen soft. Continue to extend your spine. Breathe here for as long as it's comfortable (ten to twenty seconds).
7. On an inhale, lift up, turn your feet back to parallel, and repeat on the other side.

Downward facing dog pose with head supported (*adho mukha svanasana*):
1. Have a folded blanket, block, or book in the middle of your mat.
2. Place two books or blocks at the top of your mat, shoulder-width apart.

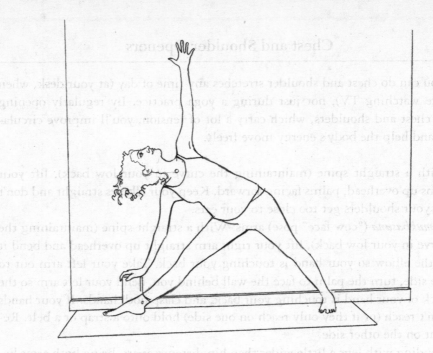

3. You're going to make an upside-down V, like a stretching dog. Begin on your hands and knees, torso over the block or book, with your hands directly under your shoulders and on the blocks, knees under your hips, toes curled under.

4. Pressing your palms into the ground, begin to straighten your legs, taking your hips back toward the wall behind you.

5. Extend your spine and press down into your heels, which may or may not reach the ground. You may need to step your feet back a few more inches if your weight doesn't feel evenly distributed on your arms and legs. As your pregnancy progresses, step your feet wider apart so there's no pressure on your abdomen.

6. As you press into your palms, let your head hang heavy and rest on the block or book.

7. Stay here for up to thirty seconds.

8. Lift up your head and slowly step your feet forward to lift up out of the pose.

Note: If it's more comfortable, particularly late in pregnancy, you can make the V by placing your hands on the seat or back of a chair (see drawing on page 273) or against a wall.

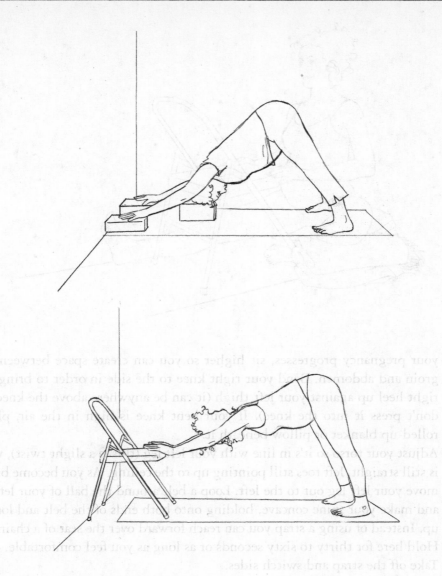

your pregnancy progresses, sit higher so you can create space between your
groin and abdomen. Bend your right knee to the side in order to bring your
right heel up against your left thigh (it can be anywhere above the knee, but
don't press it into the knee). If your spine is high in the air, place a
rolled-up blanket or pillow under your buttocks.

2. Adjust your right leg in line with your hip (with a slight twist), which
is still straight but toes still pointing up to the ceiling. As you become bigger,
move your left leg out to the left. Keep your left heel on the ball of your left foot
and make your spine concave, holding onto both ends of the belt and looking
up. Instead of using a strap you can reach forward over the seat of a chair.

3. Hold here for thirty to sixty seconds or as long as you feel comfortable.

4. Take off the strap and switch sides.

Head to knee pose *(janu sirsasana):*

Note: Make sure that your padding is high enough under your buttocks that you
have room for your stomach and to elongate your spine.

1. Sit on the floor with your legs straight in front of you, toes pointing up, back
straight. If your pelvis tips forward in this position, sit up on a blanket. As

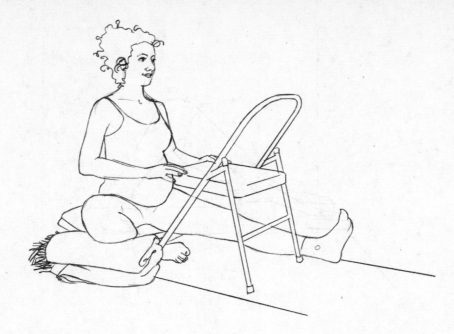

your pregnancy progresses, sit higher so you can create space between your groin and abdomen. Bend your right knee to the side in order to bring your right heel up against your left thigh (it can be anywhere above the knee, but don't press it into the knee). If your bent knee is high in the air, place a rolled-up blanket or pillow beneath it.

2. Adjust your torso so it's in line with your left leg (this is a slight twist), which is still straight, left toes still pointing up to the ceiling. As you become bigger, move your left leg out to the left. Loop a belt around the ball of your left foot and make your spine concave, holding onto both ends of the belt and looking up. Instead of using a strap you can reach forward over the seat of a chair.

3. Hold here for thirty to sixty seconds or as long as you feel comfortable.

4. Take off the strap and switch sides.

Seated forward bend (*paschimottanasana*):

Note: Make sure that your padding is high enough under your buttocks that you have room for your stomach and to elongate your spine.

1. Have a kitchen chair in front of you. Place one or two folded blankets under your buttocks.

2. Sit with your legs slightly apart and beneath the seat of the chair. Make sure that your padding is high enough under your buttocks that you have room for your stomach and to elongate your spine.

3. Reach your arms straight up, lifting your sternum to the ceiling and feeling how the top of your spine is concave.

4. Slowly reach forward, bending from the hips and keeping the spine concave. Fold your arms onto the seat of the chair and rest your head on your arms, relax your arms, neck, and head. Rest here for thirty to sixty seconds, or as long as you're comfortable. *Make sure your abdomen doesn't feel compressed in any way. If it does, come out of the pose.*

5. On an inhale, slowly lift up out of the pose.

Gentle seated twist *(bharadvajasana):*
Note: Do not do this pose after twenty-eight weeks.

1. Sit either on a chair with your legs apart or on the floor.

2. If you're seated on the floor, bend both legs and bring them to your left side, so they're folded near your left hip. Place the blankets under your right hip so both sides of your pelvis will be level (see drawing). If you're on a chair, sit sideways with a hand on the top of the chair, keeping your knees apart. If you're on blankets, make sure that the padding is high enough to give you room to turn your abdomen and to elongate your spine.

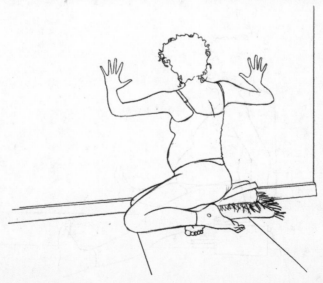

3. Keeping only one buttock cheek on the blankets, inhale and stretch up. Widen your chest, extend your spine, and draw your shoulder blades in against your back.
4. On an exhale, turn your torso to the right. Let your left hand rest on your right thigh and bring your right arm behind you. Or sit facing a wall and bring your hands onto the wall.
5. Breathe here for ten to twenty seconds, or as long as you're comfortable, relaxing into the twist and feeling that the baby is moving with you.
6. Slowly come back to center and repeat on the other side.

Seated wide-angle pose (*upavista konasana*):
1. Sit on folded blankets on the floor with your legs straight in front of you, toes pointing up, back straight against the wall.
2. Stretch your legs out to either side in a straddle split. Reach the feet away from your torso and your knees toward the ground. (Your legs should not be so wide that you can't catch hold of your big toes *comfortably* with your legs still straight.)
3. Sit up straight, making sure you're up on the sit-bones in your buttocks. Place your hands behind you, wrists next to your buttocks, and hands pressing into the floor or onto blocks or books in order to create length in the torso. As you press into the floor, don't let your shoulders creep up around your ears.
4. Breathe here for up to thirty to sixty seconds or for as long as you're comfortable.

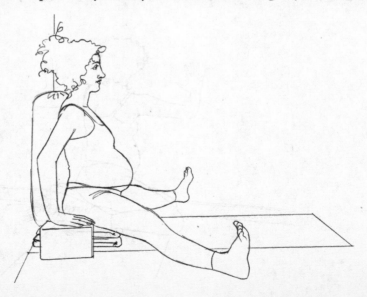

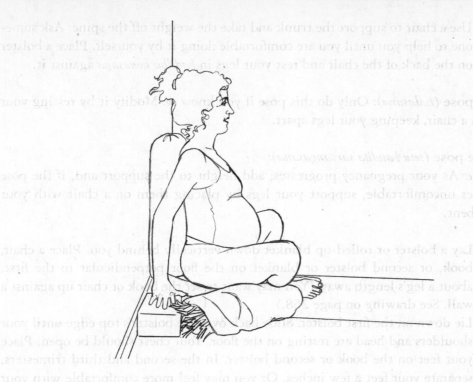

Seated bound angle pose *(baddha konasana):*
1. Sit up on folded blankets and against a wall.
2. Press the soles of the feet together, bringing them in close to your groin. Think about your thighs releasing away from each other. If this is hard on your knees, or if you're not using a belt, you can put a rolled-up towel under each thigh as support.
3. Hold onto the outside of your feet, stretch your spine, and breathe deeply.
4. *In the third trimester,* place a block or book between your feet, which will help widen the pelvis.
5. Hold this pose for a few minutes or as long as you're comfortable.

Shoulder stand *(sarvangasana):* Only do this pose if you already know it, are working with a certified teacher, and feel strong enough to support your spine and torso. Follow these modifications:
1. Place folded blankets under the shoulders so that they remain higher than the head. This relieves pressure on the lungs and abdomen.

2. Use a chair to support the trunk and take the weight off the spine. Ask someone to help you until you are comfortable doing it by yourself. Place a bolster on the back of the chair and rest your legs in *baddha konasana* against it.

Plow pose *(halasana):* Only do this pose if you know it. Modify it by resting your feet on a chair, keeping your legs apart.

Bridge pose *(setu bandha sarvangasana):*
Note: As your pregnancy progresses, add height to the support and, if the pose becomes uncomfortable, support your legs by placing them on a chair with your knees bent.

1. Lay a bolster or rolled-up blanket down vertically behind you. Place a chair, book, or second bolster or blanket on the floor perpendicular to the first, about a leg's length away. (You may want to set the book or chair up against a wall. See drawing on page 268.)
2. Lie down on the first bolster. Slide back over the bolster's top edge until your shoulders and head are resting on the floor. Your chest should be open. Place your feet on the book or second bolster. In the second and third trimesters, separate your feet a few inches. Or you may feel more comfortable with your knees bent and resting on a chair.
3. Rest here for a few minutes.
4. Gently roll onto your left side, place your hands on the floor, and slowly push yourself up.

Legs up the wall *(viparita karani):*
Note: Do not do this pose alone.

1. Place a bolster or rolled blanket a few inches from a wall with a folded sticky mat underneath it. Lay a folded blanket on the floor in front of the bolster if you'll be more comfortable lying on a blanket.
2. Kneel at the end of the bolster and lie down on your left side, so your buttocks are against the wall (stacked one on top of the other). Keep your knees bent. Have your partner help you swivel your trunk over so your back is on the floor and your legs are resting up the wall.
3. Keep your legs apart and your buttocks close to the wall. The bolster or blanket should be supporting your low back and ribs, with your shoulders on the

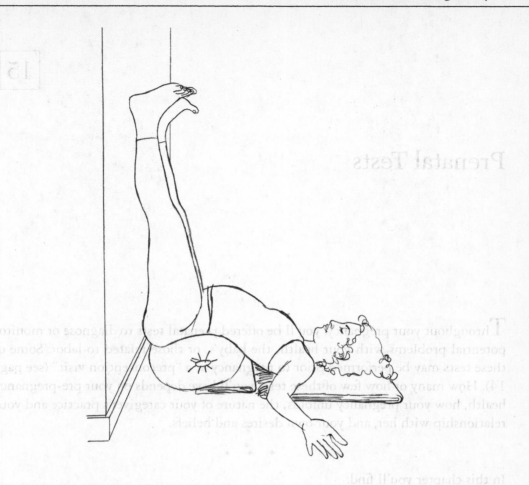

floor. You can also have your legs in *baddha konasana.* Close your eyes and put your hands on your abdomen.

4. Rest here for as long as you're comfortable.

Note: Legs up the wall pose can help relieve varicose veins and swelling in the legs. It's also good for headaches.

Corpse pose *(savasana):*

Follow the instructions and see drawing on page 269 for second and third trimesters.

Note: In appendix 3 you can find two longer, more vigorous sequences: one for the first trimester and a second that's appropriate for the second and third trimesters.

15

Prenatal Tests

Throughout your pregnancy, you'll be offered prenatal tests to diagnose or monitor potential problems with your health, the baby's, or those related to labor. Some of these tests may be performed prior to pregnancy at a "preconception visit" (see page 14). How many or how few of these tests you'll have depends on your pre-pregnancy health, how your pregnancy unfolds, the nature of your caregiver's practice and your relationship with her, and your own desires and beliefs.

◆ ◆ ◆

In this chapter you'll find:

- AFP/Multiple Marker Screen
- Amniocentesis
- Biophysical Profile
- Chorionic Villus Sampling
- Contraction Stress Test
- Cordocentesis
- Doppler Blood Flow Measurement
- Glucose Screen

- Glucose Tolerance Test
- Group B Streptococcus
- Non-stress Test
- Ultra-screen
- Ultrasound—First Trimester
- Ultrasound—Level 2
- Ultrasound—3-D

Alpha-fetoprotein (AFP)/ Multiple Marker Screen (also known as the triple screen or quadruple screen)

• *When it's done:* Fifteen to twenty weeks.

• *Why it's done:* The AFP/multiple marker screen is done primarily to assess the likelihood of certain birth defects, such as a neural tube defect, and chromosomal abnormalities like Down syndrome (trisomy 21) and trisomy 18 (a third eighteenth chromosome).

• *When it's recommended:* I recommend the AFP/multiple marker screen to all my pregnant patients because it's simple to perform and because an unexplained elevated AFP may mean we need to closely monitor a pregnancy. Plus, the new quadruple screen is much more accurate in assessing the risk of Down syndrome (about 90 percent) than the triple screen. That said, the decision whether or not to have the test is left entirely to each patient.

• *What it tests:* The test measures the presence of three (a triple screen) or four (a quadruple screen) hormones in your blood; the latter is a newer test that is fast becoming standard. The triple screen measures: (1)

PRENATAL TESTS IN CHRONOLOGICAL ORDER

First trimester tests

Complete blood count (first prenatal visit)

Genetic testing (first prenatal visit or preconception visit)

Hepatitis B screening (HBV) (first prenatal visit)

Pap test (first prenatal visit or preconception visit)

Rh factor test (first prenatal visit)

Routine blood tests (after first prenatal visit)

Routine urine (dipstick) test (every prenatal visit)

Rubella (German measles) and varicella (chicken pox) immune status (first prenatal visit or preconception visit)

Sexually transmitted disease screening (gonorrhea, chlamydia, syphilis, HIV) (first prenatal visit or preconception visit)

Ultrasound (7–9 weeks)

Chorionic villus sampling (CVS) (10–12 weeks)

Ultra-screen (aka nuchal translucency test) (11–13 weeks)

Second Trimester Tests

Alpha-fetoprotein (AFP)/Multiple marker screening (15–20 weeks)

PRENATAL TESTS IN CHRONOLOGICAL ORDER (continued)

Amniocentesis (15–20 weeks)

Level 2 ultrasound (Anatomy scan) (16–20 weeks)

Glucose screening test (25–28 weeks)

Glucose tolerance test (if necessary; 25–28 weeks)

Third trimester tests

Doppler blood flow measurements

Group B streptococcus

Preterm labor test (Fetal fibronectin)

Non-stress test

Biophysical profile

Contraction stress test (CST, aka Oxytocin challenge test)

Percutaneous umbilical blood sampling (PUBS)

alpha-fetoprotein, or AFP, a protein produced by the baby's liver that crosses into the mother's blood; (2) HCG, or human chorionic gonadotropin, a hormone the placenta produces; and (3) estriol, a type of estrogen produced by the placenta. The quadruple screen measures these three substances plus inhibin, another hormone the placenta produces.

• *How it's done:* A blood sample is drawn, often in your caregiver's office, and sent to a lab for analysis.

• *The results:* It typically takes ten to fourteen days to get results. There's no "positive" or "negative" for this test; the result you'll get will reflect the statistical probability that there's a problem with the baby (1 in 10,000, for example) based on whether AFP levels, along with those of the other hormones, are "elevated," "normal," or "low." The number you get comes from a calculation of hormone levels, gestational age, and maternal age. An AFP/multiple marker screen can *never* say definitively whether a fetus has a chromosomal abnormality or birth defect.

• *Results: elevated AFP:*

AFP/multiple marker screen results could be elevated for a number of reasons:

1. You're carrying twins. (About 10 percent of cases of elevated AFP are explained by twins.)
2. You're further along in your pregnancy than you thought. (There's more AFP if a fetus has been producing it for a longer period of time.)
3. There's an opening in the baby's spinal column (a "neural tube defect") or abdomen.
4. There's a problem with the baby's kidneys. (This is very rare.)

5. It may be unexplained. When this happens, the risk of certain pregnancy-related complications (specifically preterm labor, placental abruption, and stillbirth) goes up to some degree (how much depends on your particular results). Therefore, a caregiver may recommend some combination of third trimester testing (specifically ultrasound, non-stress test, and biophysical profile, see pages 288, 299, and 303 for descriptions of each test) to keep tabs on the baby's health.

- *Elevated AFP: follow-up tests:*
  1. A level 2 ultrasound (see page 303) is usually recommended to rule out a neural tube defect or problem with the kidneys. The ultrasound may also detect anatomical signs (sometimes called "soft markers") of Down syndrome. Finally, if you're having twins, you'll know that immediately from the ultrasound. If you haven't already had a level 2 ultrasound, your caregiver should be able to arrange the test quickly, and its results would be available immediately.
  2. If the ultrasound is inconclusive in determining if there's a neural tube defect (which rarely happens), an amniocentesis will be recommended to diagnose that condition.

- *Results: low AFP:*

A low AFP/multiple marker screen indicates a greater likelihood of Down syndrome or other chromosomal abnormalities. How much greater depends on what your particular results are. No one really knows why low AFP means a baby is more likely to have Down syndrome. All we know is that in general, fetuses with Down syndrome make less AFP and therefore less of it crosses the placenta into the

---

THE "SOFT MARKERS" OF A CHROMOSOMAL ABNORMALITY

The soft markers of a chromosomal abnormality are:

1. Choroid plexus cysts (cysts found in a particular area of the brain; most fetuses with these cysts are normal, however, a small number may have one of several chromosomal abnormalities such as Down syndrome and trisomy 18).
2. Hyperechogenic intracardiac foci (extra calcium in certain heart muscles).
3. Mild pyelectasis (fullness in the kidneys; usually this is not associated with a kidney problem).
4. A thickened nuchal fold (see nuchal translucency test, page 300).

mother's blood. But chromosomally normal fetuses can also make low levels of AFP. In fact, most often when there's a low AFP, the baby is healthy—this is why the test has the reputation of a high "false positive" rate.

• *Low AFP: follow-up tests:*

After a low AFP result, an amniocentesis can provide a definitive answer to the question of a chromosomal abnormality (see page 287). If you don't want to have an amnio, you could first have a level 2 ultrasound to look for the anatomical signs of a chromosomal abnormality and then decide what next steps make sense for you. Keep in mind that the accuracy of the results of a level 2 ultrasound depend to a great degree on the skill and experience of both the sonographer and any specialist who may review the test.

• *The risks:* There are no physical risks to mother or baby associated with the blood test.

• *With multiples:* The test may not be useful in multiple gestations (twins, triplets) and, if used, requires careful interpretation by a specialist.

REAL VOICES

The big news from my second pregnancy is that at five months my AFP tests came back positive for possible neural tube birth defects, which meant we had to see a genetic counselor, have an in-depth ultrasound, and possibly an amnio. At the time I was thirty-two years old. The news kind of freaked us out, and we read up on reasons for "false positives." We went to the genetic counselor, who suggested that the reason the numbers were high was I may be carrying twins. We thought, "No way, I must be further along." Then we went for the ultrasound, and wouldn't you know, there are twins—boys! The ultrasound technician said, "No need for the amnio!" We are shocked, elated, and in disbelief.

Hope, mom of one, pregnant

Q: How common are chromosomal abnormalities?

Dr. Evans: Because of advances in technology, we can find genetic abnormalities earlier than ever before, and that makes this a difficult question to answer. According to the March of Dimes, each year between one in eight hundred and one in a thousand babies are born with Down syndrome, the most common chromosomal abnormality.

Q: What puts you at risk for having a child with a chromosomal abnormality?

Dr. Evans: There are several risk factors for chromosomal abnormalities. First is the mother's age. As a woman gets older, the chance that she'll have a child with a

What Tests Are Right for You?

✦ Deciding whether or not to have prenatal testing to learn about your baby's health is a deeply personal process. When it comes to testing, there are no "right" or "wrong" decisions. Most often, prenatal tests bring reassuring news of a healthy fetus—but not always. Sometimes the results are ambiguous and require more tests; sometimes the results bring the news of a health problem.

When I talk with patients who know they want to have prenatal testing for chromosomal abnormalities or genetic diseases, we begin by discussing how they imagine they'd respond to the results. If the news were to come back that the fetus has Down syndrome, the parents might want to make a decision about whether or not to continue the pregnancy, or they might use the information to help themselves and family members prepare for the birth of a child who will have special needs. Also, there are times when knowing about a problem in advance can help guide prenatal care, and it can affect decisions about where to give birth and which medical professionals should be there. On the other hand many couples feel that if they know for sure that they wouldn't terminate no matter the results of either test, then the extra information isn't worth the risk. But if the need to know outweighs any risks, then testing is the right choice.

In the end, only you and your partner know what's best for your family. After weighing your personal beliefs and emotional needs against the risks to the pregnancy that testing introduces, you'll be able to decide what route to take. Your doctor or midwife can only make recommendations and help you think through the pros and cons of testing.

Finding the balance between using tests to become informed and feeling like your pregnancy hasn't become overly "medicalized" isn't always easy, but it's possible, if you give yourself the time and emotional space to examine your needs and explore the issues testing raises on your own, with your partner, and with your caregiver.

The Risks of a Live-born Child
with Down Syndrome by Maternal Age*

Mother's Age	Risk of Down Syndrome
24	1/1250
26	1/1176
28	1/1053
30	1/952
33	1/625
34	1/500
35	1/384
36	1/303
37	1/227
38	1/175
39	1/137
40	1/106
41	1/81
42	1/64

*Sources: *The Merck Manual,* Home Edition, 1997; ACOG Compendium, 2002.

chromosomal problem goes up—perhaps because her eggs, all of which were formed before she herself was born, have aged, too, and they're more likely either to contain a genetic abnormality or to divide incorrectly after fertilization. (Cell division after fertilization is known as *mitosis*; it's complicated and can go wrong for no reason at all.) Other risk factors include having already had a child with a chromosomal abnormality and having a family history (on either the maternal or paternal side) of chromosomal abnormalities.

The father's age at the time of conception isn't considered a risk factor for a chromosomal abnormality. In other words, a doctor or midwife wouldn't recommend prenatal testing solely because of the father's age. However, some studies have shown an increased likelihood of a spontaneous error in cell division, which would mean a chromosomal abnormality, when the father is fifty-one or older.

Amniocentesis ("amnio")

- *When it's done:* Fifteen to twenty weeks (usually fifteen to eighteen weeks).
- *Why it's done:* Amniocentesis can diagnose chromosomal abnormalities such as Down syndrome (trisomy 21) and trisomy 18; genetic diseases, such as cystic fibrosis and Tay-Sachs; and neural tube defects such as spina bifida. An amnio can also tell you the sex of the baby. Let your caregiver know in advance if you want to know the baby's sex along with your results.
- *Another reason it's done:* If it looks like you might need to deliver earlier than thirty-nine weeks, an amnio can determine if the baby's lungs are mature. (It detects certain substances in the amniotic fluid that are only produced by mature fetal lung cells.) You can typically get these results within a day.
- *When it's recommended:* Amniocentesis is recommended to women who will be thirty-five or older when they deliver and women who have an increased risk of a chromosomal abnormality or genetic disease. Any woman who wants the test may have it done, but check with your insurance company to be sure it's covered if you're younger than the age guidelines.
- *What it tests:* Amniotic fluid, which is basically fetal urine, contains fetal cells. By taking a sample of the fluid, the chromosomes of the fetal cells can be examined and analyzed.
- *How it's done:* Guided by ultrasound, a physician inserts a large needle through the abdomen and into the uterus to draw up about 30 cc of amniotic fluid (about two tablespoons). The site where the needle goes in may or may not be anesthetized, depending on the doctor. The needle may pinch when it enters the abdomen, but the procedure shouldn't hurt any more than getting blood taken. The biggest potential discomfort is that you *may* have a strong contraction when the needle goes into the amniotic sac.
- *The results:* It can take anywhere from seven to fourteen days to get the results, depending on the lab.
- *The risks:* Miscarriage is the biggest risk of an amnio, occurring in anywhere from one in two hundred to one in four hundred cases. Be sure to ask the doctor who will perform the test what her miscarriage rate is; it may be considerably lower—or higher—than these averages. There's also a very small risk (about one in a thousand) of developing an infection from amniocentesis. Very rarely, the needle may bump against the fetus and possibly damage an organ.

After the procedure, you'll be advised to take it easy and not lift anything requiring two hands for twenty-four hours. In the day or two following the test, you may experience some cramping or light spotting.

• *With multiples:* Amniocentesis may be performed in a multiple pregnancy. The team performing the procedure must be absolutely certain of the location of each baby so there is no confusion about which one a sample came from. If the test is being done on identical twins who share a sac, only one sample is necessary (and available).

Call your caregiver: If you start to spot; cramping becomes painful; you develop a thin, watery vaginal discharge; you develop a fever of 100.4 or higher; or your abdomen becomes sore to the touch. Also, both the doctor who performed the procedure and your own caregiver will give you specific guidelines for when to call. Follow them.

Note: If you can, have an amnio done by a team that does at least five or more procedures every week. In some rural areas, that might mean traveling, or it might not be possible. In that case, seek out the *most experienced* doctors you can find. When you call to make an appointment, especially in a group practice, feel free to ask how experienced the doctor who's scheduled to perform your test is.

REAL VOICES
I was the kid who would run naked through waiting rooms when it was time for a shot, so the idea of getting an amnio was extremely unappealing, but I felt like I should do it in my second pregnancy because of my age. It turned out that it was barely a pinprick at all, and I felt a little silly for having been anxious for weeks in advance.

Allison, mom of two

Biophysical Profile (BPP)

• *When it's done:* Third trimester, usually close to, at, or after your due date.

• *Why it's done:* The test is done to evaluate the health of both the baby and the environment inside the uterus.

• *When it's recommended:* A biophysical profile is usually done after a non-stress test (see page 299) or instead of a contraction stress test (see page 294) if a mother has a specific medical or obstetric complication or if there's any reason to think the baby is not thriving in the womb. Specifically, you may have a BPP if:

— You've been diagnosed with intrauterine growth restriction (IUGR), which means the baby appears to be too small. (For more on IUGR, see page 345.)

Preparing for an Amniocentesis

✦ Physically, there's nothing you need to do to prepare for an amniocentesis. But you can try to prepare yourself emotionally. Here are two exercises that I offer to the women I work with before the test—your partner can also do them.

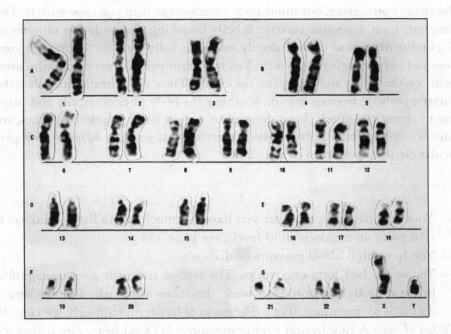

• *Visualization and affirmation:* Begin with belly breathing, inhaling and exhaling slowly and deeply for several minutes to create a relaxed state. (For a full description of belly breathing see page 63.) Use a picture of, or imagine in your mind's eye, a normal set of human chromosomes (see figure above). Focus intently on the image, imagining that this is what your child's chromosomes look like. As you're picturing the chromosomes, communicate your love to your child. After focusing on the image for several minutes, gently shut your eyes and repeat to yourself three times (or as many times as you like): "Everything is as it should be, and I love you." When you have completed the affirmations, once again focus on your breath, slowly open your eyes, and come back to your day. As an alternative to the chromosomes, you can do the same exercise imagining or looking at a picture of a strong, healthy baby.

• *Affirmation:* Begin by practicing belly breathing for a few minutes. Keep your eyes gently closed and repeat: "Everything is as it should be, and I love you." You can say this out loud or to yourself; keep focusing on the affirmation for at least three minutes. When you're done, focus on your breath, and slowly open your eyes.

• *Waiting for the results:* There's no way around the fact that waiting for test results means being worried about them. I don't think it's possible to get rid of the anxiety altogether, but mind-body exercises can help you cope with it. The simplest, most accessible exercise is belly breathing. Set aside five minutes to sit, undisturbed, and breathe deeply into your belly. Breathe in through your nose and out through your mouth. You may want to say in your mind the word "soft" on the inhale and "belly" on the exhale. These deep breaths stimulate the parasympathetic nervous system, soothing the body physiologically and helping to center the mind. (For a description of how belly breathing soothes, see page 63. For several other mind-body exercises that you may adapt to your particular circumstance, turn to page 262.)

— Your caregiver suspects that you have too much or too little amniotic fluid. (For more on amniotic fluid levels, see page 334.)
— You have high blood pressure or diabetes.
— You've reached forty-one weeks. The risk of stillbirth goes up significantly halfway through the forty-first week; this is one reason why accurate pregnancy dating is so important. (For a discussion of late-term stillbirth, see page 383.)

• *What it tests:* A biophysical profile measures: (1) fetal heart rate (using a non-stress test; see page 299); (2) fetal breathing movements (with ultrasound); (3) fetal movement (with ultrasound); (4) fetal muscle tone (with ultrasound); and (5) volume of amniotic fluid (with ultrasound).

• *How it's done:* First you have a non-stress test (see page 299), and then you have an ultrasound to measure the amniotic fluid and the baby's muscle tone and movements. How long the test takes depends on how active the baby is. If the baby's asleep, you'll probably have to wait about twenty minutes for the baby to wake up.

• *The results:* Every provider scores biophysical profiles differently. Some use all five variables; others follow an abbreviated scoring system using only the results of the non-stress test and the amniotic fluid volume. If your practitioner uses all five variables, then each one is assigned a score of 0 to 2. An overall score of 8 to 10 is considered normal, 6 to 8 is borderline, and below 6 is cause for concern.

Regardless of how it's scored, you should get your results at the time of the test. When you do, ask for a detailed explanation of your score, what was measured, and the score's implications. This may be the only time you have a BPP, or your caregiver may ask you to repeat it once, twice, or even three times a week until you give birth. Another possibility is your caregiver may recommend inducing labor based on the results of the test.

- *The risks:* There are no physical risks to mother or baby from this test.
- *With multiples:* This test may be performed with multiples.

Chorionic Villus Sampling (CVS)

- *When it's done:* Ten to twelve weeks.
- *Why it's done:* CVS can detect genetic diseases, such as Tay-Sachs, and chromosomal abnormalities, such as Down syndrome and trisomy 18. Because it's done much earlier than amniocentesis, it can alleviate anxiety sooner, and if termination is an option with a positive result, the termination is easier this early in pregnancy. The test can also tell you the sex of the baby, though it's never performed for this reason alone. Let your caregiver know before getting your results if you want to be told the baby's sex. CVS doesn't diagnose neural tube defects.
- *When it's recommended:* I recommend CVS when the risk of a chromosomal abnormality or genetic disease (see page 17) is greater than the risks associated with the test (see page 293). Or if you feel that your need to know about the health of the baby earlier in the pregnancy outweighs the risks of the test, then it's worthwhile to consider it seriously.
- *What it tests:* CVS collects and analyzes samples of chorionic villi—tiny, finger-like projections from the placenta. Because the placenta develops from the fertilized egg, its cells have the same chromosomes as the baby, meaning that a chromosomal abnormality or genetic condition that affects the child will appear in the cells of the villi.
- *How it's done:* The tissue is collected from the placenta two different ways—either through the vagina or abdomen.

In a *transvaginal* procedure, you lie back, usually with your legs in stirrups, while a doctor, guided by ultrasound, threads a catheter through your vagina, cervix, and up to the placenta, from which the samples are taken.

For a *transabdominal* procedure, a site on the abdomen is anesthetized and a needle is inserted. Using ultrasound, a doctor guides the needle to the placenta and draws out a tissue sample. Either way, it may take a few minutes to collect the tissue. The

Choosing a Test: Amnio or CVS?

✦ When a pregnant woman or couple is certain about prenatal chromosomal testing, we'll discuss the risks involved with amniocentesis and CVS. First, we talk about the local medical practices that perform both tests and look at their miscarriage rates. (In some parts of the country, there may not be a practice that regularly performs CVS, and this alone might answer the question of which test is most appropriate.) Second, we evaluate the risks a particular couple faces of a serious complication that CVS would reveal (e.g., Tay-Sachs or a chromosomal abnormality).

As a starting point for this discussion, we look at the risk of a problem and compare it to the risk of miscarriage from the procedure. If, for example, both parents are carriers of a recessive gene for a serious disease like Tay-Sachs (see page 17), the risk that the child will have the disease is one in four. If one parent is the carrier of a dominant gene for a serious disease (see page 17), the risk to the child is one in two. In either instance, CVS makes sense because the risk of disease is greater than the risk of miscarriage from the procedure.

This same process of evaluating the risk level can be used if you're older, have a family history of chromosomal abnormalities, or if you've already had a child with chromosomal abnormalities. If, however, there's nothing in your medical history that increases the risk of Down syndrome or another genetic disease, then it's likely that the risk of miscarriage from CVS is greater than the risk of a problem. When this is the situation, I typically recommend choosing amniocentesis because it's the safer route.

Ultimately, though, statistics can't measure the need for reassurance. If you and your partner want or need to know the health status of the fetus in the first trimester, and for you the risks are justified, then CVS makes sense. On the flip side, if you want the information and reassurance that testing brings but you want to keep the risks low, then amnio may be the better choice.

Note: The ultra-screen (aka nuchal translucency test) is a new, non-invasive, risk-free first-trimester test for certain chromosomal abnormalities. Combining special ultrasound and bloodwork, it can be extremely accurate (around 90 percent) in ruling out chromosomal abnormalities. Recently approved by the FDA, it's rapidly becoming widely available. If you're interested in this test, ask your doctor or midwife about availability in your area. (See "Ultra-screen," page 300, for a description of the test.)

whole procedure may take up to an hour to complete.

• *The results:* It can take one to two weeks to get results, depending on the lab. Very rarely, an amnio will be recommended as a follow-up.

• *The risks:* The miscarriage rate with CVS is about one in a hundred to one in two hundred, although your risk depends entirely on the doctor performing the procedure (who may have a much lower miscarriage rate than the national average). Infection, while rarer than miscarriage, is another serious risk. Occasionally, a woman may experience light bleeding, spotting, or cramping following the procedure. Also, if a woman is Rh-negative, amniocentesis is preferred. (For more on being Rh negative, see page 93.)

• *With multiples:* CVS may be used with multiples; an experienced practitioner should do the procedure because there's a small risk that the tissue from one baby will contaminate the tissue from another. Very rarely (about 1 percent of the time), it's possible to collect only one sample. The team doing the test must be absolutely certain of where each baby is so there is no confusion about which one a sample came from. (If the test is being done on identicals, only one tissue sample is necessary since identical twins have identical genes.)

Call your caregiver: Both the doctor who performed the test and your caregiver will have guidelines for when to contact them. Follow them. Generally speaking, after the procedure you should call if you develop a fever; you have worsening pain; bleeding and cramping become more severe; or bleeding seems at all unusual.

Note: It's extremely important that an experienced team performs this delicate procedure. If you plan to have the test, seek out a doctor or practice that does it *often,* even exclusively. When you make an appointment, feel free to ask about how experienced individual doctors are, as well as their miscarriage rates. If you live in a

---

QUESTIONS TO ASK ABOUT PRENATAL TESTS

• Why do you recommend this test for me?
• What are the risks associated with the test? Are there any alternative tests?
• Given my medical history, family history, and age, can you tell me, approximately, my risk for having a child with a chromosomal abnormality or genetic disease?
• Who would you recommend perform the test? How regularly do you work with this doctor or practice?
• How long do results typically take to come through from this particular group and the lab they work with? Will you call with the results?
• Are the results of this test ever confusing or ambiguous? If it turns out mine are, what happens next?

rural area, I would recommend traveling to the nearest major medical center to have the test.

Contraction Stress Test (CST)
(also known as an oxytocin challenge test)

This test is relatively uncommon. It's used to assess how well the baby will respond to the stress of labor by measuring her heart rate during contractions. It's recommended when a doctor or midwife is concerned enough about the baby's well-being to consider an early delivery either by induction or C-section.

• *When it's done:* During the third trimester, usually close to your due date.

• *Why it's done:* This test may be done instead of a biophysical profile to follow up a non-stress test that had ambiguous results.

• *When it's recommended:* This test is prescribed only in high-risk situations where a decision has to be made immediately about whether a baby needs to be delivered by Cesarean section or can tolerate the trial of labor. An example would be if the fetus is small (see IUGR on page 345) and the non-stress test results are ambiguous. A CST would give a doctor more information about the best way to approach delivery.

• *What it tests:* A CST assesses the baby's heart rate in response to contractions.

• *How it's done:* First you empty your bladder, then you lie on your left side and two monitors are hooked up to your abdomen. One monitor (an ultrasound Doppler transducer) follows the baby's heart rate while the other (a tocodynamometer) follows contractions. (You'll probably be asked not to eat for eight hours before the test just in case contractions progress, the baby shows signs of distress, and you need an emergency C-section.) To initiate contractions, which mimic those of early labor, you either receive a dose of a synthetic form of the hormone oxytocin (aka Pitocin, a drug that brings on contractions) or you're asked to stimulate your nipples (which triggers the release of oxytocin). You're tested until you have at least three forty-five-second-long contractions within ten minutes. These contractions should be relatively mild. (Women sometimes describe them as being like menstrual cramps.) You'll stay in the test room until all contractions have stopped, which may take a couple of hours.

• *The results:* If the baby's heart rate doesn't decrease immediately after the three contractions, the result is considered negative, which means that the baby is fine and should respond well during labor. If the baby's heart rate decreases after all three contractions, it's considered a positive result, which means that the baby *may* be under stress. If this happens, you may be asked to deliver relatively soon (how soon depends on your caregiver and the test results), possibly by Cesarean section. There isn't a lot of agreement about what to do when the baby's heart rate slows after one or two (but not all three) contractions; whether or not you'll be asked to repeat the test or consider being induced will depend on your own situation as well as your caregiver's clinical tendencies and experience. Keep in mind that a CST can be a little difficult to interpret, so whatever the result, feel free to ask a lot of questions about your test and your options.

Note: Second opinions aren't practical or all that common in this situation. That said, if you're *ever* uncomfortable with your treatment, you can pursue a second opinion.

- *The risks:* There is a small chance that labor will begin following a CST.
- *With multiples:* This test may be performed with multiples.
- *Follow-up options:* If the test results are normal, you may be asked to have another CST or biophysical profile to be sure the baby continues to thrive in the uterus. If the test results are positive or ambiguous, your doctor may recommend another CST, biophysical profile, or childbirth through induced labor or a Cesarean section.

Cordocentesis (also known as percutaneous umbilical blood sampling, or PUBS)

- *When it's done:* At any time after eighteen weeks.
- *Why it's done:* This test, which is done only in extremely high-risk situations, is used when an actual fetal blood sample is needed; neither amniocentesis nor CVS collects fetal blood.
- *When it's recommended:* Fetal blood would be necessary to see if a fetus has been affected by a serious infection, such as toxoplasmosis or German measles (rubella). Other examples include checking for fetal anemia in the case of unusual immune disorders or Rh incompatibility.
- *What it tests:* Fetal blood is analyzed for the presence of specific substances or signs of infection.
- *How it's done:* Using ultrasound, a needle is put into the abdomen and through the uterus, until it reaches the umbilical cord, from which a blood sample is drawn.
- *The results:* Results are usually available within seventy-two hours.
- *The risks:* The miscarriage rate from this procedure depends to a large degree on who's performing it. In general, it's one to two in a hundred. The mother is also at risk for infection, premature rupture of the membranes, and an emergency C-section.

Doppler Blood Flow Measurement

- *When it's done:* Typically in the third trimester.
- *Why it's done:* This test measures blood flow through the placenta to the fetus. The test is done when there's a reason to worry about either how the fetus is doing or how well the placenta is working. If the blood flow is strong, the fetus is getting enough oxygen and food; if it's weaker, the level of nourishment the fetus is getting may be compromised.
- *When it's recommended:* This test might be done if, for example, the fetus appears small in an ultrasound (the fetus may have IUGR, see page 345), or after a biophysical profile or non-stress test with results that were not reassuring (see pages 288 and 299), or if the mother has preeclampsia (see page 357), placenta previa (see page 350), or chronic hypertension.
- *What it tests:* The Doppler measures the rate of blood flow through a blood vessel. It can measure blood flow through the umbilical veins and arteries as well as in the fetus's heart and brain. If the blood flow is lower than expected, it may mean the fetus isn't getting enough blood, nutrients, or oxygen.
- *How it's done:* A doctor (usually a perinatologist) performs this test by passing the transducer (or wand) of a sophisticated ultrasound machine over the mother's abdomen.
- *The results:* The results should be available immediately.
- *The risks:* There are no risks to mother or baby from this test.

Glucose Screen

- *When it's done:* Twenty-four to twenty-eight weeks.
- *Why it's done:* This test is a standard element of prenatal care. It tests the possibility of gestational diabetes. When a glucose screen is positive, a follow-up test called a glucose tolerance test is done to determine if you have gestational diabetes. (See "Glucose Tolerance Test," page 297; for more on gestational diabetes, see page 340.)
- *When it's recommended:* Every pregnant woman should have this test. Even though gestational diabetes occurs in only about 5 percent of pregnancies and it can have no symptoms, it can have serious consequences for both mother and baby if it's not detected and controlled—and it's easily controlled once diagnosed.
- *What it tests:* Your blood sugar levels.
- *How it's done:* You drink a mixture called *Glucola,* which contains 50 grams of

glucose (sugar) in 10 ounces of liquid. After about an hour, during which you'll be asked not to eat or drink, a blood sample is drawn and sent to a lab.

• *The results:* Test results are usually available within a day or two, depending on the lab. If your blood sugar comes back at or above 140 (some providers use 130 or 135 as a cutoff), the results are considered abnormal and your provider will recommend a glucose tolerance test. Don't assume you have gestational diabetes if your blood sugar levels are elevated; only around 15 percent of women who test positive in the glucose screen are found to have gestational diabetes after a full glucose tolerance test.

ARE YOU AT RISK FOR GESTATIONAL DIABETES?

Certain women have a higher risk of developing gestational diabetes, and they may be screened as early as twelve weeks. The risk factors are:

• A previous case of gestational diabetes
• A family history of diabetes
• Having already given birth to a very large baby (bigger than 8.8 pounds, or 4,000 grams)
• A body mass index (BMI) over 29, which indicates obesity. (To determine your BMI, see appendix 4.)

• *The risks:* There's no risk to the mother or the baby from a glucose screen.
• *With multiples:* The test is the same.

Glucose Tolerance Test

• *When it's done:* Following an abnormal glucose screen (ideally before or around the twenty-eight-week mark).

• *Why it's done:* To diagnose gestational diabetes, a common, controllable pregnancy complication. (For more about gestational diabetes, see page 340.)

• *When it's recommended:* The test is recommended if a glucose screening test shows you have elevated blood sugar.

• *What it tests:* The test measures blood sugar levels. If they're high, it means that because of the hormonal changes of pregnancy, insulin, a hormone produced by the pancreas, isn't effective enough in turning sugar into fuel, leaving you with extra sugar in your blood.

• *How it's done:* The test is typically done in the morning. You need to fast—no food or drink except water—for at least eight hours before. The test has three steps: (1) You have a blood test to measure your blood sugar levels after fasting; (2) you drink a special liquid with 100 grams of glucose (This may make you queasy. Some women can't tolerate the sweet drink at all, in which case you'll be asked to try again, either that morning or at a different time.); (3) you have a blood test every hour for three hours after finishing the drink.

• *The results:* Results take two to three days, depending on the lab. Criteria for blood sugar levels vary. Some providers use lower levels to diagnose gestational diabetes. In my practice, if your initial fasting blood sugar is 105 or above, or if two out of the three other blood tests are above the cutoff (190 at one hour, 165 at two hours, 145 at three hours), I consider the results positive for gestational diabetes.

• *The risks:* There are no long-term risks to mother or baby from this test. Very rarely, a woman might throw up or have a hypoglycemic (low blood sugar) reaction during which she might feel very dizzy or faint.

• *With multiples:* The test is the same.

Group B Streptococcus (GBS)

• *When it's done:* Thirty-five to thirty-eight weeks.

• *Why it's done:* GBS bacteria sometimes live in the vagina and rectum. Almost 20 percent of all women of childbearing age have these bacteria in their ano-genital tract during pregnancy. GBS is usually harmless in adults, but it can be dangerous to a newborn if it's transmitted during childbirth.

• *When it's recommended:* GBS screening is recommended for all pregnant women. A newborn exposed to GBS could develop pneumonia, sepsis (blood infection), or meningitis (inflammation of the brain that can cause long-term damage to hearing, vision, and learning ability, and, in about 5 percent of cases, death).

• *What it tests:* Cells taken from the vagina and rectum.

• *How it's done:* Your caregiver will use a swab to collect a sample of cells from your vagina and rectum. This is not unlike a Pap smear.

• *The results:* The sample will be sent to a lab and results should come back within five days. If you test positive for GBS, you'll be treated with antibiotics (administered through an IV drip) during labor. (This shouldn't interfere with a drug-free birth plan.)

• *The risks:* There are no risks to mother or baby from this test.

• *With multiples:* The test is the same.

Note: When I prescribe antibiotics to a pregnant woman for GBS, I always recommend she take a probiotic, such as lactobacillus (aka acidophilus), to insure she has "good bacteria" in her digestive tract. When I help deliver a baby to a mom who's been on antibiotics, I recommend the mom dip her pinkie in a little lactobacillus and give it to her child to help support the baby's digestive tract as well.

Non-stress Test

• *When it's done:* Typically from thirty-five weeks forward, although it may be earlier in certain cases.

• *Why it's done:* The test is given to monitor the baby's heart rate and check his overall condition if your doctor or midwife is concerned about how well the baby is doing. It's also done if a baby is known to have a physical or genetic problem.

• *When it's recommended:* A caregiver may suggest a non-stress test if:
  – You've reached forty-one weeks or more, at which point the risk of stillbirth goes up significantly.
  – The baby seems less active than usual.
  – You've been diagnosed with intrauterine growth restriction (IUGR), which means that the baby appears to be too small. (For more information, see page 345.)
  – There appears to be too much or too little amniotic fluid. (For more information, see page 334.)
  – You have high blood pressure or diabetes.
  – You're in a higher risk category for a late loss because of an unexplained elevated AFP or because you've suffered a stillbirth in the past.
  – You're having preterm contractions or labor.
  – You're Rh negative or there's another substance in your blood cells that could trigger an allergic reaction (immune response) that could destroy fetal tissue. (This is rare.)

• *What it tests:* The test measures the baby's heart rate while active and at rest. If within a twenty-minute period the baby's heart rate accelerates at least twice for fifteen seconds, the result is considered "reactive," which means the baby's condition is considered relatively stable for the next three to seven days. (Whether it's three days or longer depends on the mother's and the baby's condition.)

• *How it's done:* After going to the bathroom, you lie back, usually on your left side, and a technician hooks up two monitors to your abdomen: one (an ultrasound Doppler transducer) monitors the baby's movements and heartbeat; the other (a tocodynamometer) monitors any contractions you may have. The test could last anywhere from ten minutes to an hour, depending on the baby's sleep patterns.

• *The results:* You should have the results at the time of the test. About 85 percent of the time, babies are reactive immediately; 15 percent of the time, they're not. The great majority of nonreactive babies are asleep. You may have to continue monitoring for about twenty minutes, until the baby wakes up, or you may be asked to drink orange juice or another sweet drink to help stimulate the baby. (There's actually no scientific evidence that drinking orange juice stimulates the baby, but it can't hurt and may help.) If your caregiver is concerned about the results, she may order a biophysical profile or contraction stress test as a follow-up (see pages 288 and 299). Sometimes, a caregiver will recommend repeating a non-stress test at regular intervals until childbirth, even when the first test has a normal result.

• *The risks:* There are no physical risks from this test to the mother or the baby.

• *With multiples:* This test may be performed in a multiple pregnancy.

REAL VOICES

Near the end of my pregnancy, they started doing non-stress tests. I wasn't really jazzed about them because one of my daughters—I was pregnant with twin girls—really hated them. She'd be very calm, and as soon as that thing went on she'd start jumping around like a football player. She'd try to duck the monitors all the time and they kept repositioning them. But my midwife and doctor really wanted them, so . . .

Rochelle, mom of three

Ultra-screen
(also known as nuchal translucency test or early screen)

• *When it's done:* Eleven to thirteen weeks.

• *Why it's done:* This is a relatively new, noninvasive method for assessing the risk of Down syndrome and other chromosomal abnormalities, specifically trisomy 18, trisomy 13, triploidy (three copies of every chromosome), and Turner's syndrome.

• *When it's recommended:* This screen is a good choice for anyone concerned about a chromosomal abnormality. Unlike amnio and CVS, it poses no risks to the baby or pregnancy. Unlike an AFP/multiple marker screen, it can be done in the first trimester. If the results are questionable, CVS and amnio are both still options.

• *What it tests:* The test has two parts: an ultrasound exam and a blood test. The ultrasound measures the thickness of a layer of skin on the back of the baby's neck (known as the nuchal fold). If the fold is more than 3 mm, it suggests the *possibility* of a chromosomal abnormality.

The blood test measures free beta HCG, a hormone produced by the placenta, and pregnancy-associated plasma protein (PAPP).

Note: You may have the ultrasound screening without the blood test.

• *How it's done:* A doctor or ultrasound technician will perform a transabdominal ultrasound exam, and blood may be drawn at that time.

• *The results:* How long the results take depends on when the bloodwork was done. If the bloodwork is done in advance, you should get the results at the time of the test. If the bloodwork is done the day of the test, it can take up to ten days to get the complete results, depending on the lab. However, you'll have some idea of your situation after the ultrasound. You'll get a number, like one in four thousand, that reflects the statistical probability of a chromosomal abnormality. The number is calculated by comparing risk factors from personal and family history with the results of the bloodwork. The test is considered about 90 percent accurate.

• *The risks:* There are no physical risks to mother or baby associated with either the ultrasound or the blood test.

• *With multiples:* The test is used with multiples, but the bloodwork might not be used. Check with your provider to find out whether the test is applicable.

Note: Ultra-screen is a new procedure. Ask your doctor or midwife where it's performed in your area.

REAL VOICES
A friend of mine in New Mexico who just had a baby referred me to a test called the ultra-screen, which I hadn't heard of before. I decided to do that instead of an amnio because it felt less invasive to me. It was great. I did the blood test at home and sent it in, and then we went to a hospital where I had the high-resolution ultrasound. After the test, we were there for about five minutes and they came back and gave us the results; they'd run the sonogram on the computer and matched it with the bloodwork. It came back with really good results in terms of my risk of Down syndrome and trisomy 18 and then we just had the regular ultrasound at nineteen weeks.

Michelle, mom of one, pregnant

Testing for Preterm Labor*

✦ Preterm, or premature, labor means labor that begins anytime before the thirty-seventh week of pregnancy. No one knows exactly why a woman goes into labor at a particular time, but the body does give subtle signals that labor may begin within a specific time frame. If you're having preterm contractions or are at risk for preterm labor, the following tests may be performed:

• *Fetal fibronectin (FFN):* If you've had a lot of uterine activity (such as contractions) or if the pregnancy membranes have ruptured (even slightly), a protein called fetal fibronectin leaks into the vagina. If you're at risk for preterm labor, your caregiver will test for fetal fibronectin by swabbing the cervix, which is just like having a Pap smear. Results can come back in one hour or twenty-four hours, depending on the lab. If the test is negative, it's extremely unlikely that you'll go into labor during the next two weeks. Two weeks after the initial test, your caregiver may want to repeat it. If the test is positive, your caregiver will want to do something to try to prevent preterm labor from starting. For example, you may be put on bed rest and asked to stay well hydrated; you may be given medications to stop contractions (for example, terbutaline or magnesium sulfate); you may need to have an amnio to see if the baby's lungs are mature and be given medications to mature the baby's lungs if necessary; or you may be hospitalized. The test is typically done between weeks 24 and 34.

• *Bacterial vaginosis:* The presence of an assortment of specific bacteria in the vagina may increase the likelihood that either preterm labor will begin or the membranes will rupture. A simple cervical swab, like a Pap smear, can be analyzed for the bacteria. If it's there, you can be treated with antibiotics, either orally or in a vaginal suppository.

• *Cervical length:* Performed anywhere from sixteen to thirty-two weeks (depending on the mother's situation), this test involves an ultrasound probe being placed in the vagina to measure the length of the cervix. If the cervix is "short" (less than 2.5 cm), the risk of preterm delivery is higher. Treatment in this situation varies—bed rest or a cervical stitch (cerclage) may be appropriate—and depends entirely on the individual situation.

*For a discussion of preterm labor and its symptoms, see page 363.

Ultrasound—First Trimester

- *When it's done:* Five and a half to twelve weeks.
- *Why it's done:* The image (sonogram) generated by an ultrasound in the first trimester can confirm the health of a pregnancy by detecting a fetal heartbeat—usually at around seven weeks, but sometimes as early as five or six weeks. It's also used to see if you're carrying twins or to help determine your due date.

Between weeks 7 and 13, a fetus grows at a very predictable rate. By using ultrasound to measure the head-to-rump length of a fetus, a caregiver can estimate the fetus's gestational age to within a few days. This is particularly helpful for women with irregular periods or those who are unsure of when they conceived.

- *When it's recommended:* Early ultrasounds are standard for women with high-risk pregnancies, and for those who become pregnant after fertility treatments. Some, but not all, practices recommend early ultrasounds for all of their patients.
- *How it's done:* Ultrasounds done before week 9 are usually transvaginal. A doctor or technician will gently insert into the vagina a long, wandlike probe that emits sound waves that bounce off the surfaces of the organs. An image, known as a sonogram, then appears on a TV-like screen.
- *The results:* You will most likely get all the information during the office visit. No lab work is involved with the test.
- *The risks:* Ultrasounds performed early in pregnancy have been studied extensively, and there are no risks associated with them. Ultrasound doesn't involve X-ray technology.

Note: An ultrasound may be performed earlier than seven to nine weeks to rule out an ectopic pregnancy. Also, if you have any spotting or bleeding at any point in your pregnancy, but especially during the first trimester, you may have an ultrasound to make sure that you aren't miscarrying.

Ultrasound—Level 2
(also known as "anatomy scan" or "targeted ultrasound")

- *When it's done:* Sixteen to twenty weeks.
- *Why it's done:* An anatomy scan gives a picture of the general health of the fetus and pregnancy. It carefully evaluates the fetus's major organs to confirm they've

---

When Images Aren't Clear

✦ Ultrasound technology relies on an image that may be more or less clear, depending on the position of the baby as well as the transmission of the sound waves. Sometimes an ultrasound *suggests* a problem (for example, if there's a shadow somewhere). In a case like this, your caregiver may recommend further tests to shed light on the potential problem. Ask your caregiver any questions you want and do whatever research you can. For example, ask what your caregiver suspects after looking at the sonogram, why, what kind of follow-up testing is recommended, what the statistics show, and what the treatment plan might be if there is a problem.

---

formed properly. The test is also used to measure the level of amniotic fluid and locate the placenta. (A placenta that's covering the cervix is known as a "placenta previa." For more on this, see page 350.) During the ultrasound exam, your cervix will be checked to make sure it isn't opening prematurely.

In addition to checking the fetus's anatomy, the doctor or technician will look for the "soft markers," or anatomical signs of a chromosomal abnormality (see page 283). If you didn't have an ultrasound in the first trimester, the anatomy scan will show if you're carrying multiples, and if your due date is uncertain, it can date the pregnancy to within five to ten days.

REAL VOICES

In my second pregnancy, I had the triple screen, which was fine. At around week 18, I went in for the ultrasound. It's a happy time because I was going to find out what sex the baby was and see her for the first time, and it would be great. So we went in, and the nurse does the ultrasound. At first she was chatty, then not so chatty—there was something a little off about it. Then the doctor came in, and he did the ultrasound, and he said, "Okay, I want to tell you that we've found something on the membrane around the tissue of her brain—a little cyst." I thought, "Okay, a cyst. Interesting." And he said, "In and of itself, it's nothing to worry about—it'll go away. But it *is* an indicator for something called trisomy 18." Oh, we asked, what's that? "It's three number eighteen chromosomes (instead of two)," he said, "and the cyst is a one percent indicator of this, and you can decide whether or not you want to have an amnio and find out for sure if she has this, but I'd like you to meet with the genetic counselor." So, while we were waiting to meet with the genetic counselor, I said to my husband, "Why are we going to risk a miscarriage if it's a one percent chance—why would we do that?" and he agreed.

Then we went in to talk to the genetic counselor. She started talking, and remember those ads when the guy's sitting in the chair and his head is thrown back by a big gust? That's what I felt like. She describes trisomy 18 and said basically that the baby would live maybe a week after the birth and that she would have horrible internal and external deformities. And I said, "Well, wouldn't you know as the baby's developing? I mean, we don't have to make a decision right now?" She said, "No. Sometimes it's not until week thirty or thirty-one that you would know." I kept looking for an out. But there wasn't one. So we decided to have an amnio, which I was able to have that day. I just wanted to know for sure what we were dealing with and then be able to make a decision with all the information. After the amnio it was really a waiting game—a week of worries and prayer and trying to focus on my older daughter. And all the time, I can feel the baby. She's moving around, and I know it's a girl and I have a name for her, and I couldn't in my head say, "If she has this, then I will have an abortion." I couldn't do that. It was my daughter now. It was a really hard, hard week. For my husband, it was completely the opposite. He said, "Why would you go through this? Why would you do this to yourself, to the family?" But he wasn't as emotionally attached to her. Thankfully it all came out okay, and she was and is perfectly healthy. But it was a hard, hard week.

Suzanne, mom of two

Finally, you can learn the baby's sex during an ultrasound; the accuracy of this depends on the baby's position during the scan. Let your caregiver and the technician know beforehand if you want to find out the baby's sex.

- *When it's recommended:* Most practitioners consider it a standard test in every pregnancy.
- *How it's done:* Because the anatomy scan is so thorough, it can take up to an hour to perform. Gel will be put on your abdomen and a doctor or technician will run a transducer over your abdomen. The transducer will emit sound waves that bounce off the baby's organs, and an image (a sonogram) will appear on the screen of the ultrasound machine. You may be asked to drink fluids before the exam because a full bladder can give a better image.
- *With multiples:* The test is the same with multiples but will take longer to perform.

Is a "First Look" Safe? Commercial Use of 3-D Ultrasound

✦ In medical settings, 3-D ultrasounds are used to investigate potential problems that were either found during "regular" (2-dimensional) ultrasound exams or suspected based on a woman's symptoms and other test results. But 3-D and 4-D ultrasounds are now also given at independent shops, to give you snapshots and "keepsake" videos from the womb. While the pictures from these advanced ultrasounds are truly extraordinary, their safety is unknown. The question becomes: Is it worth the risk?

Ultrasound transmits energy waves into the womb. When a doctor or trained technician uses the technology in a medical setting, he follows FDA regulations, using the machines for limited periods of time at relatively low settings. In a store that sells 3-D prenatal imaging, the people providing the service (or taking the pictures) may not have any specialized training or any supervision by a medical professional. And in a nonmedical setting, the 3-D and 4-D machines can be used at higher energy levels for as long as the "technician" needs to get the images she wants—even if it takes an hour.

Then there are the emotional risks. For example, if you see a problem, or what you think might be a problem, with your baby when you're in a 3-D/4-D ultrasound store, there won't be a medical professional on hand with whom you can discuss what you've seen.

In the end, only you can decide if the unknown safety risks posed by commercial 3-D imaging are worth the pictures that you get. (The FDA says they aren't.) My own recommendation to parents who really want to experience 3-D/4-D technology is to do so at a medical center that uses 3-D ultrasound machines for diagnostic purposes. While your insurance may not cover it (you'd pay out-of-pocket at the mall, too), you can at least rest assured that the technology is being administered by a trained professional and set according to the latest and best safety standards.

• *The results:* The test doesn't involve labwork, so you should get all the information during the office visit. If the ultrasound is done somewhere outside of your doctor or midwife's office, you may have to wait for your caregiver to see the images before you learn all the results.

• *The risks:* There are no known risks from an ultrasound. It doesn't involve any X-ray technology.

Note: An ultrasound may be recommended at any time in your pregnancy when it's important to get detailed information about the fetus. For example, ultrasound will be used during an amniocentesis or CVS. If an initial level 2 ultrasound shows that the placenta is relatively close to the cervix, you'll have follow-up ultrasounds to see if the position changes as your pregnancy progresses. (For more, see "Placenta Previa" on page 350.) You may have an ultrasound to confirm a suspicion that the baby is breech (your caregiver may suspect this after examining your abdomen), and likewise the technology may be used if you have a procedure to turn a breech baby (the most common of these is known as "external version," see page 432). For example, in our office, we try to turn breech babies through a combination of exercise and Chinese medicine (see page 431). Throughout the treatment, we monitor the baby's position with ultrasound. Rarely, an ultrasound exam is given during labor, when a caregiver needs some extra information.

Ultrasound—3-D

• *When it's done:* A 3-D ultrasound may be performed at any point in a pregnancy.
• *Why it's done:* When a serious complication, such as spina bifida or a specific anatomical abnormality, is suspected based on a level 2 ultrasound, a 3-D ultrasound can give a very clear picture of the baby and offer parents more information about their situation and options. It's also used when some sort of abnormality is detected on the surface of the fetus's body during an anatomy scan.
• *How it's done:* A 3-D ultrasound is done just like a regular ultrasound.
• *The results:* You should get the results at the time of the test.
• *The risks:* There are no physical risks to the mother or baby from a 3-D ultrasound. Like a regular ultrasound, it doesn't involve X-ray technology.
• *With multiples:* The test is the same.

Note: The medical material in this chapter was reviewed by Dr. Cynthia Chazotte, professor of clinical obstetrics and gynecology and women's health and director of obstetrics and perinatology, Weiler Hospital of the Albert Einstein College of Medicine/Montefiore Medical Center.

16

Living and Working

When you're pregnant, you may find yourself wondering if everyday activities like having your hair done or gardening are safe for you and your baby. Here I review a range of everyday safety-related questions that might come up over the course of a pregnancy. I also provide an overview of pregnant women's rights in the workplace.

✦ ✦ ✦

In this chapter you'll find:

- Sex and Pregnancy
- Beauty and Spa Treatments
  - Body treatments: scrubs and wraps
  - Color processing hair
  - Facials
  - Hair removal: waxing and electrolysis
  - Manicures and pedicures
  - Massage
- Traveling While Pregnant
  - Air travel
  - Road travel
- Environmental Hazards
  - New carpets, new furniture, paints, varnishes, and stored fuels

- Cats/toxoplasmosis
- Cleaning products
- Computers
- Lead
- Microwave ovens
- Mold
- Pesticides
- Pressure-treated wood
- Workplace concerns
• Workplace Rights
- Hiring and promotions
- Pregnancy and maternity leave
- Health insurance
- Fringe benefits

Sex and Pregnancy

- *Safety:* In most pregnancies, it's perfectly safe to enjoy a rich and varied sex life. Vaginal, oral, and anal sex are all safe (though anal sex may be more uncomfortable as your pregnancy progresses), as is stimulation from a vibrator. During oral sex, your partner should not blow into your vagina—it can send air into the blood, create an embolism (air bubble), and put you and the baby at serious risk. (There are a few case histories in the medical literature where women actually died from this.) After an orgasm, you may have contractions for around ten to fifteen minutes; once the contractions stop, you may notice a change in your baby's movement. Some babies will respond to the contractions by resting; others will become more active. Either way, your sexual activity won't affect or hurt the baby, who is well protected by the fluid in his amniotic sac.
- *When to be cautious about sex:*
  - *If you experience spotting or bleeding at any point in your pregnancy:* Contact your care provider and refrain from having sex until you discuss it with her. If this happens during the first trimester and the bleeding is light (like spotting), a middle-of-the-night phone call probably isn't necessary (unless you have other symptoms like dizziness or pelvic or shoulder pain; see ectopic pregnancy on page 125). During the first trimester, if the bleeding is steady or heavy, or if you bleed even a small amount in the second or third

trimester, call your doctor or midwife right away. Once you've been examined and given a clean bill of health by your caregiver, she'll tell you when you can resume sexual activity.

— *If you experience spontaneous spotting after intercourse:* It's a good idea to go in for an examination. Sometimes the cervix turns a little "inside out" during pregnancy, and intercourse irritates the cells that now face out. Or you may have a vaginal infection. Either way, once you've had things checked out, you should be able to resume sexual activity after about a week or once the infection is treated (if that's necessary).

— *If you're at risk for preterm labor:* Discuss the particulars of your situation with your care provider. He might recommend you refrain from vaginal or anal intercourse because both nipple stimulation and getting semen on the cervix can trigger contractions. (Nipple stimulation can cause the release of oxytocin; semen contains prostaglandin. Both substances stimulate contractions; see page 438.)

• *When to avoid sex:*
— *If you have a weak ("incompetent") cervix:* when the cervix opens early in the second trimester (see page 343).
— *If your placenta is very near or over the cervix:* known as placenta previa (see page 350).
— *If your membranes have ruptured.*

• *Shifting sexual desire:* Women have different levels of sexual interest at different points in pregnancy. Some women find that between nausea and fatigue, they're not at all interested in sex during the first trimester. Others find they're *very* interested from the get-go. Many women find that the second trimester is a time of particular sexual satisfaction, and then interest wanes again in the third trimester, as they get bigger and less physically comfortable.

Libido is not the only thing that can change. Your responses to sexual stimulation can change as well. What you enjoyed before you were pregnant, or even last week, might not be as pleasurable now. Try to be open with yourself and your partner about what feels good and what doesn't. Talk to each other about what's satisfying for each of you. You may want to explore different positions and adapt familiar ones to your changing body.

For example, the classic "missionary" position can be modified by the man propping himself up on his hands and knees so there's no pressure on the woman's abdomen. Sometimes intercourse is significantly more pleasurable when the woman can control the depth of penetration, which is easier when she's on top, when spooning, or side to side (while she still can do this), or from behind where the man remains stationary as the woman moves back and forth.

What's important is that there's no one way you're supposed to feel about sex during pregnancy (or ever). Every woman will have unique experiences and desires. You and/or your partner may find your shifting interest in sex disconcerting, but you also may find that even if you're not being explicitly sexual, you can discover different kinds of emotional and physical satisfaction by being physically intimate and engaged, through nurturing touch, massage, or simply holding each other.

REAL VOICES

The first time I was pregnant it was really hard to have sex. One of my new friends said she thought she must be so vain because sex is so wrapped up in how she feels about her own body—but I definitely feel that way. If I feel good about myself, then I feel good about sex. In my first pregnancy it was all so foreign to me, and having this big belly in between me and my husband was hard . . . it made me feel kind of out of control. On the other hand, being pregnant the second time, I loved to have sex anytime, and anytime I could I would.

Glenda, mom of two, stepmom of one

Certainly during the first trimester when I had all the morning sickness it was like, "Sex? Ick. Forget it." Second trimester it came back pretty strong, which was nice. And now at the end of the third trimester it's waning again—but it's not even a question of drive sometimes. Like I might think, "Yeah, sex sounds like a really nice idea," but it's harder to get the sensation in my genitals; they're just sort of numb. Also you know if you stimulate your nipples, you'll have a contraction. If you have an orgasm, you'll have a contraction. So it's much more complicated than just drive.

Michelle, mom of one, pregnant

Beauty and Spa Treatments

Not only are most beauty treatments safe, but if you're feeling physically uncomfortable or somewhat less than enthusiastic about your appearance, they can be a great pick-me-up. That said, not every beauty or body treatment is a good fit for pregnancy, and there are some commonsense adjustments you'll want to make.

Body treatments: scrubs and wraps

Body scrubs and wraps are generally safe. Before you set up an appointment for a particular treatment, talk with someone on the spa staff who knows what it entails, to see if it sounds appropriate for you in your pregnancy.

• *Make sure it's gentle:* Some body scrubs can be vigorous.

• *Stay cool:* If a treatment involves spending time in a warm tub or steam room, skip it.

Color processing hair

Traditionally, pregnant women have been discouraged from dyeing or highlighting their hair, for fear that the chemicals from the dye would enter the bloodstream through the scalp. However, there are no scientific data to support that claim. To err on the side of caution, I used to recommend that women avoid color processes that brought chemicals directly in contact with the scalp. But some were still unhappy about how they looked. Considering that there's so much about your appearance that's changing and that there's absolutely no evidence linking hair dye to birth defects, I now recommend that you do

---

STEER CLEAR OF STEAM

Whether you're at the gym or a spa, avoid hot tubs, whirlpools, steam rooms, and saunas. Fetuses are very sensitive to heat, especially in the early part of pregnancy, and your body temperature should not get above 102.4 for more than ten minutes at a time.

---

what feels best—and if that means coloring or highlighting your hair, then by all means do so. While this will bring you in contact with some chemicals, and I believe that pregnancy is a time to create a "toxic-free zone" in and around your body, the emotional benefits of feeling like you look your best might outweigh the undocumented risks associated with coloring your hair . . . The choice is yours.

• *Ventilation:* Make sure that the space where you're having your hair done is well ventilated to limit your exposure to airborne chemicals. In the first trimester, if you're sensitive to smells, it may be difficult to spend several hours in a strong-smelling salon.

Curling and Straightening Your Hair

- *Permanents:* There are very few studies on the effects of hair treatments in human pregnancy, but as with hair dye, permanents, which usually require a two-step chemical application process, are considered low-risk during pregnancy. In other words, the amount of chemicals that leach into the body through the scalp is thought to be too small to harm a fetus.
- *Hair straightening:* There are two different ways to straighten hair. The first involves chemical processing, and just like other hair treatments, the risk of the chemicals seeping in through the scalp is considered extremely low. The second, newer hair straightening method is known as *Japanese thermal hair straightening*, and it involves conditioning and applying a hot iron to the hair. Since the process doesn't involve chemicals, there's absolutely no risk from it. But, depending on your hair type, it can take up to six hours, and it's expensive ($300 to $1,000 a treatment).

- *Consider frequency:* Highlights tend to last longer than dye, so if you'd like to color your hair less frequently to try to limit chemical exposure, they might be a good option.

Facials

Facials are absolutely safe during pregnancy. A basic facial involves a series of cleansing and hydrating masks, a face and neck massage, and extractions of blackheads and blemishes. Since they're not explicitly medicinal (though they may be referred to as "therapeutic"), products used in a facial should not pose any risk to you or your baby.

A facial can take anywhere from an hour to ninety minutes, during

PRENATAL SPECIALS

More and more spas are offering facials, massages, and body treatments tailored to the needs of pregnant women. If you're going to treat yourself—or if someone's going to treat you—call around to several different day spas to see if any offer prenatal treatments.

which you'll be lying flat on your back. While many women find that time relaxing, be prepared for a long stretch. In the first trimester, you may need to have snacks at the ready, and later in pregnancy, you may need to talk with the aesthetician about bathroom breaks.

• *Lie at an angle:* Sometime between twenty and twenty-four weeks, depending on how quickly your abdomen grows, it will become uncomfortable and unhealthy for you to lie flat on your back. The pressure from your uterus against the vena cava, a major blood vessel, will decrease blood flow to the baby and could make you dizzy or faint. To relieve the pressure on the vena cava, place a pillow under your left hip and low back so it tilts to at least a fifteen-degree angle.

Hair removal: waxing and electrolysis

While you're pregnant, the combination of increased hormones, blood volume, and circulation stimulates hair follicles, meaning hair can grow more noticeably all over your body, including on your face, arms, and back. Hair removal by waxing or electrolysis is absolutely safe. (For more on excess hair in pregnancy, see page 163.)

> REAL VOICES
> The weirdest side effect I've had so far is every so often I notice a long white hair growing just under my eye in that delicate skin. It's easy to pluck and doesn't grow back quickly, but it's really disconcerting!
>
> Deborah, pregnant

Manicures and pedicures

Both are safe.

• *Ventilation:* The chemical smell in a nail salon can be quite strong, so look for a salon that's well ventilated.
• *Clean instruments:* Whether or not you're pregnant, look for a nail salon that either sterilizes its instruments or allows you to bring (or store) your own. You definitely want to avoid an infection or fungus on your nail bed.

Massage

Prenatal massage can be used to relieve everything from headaches to sciatica to general fatigue. It's also wonderful if you just want to treat yourself to an especially relaxing afternoon. During the massage, you'll probably lie on your side propped up by pillows. There are special prenatal massage tables that have holes cut into them and bands to hold your abdomen, but many find that those tables put too much strain on the uterine ligaments and back. Finally, don't expect to get a foot, ankle, or hand massage unless you're at the very end of your pregnancy. Those areas contain pressure points that could stimulate labor and most prenatal massage therapists avoid them.

• *Look for experience:* Even at a day spa, your massage therapist should be licensed in prenatal massage.

• *Ask for special oils:* If your massage therapist will use aromatherapy massage oils, ask that she mix them at about half their usual concentration, which is safer for prenatal massage. Also, make sure that the scent she's using is safe for pregnancy. (For a list of these, see page 103.)

• *Speak up:* If a therapist is working too deeply or if massaging a specific area feels too intense, let her know. You should be absolutely comfortable throughout.

Q: I'm in my first trimester and I have a belly button ring. Should I take it out?

Dr. Evans: Unless the area around the piercing becomes irritated, there's no reason to take it out now. But you'll want to remove it by early in your third trimester.

REAL VOICES ON MATERNITY CLOTHES

I wish I had succumbed to maternity clothes earlier. Why suffer through fifteen weeks with stomach cramps from how tight the waist is, when you could be breathing easy in elastic from the get-go?

Dorothy, mom of two

Stay away from maternity clothes for as long as possible. Just buy big and loose. (I like elastic-waist pants, X-large T-shirts, and big tunics.) That way, you don't buy for a limited amount of time and you can always wear these clothes again in the post-birth period, during which you still can't fit into your old clothes.

Asha, mom of one, pregnant

At 2.5 months you go strap on that cute little pregnancy pillow they have in maternity stores so you can guess how big you'll be when you can finally fit into those cute maternity capris you're trying on. But they don't tell you it's how you'll look at five months, and by the time you're eight months along those #@%! capris will be a memory and that pillow will taunt you with its daintiness. Not that I'm bitter.

Marjorie, mom of one, pregnant

When you're shopping for maternity clothes, always look at your butt. I would try stuff on and it would seem to fit and I'd think it was so cute, and then I'd turn around . . .

Johanna, mom of one

Buy things that make you look pregnant rather than things that make you look like you've just gained fifty pounds on your own. Fitted is actually better!

Invest in (or borrow) one good "suit" you can wear through a few seasons. A sleeveless dress with a matching jacket will get you from winter into summer.

Don't buy maternity underwear under any circumstances. It will make you cry just looking at how huge they are. Buy low-cut undies that will sit below your belly and maintain the illusion that nothing has changed—after all, you're still the same sexy woman you always were.

Finally, don't buy everything at once. Hold out and get something new at about month 7. You'll feel very excited by your new outfit, and it will be a great pick-me-up.

Suzanne, mom of two

Borrow. Don't buy.

Elsie, mom of one

I would suggest going right for the pouch. It's just so much more comfortable and practical.

Beth, pregnant

Don't get anything that has a "pouch" if you can avoid it. It makes you feel like a kangaroo and you can't wear any short shirts with them—the pouch fabric will show and it's ugly. Side panels are much better.

Suzanne, mom of two

I hated anything with a panel and loved anything with an adjustable waist.

Dorothy, mom of two

I invested in one really great, really expensive pair of jeans. I thought I was nuts when I bought them, but then I literally wore them every day until, by the end of my eighth month, I couldn't wear them anymore.

Johanna, mom of one

I couldn't have lived without black stretchy pants.

Dorothy, mom of two

Late in my pregnancy, I bought camisoles with a support bra built in and I love them!!

Beth, pregnant

My husband's elastic-waist gym shorts, Oxford shirts, and flannel pajamas were lifesavers.

Suzanne, mom of two

If I had known that I'd still be wearing my maternity clothes for two months after I had my baby, I never would have started wearing them as early as I did—nor would I have been so excited about my new clothing! For some reason, I was under the hopeful, yet completely delusional, idea that as soon as I had the baby, my stomach would be flat again!

Sarah, mom of two

I wouldn't buy anything white. By late in the second trimester, my belly caught every little drip and drab that used to land on a napkin.

Rebecca, mom of one

Traveling While Pregnant

Generally speaking, it's safe to travel while you're pregnant. Decisions about where to go, what to do, and how to be away can be made based on how you feel. Whether you're traveling for business or pleasure, and whether you'll be in a city or a more remote location, it's worth doing a simple Web search to learn what medical facilities are available at your destination. Also, check with your insurance company to confirm coverage. If you're considering traveling close to your due date, you need to think about whether you'd be comfortable giving birth away from home.

Air travel

• *Timing:* The second trimester, especially weeks 18 to 24, is widely considered the best time to fly. Airlines typically permit domestic travel until thirty-six weeks and international travel until thirty-five weeks for singleton pregnancies.

• *Move around:* Plan on an aisle seat and get up every hour or so to walk around for ten to fifteen minutes—especially on a long flight. Because of the changes in circulation during pregnancy, sitting for extended periods on a plane increases the risk of developing a blood clot in your leg (deep vein thrombosis), which could create a serious threat to your health.

• *Support hose:* If your flight will be longer than three hours, get a pair of compression hose (very strong support hose) at your local pharmacy. The hose, combined with walking around during the flight, will help keep blood from pooling in your legs and forming a clot.

• *Stay hydrated:* It's easy for any traveler to become dehydrated during a flight, but pregnant women are especially prone to dehydration. Travel with your own supply of bottled water, and don't be shy about asking a flight attendant for more to drink. You may find your nose is stuffy or dried out. Bring along some vitamin E oil to keep your nostrils moist. If your nose is especially irritated, ask for a cup of hot water and use the steam to soothe the dried membranes.

• *Manage gas and bloating:* During takeoff and landing, you may feel more bloated and uncomfortable than usual because of changing air pressure and your (possibly) slow-moving digestive system (see page 160). Before and during your flight, avoid foods that you know make you gassy, wear loose clothes, and, as always, keep drinking water.

• *Wear your seat belt:* Clip it under your abdomen.

• *With multiples:* If you're pregnant with twins or more, the safety of air travel depends on how your pregnancy is progressing. If a twin pregnancy is going smoothly, air travel through the twenty-eighth week is fine. With triplets or higher-order multiples, decisions about travel must be made on a case-by-case basis. If you're carrying multiples, talk to your caregiver before finalizing travel plans.

• *Avoid flying if:*
  – *You're at risk for preterm labor* (see page 363).

- *You have a weak (incompetent) cervix* (see pg. 343): In certain situations, it may be safe to travel if you have an incompetent cervix, but your care provider should examine you, and you should discuss the risks thoroughly before finalizing your plans.

- *You have placenta previa* (see page 350): It may be safe, but talk to your care provider first.

- *You have a medical or obstetric complication:* Such as pregnancy-related high blood pressure, which could result in an emergency. (*Note:* If you have gestational diabetes and it's under control, you can travel.)

Note: Because pregnancy is so unpredictable, look into travel insurance for trip cancellation if you're planning a big trip. That way, if you have to cancel at the last minute, you're somewhat covered.

REAL VOICES

Make sure you drink plenty of water on the airplane and bring a lot of snacks, particularly those that help with morning sickness. Also bring along plenty of your favorite snacks for once you're at your destination, because you may not be able to get them.

Tina, mom of one

I always brought healthy snacks, like a big bag of almonds, because it can be really hard to find anything besides junk food in airports and hotels. Also, whenever I was about to walk through the metal detector, I would take a minute to collect myself and imagine making a protective shield for the baby.

Cindy, mom of three

I traveled alone, and even though it was just domestic, the actual traveling was exhausting. The vacation itself was great, but I'd recommend traveling with a partner or a friend if you can.

Michele, mom of one, pregnant

Q: Is it safe to travel to high altitudes?

Dr. Evans: There's no simple answer to that question. If you're not used to being at high altitudes, or you don't exercise regularly, then the thinner air, even in a place like Denver or Santa Fe, can mean you'll feel the effects of altitude more strongly. For example, your heart rate will go up and you'll absorb less oxygen (because there's less in the air), which means the baby will get less oxygen. Therefore, if you tend to be sedentary or live at sea level, you might want to avoid a trip to high altitudes because you may be uncomfortable there. If you have a very bad reaction to the altitude, it could become an issue for the baby. If you're in relatively good shape, however, and especially if you're not planning to do any vigorous activities, it shouldn't be a problem.

Q: I've been planning to go to Australia and possibly Thailand when I'm five months pregnant. Is that a problem?

Dr. Evans: The major problem with a trip to Australia from the U.S. is the length of the flight. I tend to be cautious about flights that are longer than eight hours, but talk with your caregiver about it. If you wear compression hose during the flight and make sure you stretch out and walk around for a solid ten minutes every hour, you'll probably be fine.

If you plan to travel in the Far East, the biggest threat would be from infectious diseases. Now more than ever you want to avoid getting a parasite or a high fever. Consult with a travel medicine specialist (your caregiver can recommend someone, and many hospitals now have them on staff) and search the Centers for Disease Control Web site (*www.cdc.gov*) for information about standard immunizations and precautions for the country you plan to visit. Once again, consider what medical facilities will be accessible to you when you're traveling, in case you become ill or an unexpected complication develops.

Road travel

If you're planning a road trip, schedule frequent stops. You'll probably want (and need) to stop every hour and a half or so to go to the bathroom. When you do stop, take a few minutes to walk around, stretch your back, chest, and shoulders (see "Chest and Shoulder Openers" on page 271), and breathe in some fresh air.

Caution: Car accidents are a major threat to the health of both mother and baby. Always wear your seat belt and go see your doctor or midwife after any accident, even a minor fender bender.

Environmental Hazards

• *At home:* When it comes to environmental hazards in the home, there's one good rule of thumb: If it has an odor, proceed with caution.

New carpets, new furniture, paints (wall paint and spray paint), varnishes, and stored fuels

The reason these smell is they emit organic compounds, which should be avoided. To reduce exposure:

- *New carpets:* Unroll them outside to air them out. If that's out of the question, open the windows when the carpets are installed and try to stay out of the house until the smell dissipates. If you can stay overnight somewhere else, all the better.
- *New furniture:* When it arrives, stay out of the house for the day and allow as much fresh air through the house as you can. With both new furniture and carpets, you want to steer clear until the smell dissipates. Also, if you want to move furniture around, ask friends to help out and don't do any heavy lifting yourself. (When you're pregnant, don't lift anything by yourself that's heavy enough to require two hands to lift off the ground.)
- *Painting, varnishing, or spray painting:* Don't do it yourself. Once the painting is complete, try to stay away until the paint no longer smells.
- *Stored fuels:* Avoid them.

Note: Houseplants will not reduce the level of indoor airborne toxins, but they're great to have around. They bring oxygen and color into your home, and, if you're open to it, they can enhance your connection to nature.

Cats/toxoplasmosis

Cat feces can carry *Toxoplasmosa gondii*, a parasite that causes the infection toxoplasmosis, which is relatively mild in adults but quite dangerous to a developing fetus. You can also get toxoplasmosis from raw and undercooked meat, raw eggs, and unpasteurized milk. Fruits, vegetables, and herbs from home gardens, where cat feces can end up in the soil, can also carry the parasite. A blood test at a preconception (ideal) or prenatal visit can determine if you've had toxoplasmosis in the past; but you can't develop immunity to it. Exposure to the parasite is most dangerous when it occurs between weeks 10 and 24. Outdoor and newly acquired cats, along with the raw foods listed above, pose the greatest danger.

If you suspect you've been exposed to a live toxoplasmosis infection because you've changed the litter for a cat that's new to you, or you may have been exposed through food and now have mild flu-like symptoms, see your care provider as soon as possible. You'll have various tests. If they are positive, early treatment with medication can reduce the chance that the fetus will be exposed to the infection.

Precautions for toxoplasmosis:

• *Avoid the litter:* While you're pregnant, have your partner or a friend clean out the cat litter. If no one else can do it, wear gloves, clean the litter daily, throw it away outside of the house, and wash your hands thoroughly with soap and warm water afterward.

• *If you garden:* Wear gloves and wash your hands thoroughly afterward.

• *Don't eat undercooked or raw meat:* And wash your hands after handling raw meat.

• *Wash fruits, vegetables, and herbs* from any home garden thoroughly by soaking them for ten to fifteen minutes in cold water mixed with one drop of dishwashing soap. Rinse them completely, until no soap bubbles remain.

Cleaning products

While these have a strong smell, there's no evidence that the regular use of household cleaning products will harm a developing fetus. Still, to be on the safe side, keep rooms well ventilated while you're cleaning and wear rubber gloves.

Computers

Concern about the effect of prolonged computer use on pregnancy, particularly on early pregnancy, isn't uncommon, but it seems to be unnecessary. As of this writing, large-scale studies show no relationship between computer use and miscarriage or birth defects.

Lead (paint, pipes, ceramics, at work, in hobbies)

Lead crosses the placenta, and exposure to it during pregnancy poses many dangers. It can lead to miscarriage, low birth weight, and preterm labor (see page 363). And a child exposed to even low levels of lead in the womb can experience cognitive delays and developmental problems.

• *Lead in paint:* If your house or apartment was built before 1978, the year the government banned lead-based paint, there's a chance there could be lead paint in your home. Lead-based paint is usually not a hazard unless it's deteriorating or on a surface where there's friction, like a window or a door. To determine if your home is at risk, you need to hire a professional lead inspector for an inspection and risk assessment. (Call 1-800-242-LEAD for a local inspector.) To remove a lead hazard permanently, hire a certified lead "abatement" contractor. (Regional EPA offices will have listings; for the contact information of regional offices go to: *www.epa.gov/epahome/ whereyoulive.htm#regiontext*.)

Precautions for lead paint:

— *If you rent and there's chipping paint,* contact your landlord and let him know that you suspect a problem and you're expecting a baby.
— *Clean windowsills, door frames, and floors weekly* using warm water and an all-purpose cleanser or one especially made for lead (dust can recirculate after vacuuming). If you can't have someone else do this task, wear gloves while you're cleaning and wash immediately afterward. Also wash any sponges thoroughly after cleaning.
— *Wash your children's hands thoroughly* before they eat, nap, or go to sleep at night.
— *Keep play areas clean* and keep toys, bottles, and cups off the windowsills.
— *Take off your shoes* when you come in.

• *Lead pipes:* If you don't know if you have lead piping bringing water into your house, your local health department or water supplier can help you find out.

Precautions for lead piping and tap water:

— *Let the water run* for fifteen to thirty seconds before using it, especially if you haven't turned on the faucet for a few hours.
— *Use only cold tap water* for cooking and drinking. If you need hot water, heat up cold tap water.
— *Consider installing a carbon filter* on your faucet or buying bottled water.
— *If you're concerned about the quality of the plumbing* that leads to your house or water quality in general, contact your local EPA office or health department to learn more about it.

• *Lead in ceramics:* Earthenware, pottery, and china that's handcrafted, imported, or made before 1951 can leach lead into food. If you're concerned about a plate or bowl you own, don't use it for serving or storing food.

• *Lead on the job:* If you work with lead, you should have a preconception blood test to measure your blood lead levels. If you haven't been tested and you're already pregnant, let your caregiver know. She'll want to test your blood levels to determine what risk there might be to the fetus. If your partner works with lead, he or she should shower after work and wash work clothes separately.

• *Hobbies:* Ceramics, stained glass, and finishing furniture are hobbies that bring you in contact with lead. If you do them regularly, it's a good idea to get your lead level checked by a blood test and to stop while you're pregnant or nursing.

Note: If you think you're at risk from any of the factors listed above, consider having a blood test to measure your lead exposure. Also, make sure you're getting 1,500 mg of calcium a day; the body absorbs more lead when calcium levels are low. (For more on calcium in pregnancy and calcium-rich foods, see page 220.)

Microwave ovens

Microwave ovens heat food with electromagnetic energy waves. The microwaves make water molecules vibrate, which causes friction between the water molecules and other molecules, and with friction, there's heat. The heat microwaves create is a form of radiation, and while technically it could heat human tissue, in practice, something has to be *inside* of a microwave oven in order for it to be affected by the radiation. If a microwave oven has a working seal on the door, then all the microwave energy stays within the oven and there's no risk to you.

If you're concerned that your microwave is leaking—because the door is warped, you can feel air coming out of it when it's on, or it works with the door open—have it tested, otherwise it's best not to use it. Alternatively, when you use it, you could stand on the other side of the room (usually you have to be within six feet to experience any effects from the microwaves), or ask your partner to use it when you're not in the room.

There are professionals who can check for "leakage" around the microwave. Ask your home insurance broker, a local homeowners or renters association, a real estate broker, or your care provider if he knows of anyone who can do this. In fact, we had this done in our home and now always stand at least three feet from the microwave when it's on.

Note: Avoid microwaving foods in plastic containers or plastic wrap. The heat can cause dioxins to seep out of the plastic and into the food.

Mold

Humidifiers, central air-conditioning, leaks, and carpets over concrete floors that have been wet can all create mold that can aggravate runny noses and allergies and irritate eyes and skin.

To reduce irritation:

- *Clean and disinfect humidifiers and cooling systems regularly.*
- *Repair leaks and take up carpets* that have been laid on concrete floors if you've had any flooding or excessive moisture.

Pesticides

These chemicals are part and parcel of our daily lives. They're on our food, and we use them inside our houses as well as for gardens and on lawns. How much of a threat they pose in general (not just when you're pregnant) really depends on the nature and length of your exposure as well as your genetic susceptibility (each of us will respond differently to the same pesticide exposure). While you're pregnant, it's important to take precautions to limit your exposure to and risk from pesticides.

- *Outdoor spraying:* If you live in an area where there's insecticide spraying, and if you have any control in the matter, try to stop it. If you can't, keep the windows sealed and try to be indoors as much as possible while the spraying is going on and you can still smell the insecticide in the air.
- *Garden and lawn use:* If you use pesticides or herbicides in your garden or on your lawn, try to make it through a season chemical-free. If your garden must have pesticides, have someone else apply them. If you must apply them, be sure to wear gloves and a mask, and wash your hands thoroughly after gardening. Try to avoid the garden for a day or two after it's been treated.
- *Home use:* If you need to use any kind of pesticide in your home, follow the directions scrupulously and stay out of the house for as long as you can afterward. For example, if a roach spray recommends staying out of the house for two to three hours, think about staying away for four to six hours. If you can, have a partner or a friend do the spraying.

If your bug problem is severe, don't use "bug bombs" and other high-volume pesticide delivery systems that spray the chemicals everywhere. Instead, try to find a professional exterminator who can target his spraying so it will be as effective as possible without being overly invasive. Try to stay out of the house during the spraying and for the whole day afterward.

If you live in an apartment with regularly scheduled exterminator visits, tell your superintendent that you don't want your apartment sprayed. If you don't have a choice, make sure the apartment is well ventilated and try to stay out of the apartment the day of spraying. And find out what pesticide is being used. Recent surveys show that banned pesticides are still used frequently. Make sure your building is applying *approved* pesticides only (see *http://www.epa.gov/pesticides/*).

• *Food:* Wash conventionally grown produce thoroughly to get rid of as many surface pesticides as possible. To do so, soak fruits and vegetables for fifteen minutes in water mixed with just one *drop* of dishwashing liquid, then rinse them *thoroughly*, being sure that all soap residue is gone. Also wash organic produce well. Don't use the outer leaves of greens like lettuce and cabbage.

Note: A recent study in New York City shows that pesticide use during pregnancy is associated with smaller babies. While this change in birth weight doesn't necessarily predict or affect long-term health, it does demonstrate that pesticides can have an impact on fetal size. This new information, combined with earlier studies that show a relationship between pesticide exposure and decreased newborn performance (for example on the APGAR test, see page 488), leads me to wonder about the effects of pesticides on organ systems. There's a study under way at Columbia University to investigate the impact of pesticides on fetal development. The bottom line is that while pesticides are part of our world, it's important to take the steps described above to try to limit your exposure as much as possible.

(For information about a range of household, environmental, and health risks, see the book *Risk: A Practical Guide for Deciding What's Really Safe and What's Really Dangerous in the World Around You* by David Ropeik and George Gray; Mariner Books, 2002.)

REAL VOICES

In the beginning of my pregnancy I probably called the teratogen (chemical agents that can cause fetal malformations) hotline every other day with questions about my habits. I'm very healthy. I eat very healthy. I don't smoke. I definitely don't drink while I'm pregnant—I do otherwise. I exercise every day pretty much. Still, I was so worried about everything: the kind of shampoo I used, that I dye my hair, that I used Retin A on my eyes (see page 152).

Pregnancy is such a natural process, but we live in such an unnatural, chemically active environment—and I'm a worrier, so I just worried about everything.

Glenda, mom of two, stepmom to one

Pressure-treated wood

Until the end of 2003, wood preserved by pressure treatment with inorganic arsenic was commonly used for home decks, picnic tables, and many playgrounds. (The EPA now recommends pressure-treated wood be voluntarily phased out for home use.) The wood poses a potential danger to small children, and it makes sense to take basic precautions when around these products while you're pregnant.

• *On picnic tables:* Use a tablecloth whenever you eat on a pressure-treated wood picnic table. If you're not sure about the wood, play it safe and use a cloth.
• *After the playground:* Wash your child's hands and your own thoroughly.
• *If you have a wood deck:*
   – *Seal the deck with standard wood sealants* every six months. (Stay away until the smell dissipates if you do this during your pregnancy.)
   – *Don't let your kids or pets play beneath the deck,* and don't store toys there.
   – *If you can, stay off the deck while you're pregnant,* and if you spend time on it, wash your hands thoroughly when you come in.
   – *Wash the table and deck* with plain soap and water.

Workplace concerns

• *Artists (painters, sculptors, photographers who develop photos, stained glass artists, ceramicists):* Work in these areas can bring you into contact with a wide variety of chemicals, especially lead. If you're not yet pregnant, have your lead level tested by a blood test. If your lead levels are low, take safety precautions if you plan to continue working during your pregnancy. Wear gloves and a mask, shower as soon as you get home, and wash your clothes separately from the rest of your family's.
• *Flight attendants:* There've been a number of studies done on flight attendants to determine if the change in air pressure or increased exposure to radiation in high-altitude flights increases the risk of miscarriage. As of the latest studies, no increased risk has been detected. But if you're a flight attendant and typically work flights that are longer than eight hours, look into changing your routes to work shorter flights.

• *Horticultural and agricultural work:* Take the necessary precautions to reduce your exposure to chemicals and parasites (such as toxoplasmosis in the soil) during pregnancy. Wear gloves and a mask, shower as soon as you get home, and wash your clothes separately.

• *Manufacturing:* If you work in manufacturing, you may face a variety of safety issues during your pregnancy, including standing on your feet for long periods, ventilation, and exposure to chemicals. Your employer should be able to accommodate the physical demands of your pregnancy, and you cannot be penalized or fired because of it (see "Workplace Rights," page 329). If you're exposed to chemicals on the job, you have a right to know what they are. OSHA, the Occupational Health and Safety Administration, is an invaluable resource. On its Web site (*www.osha.gov*), you can find a wide range of resources, including "Hazard Communications," which provides specific information about chemical safety in the workplace.

• *Hair salons:* Studies of haircutters, colorists, and stylists haven't shown an increase in miscarriage rates from working in a salon, but if you work in a salon, wear gloves when coloring hair, sit as much as possible during the day, and try to work in a well-ventilated area.

• *Work with small children:* If you work with small children as a teacher, nanny, or nurse, or if you spend a lot of time with them, your risk of contracting fifth disease (aka parvovirus B19) increases. Approximately 50 percent of adults are immune to fifth disease, a relatively mild infection that occurs mostly in children and is typically accompanied by a rash. However, like other infections that are mild in adults, fifth disease poses a potentially serious threat to a developing fetus. Ideally, if you are in a higher risk category for fifth disease, your immunity will be tested at a preconception visit.

If you suspect you've been exposed to the virus and you haven't been tested, you can have a blood test that will show if: (1) you're immune because you've been infected in the past; (2) you haven't been infected recently; or (3) you have been infected recently. If you've been infected, there's approximately a 5 percent chance that the baby could develop severe anemia. While some doctors and midwives might treat an active parvovirus infection as a low-risk situation, ask for a consultation with a high-risk specialist (perinatologist) to monitor your pregnancy more closely with ultrasound and blood tests. The specialist will look for signs of fetal infection such as decreased growth or fetal swelling. (If a fetus starts to show signs of an infection, and an infection is confirmed through cordocentesis (see page 295), then, depending on how far along a woman is, a baby could be delivered early and treated in a neonatal intensive care unit. This is very rare.)

Q: When should I stop working?

Dr. Evans: That's up to you. If you can make it into work without getting exhausted, the work isn't physically demanding, and you feel relatively good, there's no reason to stop working late in pregnancy. But if you find that you're working really long hours, you're exhausted, and you have no time for yourself or your baby, think about stopping work at least a week before your due date to give yourself a little time to relax and connect with your baby.

If you have a long commute and you're having your first baby, you'll most likely still have enough time to make it home if you sense you're going into labor. But you have to be willing to leave work when you first suspect labor is starting, which means you could leave for some false alarms. If you drive yourself to and from work, as opposed to taking a commuter train, consider stopping at thirty-eight weeks and/or coming up with a contingency plan with a coworker (or be ready to call a taxi) just in case you start having regular contractions at the office. It isn't safe to drive when you're having contractions.

Talk with your care provider, your partner, and your employer about when it makes sense for you to leave work and how you can structure your maternity leave. Many of the women I work with find that while they enjoy the time off before the baby, they would prefer to have more time off after the baby arrives.

Workplace Rights

Here is a review of your basic rights in the workplace while you're pregnant and in the initial postpartum period.*

Hiring and promotions

- An employer can't refuse to hire or promote you because you're pregnant as long as you're able to perform the major functions of your job.
- An employer can't refuse to hire you because of the prejudices of coworkers, clients, or customers against pregnant women.

(*Sources: The U.S. Equal Employment Opportunity Commission, *www.eeoc.gov/facts/fs-preg.html*; the U.S. Department of Labor, Women's Bureau.)

REAL VOICES

I worked at Planned Parenthood, and there weren't very many of us in my age group. There were lots of twenty-somethings who were far from thinking of getting pregnant, and then there were a lot of older women. I was one of the first to get pregnant, and it was kind of fun for the staff. People were very supportive. They threw a huge shower for me. But I declined a lot of assistance; I didn't want to be treated differently. So I got a lot of flack from coworkers because I would still carry computers around and things like that. They gave me a hard time, but were just being protective.

Martha, mom of two

Pregnancy and maternity leave

- Pregnant employees must be allowed to work as long as they're able to perform their jobs.

- As a pregnant woman, you can't be singled out or asked to follow special procedures related to your health and ability to work.

- If you're temporarily unable to perform your job because of your pregnancy, you must receive the same treatment as any other temporarily disabled employee. For example, your employer must provide modified tasks, alternative assignments, disability leave, or leave without pay.

- If you recover after being on leave for a pregnancy-related condition, your employer must allow you to return to work and cannot require that you remain on leave until the baby's birth.

- An employer cannot prohibit you from returning to work for a predetermined length of time after childbirth.

- Employers must hold open a job for a pregnancy-related absence for the same amount of time that jobs are held open for employees on sick or disability leave.

- Under the Family and Medical Leave Act (FMLA), if you've worked for an employer with fifty or more employees or for the local, state, or federal government for one year and at least 1,250 hours during the previous year, you're entitled to up to twelve weeks total (unpaid) leave within one year of the birth (or adoption) of your child. You may begin your leave before you give birth.

- Under FMLA, men are permitted up to twelve weeks total (unpaid) leave at any point within one year of the birth (or adoption) of their child. Domestic partnerships are regulated by states, and private companies may also have domestic partnership policies; check with your local government employment bureau or your company's human resources department to see what benefits your partner is entitled to.

REAL VOICES

My entire department was laid off when I was six months pregnant. It actually worked very well. Thankfully I was in a great situation. My boss was my mentor; I had followed her to this company from another company. I had already told her that I wasn't coming back so she could start looking for someone. I was always very up front with her, even though I hadn't told anyone else that I wasn't planning on returning. And she was very up front with me when the layoffs were coming. She went to bat for me and got me a good severance package . . . when they wanted to just shove me out the door despite the fact that I was basically unemployable.

Rochelle, mom of three

Health insurance

- Health insurance provided by an employer must cover expenses for pregnancy-related conditions on the same basis as costs for other medical conditions.
- Pregnancy-related expenses should be reimbursed exactly as those incurred for other medical conditions, whether payment is on a fixed or percentage basis.
- The amount payable by the insurance provider can be limited only to the same extent as costs for other conditions. No additional, increased, or larger deductible can be imposed.
- Employers must provide the same level of health benefits for spouses of male employees as they do for spouses of female employees.

Fringe benefits

- Pregnancy-related benefits must be the same for single and married employees.
- In an all-female workforce or job classification, benefits must be provided for pregnancy-related conditions if benefits are provided for other medical conditions.

- If an employer provides any benefits to workers on leave, the employer must provide the same benefits for those on leave for pregnancy-related conditions.
- Employees with pregnancy-related disabilities must be treated the same as other temporarily disabled employees when it comes to accrual and crediting of seniority, calculating vacation, pay increases, and temporary disability benefits.

17

Medical Complications of Pregnancy

While the vast majority of pregnancies progress without any medical complications, not all do. Sometimes complications can develop unexpectedly, and sometimes a woman's medical history puts her at risk for certain complications. There's no way to know for sure who will experience a medical difficulty over the course of a pregnancy.

By following the basic guidelines for prenatal care—paying attention to your body and what it's telling you, taking good care of yourself, and getting consistent, quality care from a trusted caregiver—you're taking the most important steps you can toward preventing or managing whatever complications might arise.

◆ ◆ ◆

In this chapter you'll find:

- Amniotic Fluid: Too Much (Polyhydramnios) or Too Little (Oligohydramnios)
- Anemia
- Gestational Diabetes
- Incompetent Cervix
- Intrauterine Growth Restriction
- Placental Abruption
- Placenta Previa
- Preeclampsia
- Preterm Labor

Amniotic Fluid: Too Much (polyhydramnios) or Too Little (oligohydramnios)

Amniotic fluid not only protects and cushions your baby, it also helps in several aspects of fetal development. Because the baby moves around in it, amniotic fluid promotes normal muscle and bone growth. Because she breathes and swallows the fluid, it helps your baby's lungs and gastrointestinal system mature.

In the first trimester, amniotic fluid comes from the mother, and it's mostly water. Early in the second trimester, the baby starts to produce sterile urine and begins the cycle of swallowing and urinating through which amniotic fluid builds. While there's variation from pregnancy to pregnancy, in general the volume of amniotic fluid will increase until sometime about thirty-two weeks, when the amount of fluid plateaus at a little less than a quart. It then stays stable until around thirty-nine weeks, when it begins to decline.

• *Is there a problem?* After an examination, your care provider may suspect that you have too much or too little amniotic fluid based on two factors: (1) how your abdomen feels, and (2) how your uterus has been growing (see "Tracking Fetal Growth and Fundal Height" on page 338).

• *Diagnosis:* Both excessive and low levels of amniotic fluid are diagnosed by ultrasound. To make a diagnosis, an ultrasound technician (and/or a doctor) divides the abdomen into four quadrants, measures each quadrant by ultrasound, and adds up the measurements to calculate what's known as an amniotic fluid index (AFI). An AFI of 5 to 25 cm is considered normal, an AFI of 25 or above is considered excessive, and an AFI of 5 or below is considered low.

Excessive amniotic fluid (polyhydramnios)

According to the March of Dimes, about 2 percent of pregnant women develop too much amniotic fluid, also known as *polyhydramnios*, and most often, there's no apparent reason for the condition. The baby is healthy, you're healthy, and extra fluid has simply built up slowly over the course of the second and third trimesters. If you're carrying twins, there's a greater chance you'll develop excessive amniotic fluid.

- *Signs of too much fluid:* When you have too much fluid, your abdomen, which should feel like a full balloon, would feel almost too full and taut, and the baby will feel "bouncy" to the touch.

Other signs that you might have too much fluid:

  — Rapid weight gain

  — Your uterus appears to grow too quickly (see "Tracking Fetal Growth and Fundal Height," page 338)

  — Baby's movements feel "muffled"

  — Your back and/or abdomen hurt more

  — Your hands and ankles swell

- *Causes of too much fluid:*

  — *Anatomical problem:* If the fetus can't swallow because of anatomical problems with the esophagus, gastrointestinal tract, or central nervous system, then too much fluid may build up. This is relatively rare.

  — *Diabetes:* Fluid may increase in cases of poorly controlled gestational diabetes or preexisting diabetes. When polyhydramnios happens as a side effect of diabetes, diagnosing and treating the condition can help the amniotic fluid levels return to normal.

  — *Other causes:* Rh incompatibility (see page 93), certain chromosomal abnormalities, and in the case of identical twins who share a placenta, twin-twin transfusion syndrome (in which one baby gets too much blood and the other too little), a relatively rare but dangerous condition (see page 383).

  — *Unknown:* As noted above, sometimes there's no apparent reason for too much fluid, and mother and baby are both perfectly healthy.

- *Follow-up:* After a diagnosis of excessive fluid, your care provider may recommended a level 2 ultrasound to rule out anatomical problems, even if you've already had this test earlier in your pregnancy. Excessive fluid can be diagnosed with a level 1 or level 2 ultrasound, but only the latter can diagnose an anatomical problem. (For a description of both tests, see page 303.) If no anatomical problems are found (which is likely), your care provider may recommend closer monitoring for the rest of your pregnancy with ultrasounds and non-stress tests (see page 299) because excessive fluid puts you at risk for preterm labor.

If you haven't been tested for gestational diabetes, you may be tested now, either by blood test or glucose tolerance test (see page 297). Even if you've already had a normal, one-hour glucose tolerance test, you may have to repeat it.

• *Side effects from too much fluid:* If you have too much fluid in your third trimester, you might have some difficulty breathing (this is very rare). If this is the case, your doctor might suggest a therapeutic amniocentesis, which removes the excess fluid and relieves pressure on your diaphragm and lungs. (There is no good data on the miscarriage rate of therapeutic amniocentesis because it's so unusual, but it's thought to be quite low, and if a problem develops, the baby can probably be delivered safely. Talk with your care providers about the risks of your particular situation.)

• *Recurrence:* If you experience excessive amniotic fluid in one pregnancy, it doesn't increase the risk that you'll develop it in your next pregnancy.

Note: If you go into labor with high fluid levels and your membranes haven't ruptured, you're likely to be monitored continuously while you labor, because occasionally, when there's a lot of fluid and the membranes rupture on their own, the fluid gushes out with enough force to cause an abruption, or a separation between the placenta and the uterus. This can spiral rapidly into a serious situation for the baby. There are two other unusual, but potential, complications when the membranes break forcefully: The umbilical cord can drop into the birth canal (see "Prolapsed Cord," page 434) or a part of the baby other than the head, such as an arm, can enter the birth canal first, complicating delivery. Your caregiver will examine you shortly after your water breaks (or is broken) to make sure that these complications haven't occurred.

If the membranes don't break on their own, an obstetrician or midwife will be very careful if and when he or she breaks them. This means that there will probably be an IV running and a nurse will be in the room because of the risks introduced by breaking the membranes when fluid levels are high.

Low amniotic fluid (oligohydramnios)

About 8 percent of all pregnant women develop low amniotic fluid, or *oligohydramnios*. It's most common in the late third trimester, when amniotic fluid levels start to decrease naturally. When the condition develops slowly at the end of a pregnancy, it increases the risk of complications during delivery and the possibility of a C-section, but for the most part it doesn't indicate a problem. If your fluid levels are low, your caregiver may recommend closer monitoring of the baby's well-being through non-stress tests or biophysical profiles (see pages 299 and 288). If, however, fluid levels drop *dramatically* late in the third trimester and your water does not break, it's a sign that the placenta can no longer nourish the baby, even if you haven't yet reached your due date. In this situation, your caregiver may recommend that it's safest to plan to deliver the baby soon.

Low fluid between twenty-six and thirty-four weeks is more worrisome because it indicates how much the baby is urinating, which in turn reflects on placental function, blood flow, and overall fetal well-being. Here's why: When a baby doesn't get enough blood and nutrients through the placenta, his urine output goes down. Therefore, if low fluid develops after week twenty-six, it can be a sign of intrauterine growth restriction (see page 345).

Very rarely, low fluid develops earlier than twenty-six weeks, and if it does, it can cause birth defects, because without enough fluid to swallow, the baby's lungs can't develop properly and her organs may become compressed. Also, with less fluid, there's not enough room for her to grow and kick and develop her muscles, and the risk of miscarriage, preterm birth, or stillbirth goes up.

• *Signs of too little fluid:* If your fluid levels are low, your abdomen might feel almost bony instead of taut. Other signs include smaller than expected uterine growth (see "Tracking Fetal Growth and Fundal Height" on page 338) or feeling the baby move less.

• *Causes:*

— *Before twenty-four weeks:* If fluid is low before twenty-four weeks, an anatomical abnormality of the kidneys and urinary tract may be causing the problem. In most cases, a level 2 ultrasound can diagnose or rule out a problem.

— *Between twenty-four and thirty-four weeks:* Intrauterine growth restriction (IUGR, see page 345) could be the cause.

— *After thirty-four weeks:* When low amniotic fluid occurs after thirty-four weeks, it's usually a sign that the placenta can no longer nourish the baby as well as it once did, but frequently it's not clear what causes the placenta to fail.

— *Maternal health issues:* Certain health problems can contribute to low amniotic fluid. These include: high blood pressure (either poorly controlled or chronic), lupus, and problems with the placenta such as placenta previa (see page 350). These conditions may limit the nutrients the baby receives, and when he doesn't get enough nutrients, he can't urinate enough to keep amniotic fluids at a healthy level.

Tracking Fetal Growth and Fundal Height

✦ Starting at twenty weeks, your care provider will keep track of the baby's growth at each prenatal visit by measuring fundal height, which is the distance, in centimeters, from the top of the pubic bone to the top of the uterus (also known as the *fundus*). From about twenty weeks on, fundal height roughly corresponds to gestational age—in other words, when you're twenty-nine weeks, your fundal height would measure approximately twenty-nine centimeters. This isn't a precise measurement—factors like the position of the baby, how you're carrying, and the level of amniotic fluid all contribute to fundal height measurements.

Because you'll be measured at each prenatal visit after twenty weeks, your caregiver will be able to see trends in the growth of your uterus. If your fundal height measurements have been consistent and your caregiver measures a sudden drop or increase by two or more centimeters, she'll probably recommend an ultrasound exam within the next few days to see if amniotic fluid levels are too high or low, or to see if the baby seems either too small (see "IUGR" on page 345) or large for where you're estimated to be in your pregnancy. How quickly the ultrasound will be done depends on details such as your blood pressure, fetal movement, etc.

• *With multiples:* While fundal height helps your provider keep track of the baby's growth, it's not a useful measurement for multiples. Therefore, if you're carrying twins or more, you will probably have monthly sonograms after twenty weeks to keep track of the babies' growth.

Note: There's a difference between low amniotic fluid caused by ruptured membranes ("the waters break") and low fluid caused by a problem with the placenta, an anatomical problem with the baby, or a chronic health condition with the mother. Once the membranes rupture and amniotic fluid either leaks or gushes out, the risk of a serious infection to the mother or baby goes up, and usually it's just a matter of time before labor begins spontaneously. This isn't true for low fluid caused by any other reason.

The period between when the membranes rupture and the start of labor is known as the latency period. Its length depends on how far along in your pregnancy you are. All things being equal, the closer you are to your due date, the shorter the latency period will be. If your water breaks before thirty-seven weeks, there are many medical interventions that can be used to prolong the latency period and give the baby (and the baby's lungs) more time to mature. Whether or not those interventions will be tried depends on how early in your pregnancy the membranes rupture. It's important that a medical intervention start immediately after the water breaks, so if you suspect your membranes have ruptured and you're not yet thirty-seven weeks, call your caregiver as soon as possible.

• *Follow-up:* After an ultrasound exam to determine if amniotic fluid levels are too low, you may be closely monitored with follow-up ultrasound exams and non-stress tests (see pages 303 and 299). Often, simple measures such as taking it easy or going on bed rest combined with drinking more clear liquids improve fluid levels. Alternatively, if you have low fluid levels, your caregiver may recommend inducing labor, depending on how close you are to your due date and the results of any fetal testing (such as non-stress tests and biophysical profiles).

• *Recurrence:* If you experience low amniotic fluid in one pregnancy, it doesn't increase the risk that you'll develop it in your next pregnancy.

> REAL VOICES
>
> I was a week postdate with my daughter. They did an ultrasound to make sure she was okay, and they found *no* amniotic fluid. Then it was: Run run run run run! Do it right now! Later, before we went to the hospital so I could be induced, we went to the 2nd Avenue Deli (in New York City) because my husband said, "She needs lunch!" My father insisted that a pound of Josie, who was over ten pounds at birth, was corned beef.
>
> Marjorie, mom of one, pregnant

Anemia

In its most common form, anemia reflects a lack of iron, an important component in the production of red blood cells, which carry oxygen in the blood. During pregnancy, your blood naturally has proportionally fewer red blood cells because your blood volume increases by 40 to 50 percent, but your red blood cells don't rise at the same rate (or at all unless you consume more iron).

Typically, about 65 percent of the body's iron is in its red blood cells, so if your red blood cells are low, your iron level may be low. Your iron resources will be depleted further because the baby will always take the iron he needs from you. (This is why it's important to take in 30 mg of iron a day through food and/or supplements while you're pregnant; for iron-rich foods, see page 235.) When a pregnant woman's red blood cell levels dip below a certain point, she's considered anemic.

Because birth, whether vaginal or by Cesarean delivery, involves blood loss, most women need to take, or continue taking, an iron supplement for six weeks postpartum. Your iron levels will be checked by a blood test at your six-week postpartum visit to see if you need to keep taking a supplement. Most often, iron levels return to normal within three months of giving birth.

• *Diagnosis:* To make sure your red blood cell levels are within a healthy range, you'll probably have a blood test between twenty-five and twenty-eight weeks (often at the same time as your glucose screen), then again at thirty-six weeks to help you prepare nutritionally for the postpartum period. The blood test measures your hematocrit level; hematocrit represents the number and size of red blood cells, and it reflects your iron level.

If your hematocrit is above 35 percent at any of these tests, you may not need an iron supplement. If it's below that, you do; exactly how much supplementation you need depends on your test results.

• *Recurrence:* If you develop anemia in one pregnancy, it doesn't increase the risk that you'll develop it in your next pregnancy.

Gestational Diabetes

Gestational diabetes occurs in approximately 5 percent of pregnancies, making it one of the more common pregnancy-related health complications. If the condition is detected and managed well, it should not affect your health or that of the baby.

When you eat, food is converted to sugar (glucose), which first enters your blood and then is fed to your cells with the help of insulin, a hormone produced by the pancreas. If the body doesn't produce enough (or any) insulin, too much sugar remains in the blood instead of being delivered to the cells for conversion into useful energy. This (basically) describes diabetes.

During pregnancy, you produce a hormone called human placental lactogen (HPL), which makes the body use insulin less efficiently (a phenomenon known as an anti-insulin effect). When the body can't compensate for the anti-insulin effect of HPL, too much sugar remains in the blood after a meal. This is what's known as *gestational diabetes*. It's directly related to pregnancy and usually clears up after you've given birth. (But women who develop gestational diabetes have a greater risk of developing diabetes later in life.) The anti-insulin effect of HPL peaks between twenty-four and twenty-eight weeks, the time frame in which you'll be tested (see page 297). After it peaks, HPL levels remain constant.

• *The risks:* If gestational diabetes is left unchecked, the fetus will get extra sugar from the mother's blood (sugar crosses the placenta easily), and the fetus will respond by producing more insulin. In a fetus, insulin not only lowers blood sugar but also acts as a growth hormone. When a mother's blood sugar isn't under control, the baby will get too much sugar, produce too much insulin, and grow very large, which could lead to a complicated delivery.

Also, if a mother's blood sugar is high, a newborn's blood sugar could drop precipitously right after birth. The scenario goes like this: High blood sugar in the mother leads to high blood sugar in the baby at birth. Because of excess blood sugar, the newborn has high levels of insulin. Once born, the baby no longer gets sugar from the mother's blood, and the baby's high insulin levels will cause a quick drop in her blood sugar. This can lead to metabolic problems. Therefore, if you have gestational diabetes, it's likely your baby's blood sugar will be checked directly after birth. If it's low, you'll feed her as soon as possible with breastfeeding, formula, or a little sugar water. In some hospitals, depending on the test results, the baby is fed by IV. (Different hospitals have different protocols.) If you're concerned, ask your doctor or midwife about the procedures where you'll be giving birth.

Gestational diabetes can also lead to a high amniotic fluid level.

Most dangerous of all, though, if blood sugars are not controlled through diet and/or insulin, the risk of stillbirth goes up. No one really knows why this happens, only that it does. Because of the various risk factors gestational diabetes creates, women with it may be more closely monitored by non-stress tests and possibly biophysical profiles (pages 299 and 288) as their pregnancies near term, especially if they don't give birth by their due dates.

• *Symptoms:* The condition has no distinctive symptoms, which is why every pregnant woman is screened for it. If you have gestational diabetes, you may find you're thirsty and tired, and you have to urinate frequently. Then again, since those are symptoms of pregnancy, you might not think twice about them.

• *Diagnosis:* Between weeks 24 and 28 you'll be tested for gestational diabetes by a glucose screen (see page 296). If that test is positive, you'll have a glucose tolerance test (see page 297). Only 15 percent of women who have a positive result in the glucose screen go on to test positive for gestational diabetes.

• *Treatment:* Gestational diabetes can usually be managed through diet, regular testing, and exercise. The gestational diabetes diet I recommend is a "low glycemic" diet, meaning it's limited to foods like whole grains, proteins, and certain fruits and vegetables that the body can process slowly (as opposed to "high glycemic" foods that give the body a quick jolt of sugar). Most women diagnosed with gestational diabetes will get a home testing kit that they use to check their blood sugar throughout the day, initially four times a day, after fasting (i.e., after sleeping and before breakfast), and two hours after each meal. Depending on your situation, you may be able to test fewer times a day.

• *Recurrence:* If you have gestational diabetes in one pregnancy, you're more likely to develop it in your next pregnancy.

REAL VOICES

I had wondered about having gestational diabetes in my first pregnancy because every morning at eleven I would get dizzy and disoriented and shaky. I didn't have any other symptoms, and I knew that most women don't. I got tested at twenty-eight weeks, and I failed the first test. Then I went back for the next test, which confirmed that I had gestational diabetes. By the time I actually got the results back and met with the nutritionist, I was almost thirty-two weeks, and I delivered at thirty-seven—so I only had five weeks on the diet. With the diet I was on, you eat six times a day, and it's all the foods I normally eat, thankfully. I could even have a tiny portion of frozen yogurt at night. Those first couple of days, though, I was so upset! I felt so hungry all the time and so deprived because I couldn't snack the way I wanted to. Once I got past the feeling that I would be hungry all the time, the diet actually sustained my sugars really well. I never felt shaky—it was great.

Mary, mom of two

Incompetent Cervix

This poorly chosen term refers to a cervix that opens up too early in a pregnancy. The cervix is the lower end of the uterus; it is made mostly of connective tissue (collagen) and about 10 percent muscle. The cervical canal connects the cervix and the vagina. (The opening into the uterus is known as the "internal os"; the opening into the vagina is the "external os.") Your menstrual flow—and baby—passes through this canal. When you're not pregnant, the cervix is rigid. During pregnancy, it softens slowly over the course of the forty weeks and opens toward the very end.

If, however, the cervix softens and begins to open between fourteen and twenty-four weeks, the softening may, tragically, cause the baby to be born extremely early. This is what's meant by the term "incompetent cervix." The cervix opens prematurely, and the membranes either rupture or press into the vagina. Then there's a very mild labor with little or no cramping or contractions. The baby just seems to "fall out" with a gush of fluid or a feeling of fullness in the vagina. It's a relatively uncommon event (good statistics of its frequency are hard to come by for a variety of reasons having to do with reporting and assessing the condition), but, unfortunately, there's no way to predict whether or not it will happen in a first pregnancy. That said, there are situations in which the risk is greater. These include: if your mother took DES (diethylstilbestrol, a synthetic form of estrogen that was prescribed until 1971) during her pregnancy with you; if you've had surgery on the cervix (such as a cone biopsy or LEEP, a treatment for cervical dysplasia); or if you've already suffered a miscarriage due to an incompetent cervix.

• *Interventions:* Unfortunately, if a woman goes into labor in the first half of pregnancy, there's little that can be done to stop it from progressing to miscarriage. Before her next pregnancy, though, her care provider will try to figure out if the loss was in fact due to an incompetent cervix, or to another cause. Was her labor really painless? Had cramping preceded it, or was it very sudden? If it was painless and sudden, then in all likelihood an incompetent cervix caused the loss and not another issue, such as an anatomical malformation of the uterus, which would be treated by surgery between pregnancies.

In her next pregnancy, a woman with an incompetent cervix (or any of the risk factors described above) would be watched very closely for signs of preterm labor. For example, she would have weekly or biweekly sonograms of her cervix starting at twelve weeks to see if it's shortening or if the pregnancy sac is descending in the uterus. Often, close monitoring is enough to prevent another loss.

If the cervix starts to shorten and/or if the pregnancy sac presses into the top of the cervical canal, then a stitch, called a cerclage, might be put into the cervix. (There are a number of different stitch techniques that might be used, depending on the patient's history.) Bed rest may be prescribed, but this, too, depends entirely on the patient's particular situation and history. Typically, the stitch is removed around thirty-six to thirty-seven weeks.

• *Nutritional note:* Vitamin C is essential to the production and maintenance of collagen, the connective tissue that makes up 90 percent of the cervix. Therefore, when I'm working with a woman who may have an incompetent cervix, I recommend she take extra vitamin C—up to 3 grams a day, as long as she doesn't develop diarrhea.

This nutritional strategy isn't widely embraced in the conventional medical community and, admittedly, there are not data to support it. But theoretically it's possible that it could help, and it can't hurt.

Depression in Pregnancy

✦ The enormous emotional, physical, and hormonal changes of pregnancy create a risk of depression, particularly in women who have a history of depression. The noticeable symptoms are similar to those of depression at any time in life: not eating enough or eating too much, not sleeping (and not because of the need to go to the bathroom frequently), having low energy or feeling distracted, an inability to get out of bed and face the day, feeling worthless or guilty (sometimes women may despair because they don't think they can be good parents), having difficulty enjoying activities (especially those a woman used to enjoy), tearfulness (sometimes a woman's partner will call because he's concerned that she seems to be crying a lot), or repeatedly thinking about death. If it's not treated, depression in pregnancy increases the risks for a low-birth-weight baby and postpartum depression.

When a pregnant woman I'm working with develops depression, I most often suggest consulting with a psychologist, psychoanalyst, or psychiatrist to explore talk therapy and/or medication. It takes a trained mental health professional to decide if medication is necessary and which of the many antidepressant medications that are safe in pregnancy is most likely to be successful for a particular person.

Once the need for medication has been addressed, simple interventions that I've seen improve mood, particularly with milder depressions, include setting up, and sticking to, a schedule of both moderate exercise (such as walking) and regular outdoor activity (such as gardening). Many patients find being in the sun helpful, especially those struggling with seasonal affective disorder (sadness during the darker winter months). If you find sunshine helpful *for you,* I would strongly consider buying a full-spectrum-light lamp.

Although it's not a standard therapy, I suggest taking 1,000 mg a day of DHA, an omega-3 essential fatty acid that has been shown to improve mood. In addition, I have seen acupuncture help in managing depression during pregnancy. Other types of body work (especially massage) or energy work (such as craniosacral therapy) can be useful as well.

Finally, since protein serves as a building block for the brain chemicals that prevent depression (neurotransmitters), low protein levels can contribute to depression. Consider discussing with your care provider whether or not you should have a urinary amino acid analysis done. The test, which falls under the category of "functional medicine" (see page 56), determines whether or not you're eating the right amount and type of protein to meet your particular needs. It's offered by Great Smokies Diagnostics Laboratory (*www.gsdl.com*), and it may not be covered by your insurance. Whether or not you decide to have the test done, sometimes simply eating more protein (especially when combined with increasing omega-3 essential fatty acids) can improve mood. (For a list of protein-rich foods, see page 229.)

Intrauterine Growth Restriction (IUGR)

IUGR is a condition in which a fetus doesn't grow at the expected rate, which creates the potential for certain health complications both in utero and shortly after birth. The term "IUGR" is commonly used for a fetus that appears to be in the bottom tenth percentile or lower for weight. This doesn't mean all small fetuses have IUGR or are at risk for complications once they're born. (After all, you'd expect 10 percent of infants to be in the bottom 10 percent for size. Some infants are simply small.) Complications are more likely in infants born below the bottom fifth percentile, and especially in those below the bottom third percentile, for size.

- *Causes:* A variety of factors may cause IUGR. These include:
  - – *Contact with toxins:* Through smoking, drug or alcohol abuse, and exposure to teratogens (chemicals or drugs that cause fetal malformations).
  - – *Weight and nutrition issues:* Such as a mother's failure to gain sufficient weight during pregnancy, being significantly underweight before pregnancy, or malnutrition.
  - – *Maternal medical conditions:* Including hypertension (both preexisting and from preeclampsia, see page 357), diabetes (preexisting, not gestational), and kidney disease.
  - – *Problems with the placenta:* Such as placental abruption and placenta previa (see pages 349 and 350), which potentially limit the flow of blood and nutrients to the fetus.
  - – *Multiple gestation:* Particularly when a woman's carrying more than two fetuses or when identical twins share a placenta.
  - – *Infections:* Including German measles, chicken pox, and toxoplasmosis.
  - – *A genetic disorder* in the fetus.
- *Diagnosis:* If, when measuring fundal height (see "Tracking Fetal Growth and Fundal Height" on page 338), your caregiver notices a surprising drop of two centimeters or more, he'll probably order an ultrasound to assess both the baby's growth and amniotic fluid levels. During the ultrasound, the baby's head circumference and diameter, abdominal circumference, and femur length will be measured, and the amniotic fluid level will be evaluated. (Either IUGR or low amniotic fluid levels— see pages 345 and 336—may have caused the change in fundal height. With IUGR, amniotic fluid levels might be low, but they can also be normal or high.) Finally, a weight estimate will be calculated, although by the end of a pregnancy, fetal weight is difficult to measure accurately.

IUGR would be suspected if the baby appears small overall, or if the baby's head is much larger in proportion to her body, measured as the ratio of head circumference to abdominal circumference. This ratio is useful because a fetus reacts like an adult when food is scarce—the nutrients will go to the fetus's most vital organs, primarily the brain, and as a result, if the fetus is not getting enough food, the head circumference will be that much greater than the abdominal circumference.

- *Follow-up:* After a diagnosis of IUGR, or if it's strongly suspected, a Doppler may be used to measure how well blood is flowing through the placenta (see

How to Track Fetal Movement

✦ Fetal movement is one of the best indicators of fetal well-being we have—a baby that moves consistently is a healthy baby. Starting somewhere between thirty-two and thirty-four weeks, it's helpful to set aside some time each day to check in with your baby and his movements. (This is good for you and the baby in many ways; see "Connecting with Your Baby Before Birth" on page 405.) When you do this, you develop a sense of your baby's habits. Even though their routines are likely to vary, babies tend to be active after you eat. (Some moms swear by chocolate to get their kids moving; others say a glass of ice water does the trick.) It's also useful to develop a sense of the type of movement you tend to feel. For example, if the movements are more often rapid kicks or long pulls, if they come in clusters or one at a time.

Caregivers give a range of the number of movements they recommend detecting within an hour each day—anywhere from six to ten. If you start to count movements, decide how many movements you'll count and use that number each time you do it (it may be daily). Use the following chart below or make one like it.

A movement may be short or long, but you know it's complete when there's a pause. Notice if there's a change in the type of movement you feel, for example if the movement feels less vigorous or just somehow different. If it does, put a call in to your care provider. If you don't feel the usual number of movements within an hour, eat something and keep track for a second hour. If you still don't feel enough movement, or if something seems off, call your caregiver.

Most of the time, when someone reports that the baby isn't moving, everything is fine. The mother may be working or taking care of other children, or just too busy to pay close attention.

Fetal Movement Chart

Instructions:

1. Count six movements from your baby, three times daily, after each meal.
2. Place your hands on your abdomen.
3. Record: (a) the time of the first movement: (b) the time of the sixth movement. If you feel lots of movement in the first minute, it counts as one movement.

4. If you do not feel six movements in one hour, begin hour #2. You must now start counting from one and get six new movements.
5. If you do not feel four movements at the end of the second hour, call your caregiver.

Tricks: (a) Count movements after you eat a meal.
      (b) Eat something sweet if you are not a gestational diabetic.

| | Morning | | Afternoon | | Evening | |
Date	1st Movement	6th Movement	1st Movement	6th Movement	1st Movement	6th Movement

"Doppler Blood Flow Measurement" on page 296). Other follow-up tests might include a biophysical profile and a non-stress test (see pages 288 and 299). Any or all of these tests may be repeated at regular intervals in order to keep track of how the baby is doing. Depending on your health, how near you are to your due date, and if the baby seems to be in some distress, your caregiver may recommend inducing labor or scheduling a C-section.

• *Recurrence:* Having had one baby who experienced IUGR does slightly increase your risk of having a second with IUGR. Therefore, in your next pregnancy you may have an eight-week ultrasound to get a better measurement of gestational age, and if smoking, high blood pressure, or a chronic health issue increases your risk for the condition, you may have sonograms frequently throughout your pregnancy to keep close tabs on the baby's growth.

Note: IUGR is a serious condition, but it can be difficult to diagnose. In general, babies born after being diagnosed with IUGR do well, but their health depends on what caused growth restriction (if it can be determined) and how close to term they were born, among other details.

Placental Abruption

When the placenta separates from the uterus at any time before birth, it's known as a placental abruption. The separation can be mild to severe. If a relatively minor separation happens before twenty weeks, it's most likely that it will heal and you'll carry to term. However, your caregiver may recommend closer monitoring for some period of time after an abruption because it puts you at risk for IUGR (see page 345).

Most abruptions occur in the third trimester. The diagnosing and reporting of abruption isn't consistent; based on generally accepted information, they happen in one in a hundred to one in two hundred pregnancies (1 percent to 0.5 percent).

• *Symptoms:* Painful bleeding of dark blood is the classic symptom, along with a hard or tense and painful abdomen.

• *Causes:* Causes of a placental abruption include a multiple pregnancy (twins or more), preterm labor (preterm labor can cause a placenta to separate if the placenta is near or over the cervix; or an abruption may trigger preterm labor because the blood irritates the uterus, which then starts contracting), a fall, or a car accident. In fact, anytime a pregnant woman's belly hits the ground or absorbs impact, she should contact her caregiver, who will check for an abruption. Most of the time, there's nothing to worry about, but if you fall, are hit, or are in an accident, you should discuss it with your caregiver and possibly be examined. If after an accident and an examination you don't develop any symptoms of an abruption within twenty-four hours, one isn't likely to develop.

The risk of losing a baby to an abruption goes up if you smoke—yet another good reason to stop smoking while you are pregnant.

• *Diagnosis:* Sometimes an ultrasound can diagnose a placental abruption. Otherwise, a doctor or certified midwife can make a diagnosis based on the individual's symptoms. During the evaluation period—that is, from the onset of symptoms through evaluation and diagnosis—a woman with a suspected abruption will probably be put on bed rest. How restrictive the bed rest is, and if it continues after a positive diagnosis, depends on her situation. Often, once any bleeding stops and a woman has a follow-up exam, she's taken off bed rest.

• *Follow-up:* If a minor abruption happens before twenty weeks, you will have frequent ultrasounds to confirm that it heals, that amniotic fluid levels remain normal, and that the baby continues to grow at a healthy rate.

When a minor abruption occurs after twenty weeks, the procedures for tracking how it heals and how the baby is growing include: ultrasounds, non-stress tests, and biophysical profiles (see pages 303, 299, and 288).

If the abruption is severe, the baby may need to be delivered—even if it's before thirty-seven weeks. Whether a vaginal birth or C-section is safer depends on the individual situation.

Placenta Previa

Placenta previa is diagnosed when the placenta implants over or near the opening of the cervix (known as the internal cervical os). The placenta can cover the cervix completely, or some percentage of it may lie over the internal os. The biggest concerns from a previa are heavy bleeding late in pregnancy and complications during labor and birth; the latter can be avoided with a Cesarean delivery (see "Birthing Options," page 352). When you have a complete previa, a care provider may also keep a close watch on the baby's growth. Because very little blood flows through the cervix, a complete placenta previa could mean somewhat reduced blood flow to the

Second Thoughts on Bed Rest

✦ About one in five women—or 20 percent—are prescribed some degree of bed rest during their pregnancies. "Bed rest" can mean anything from not being allowed to lift your head to being allowed to sit up, go to the bathroom, and walk up and down stairs once a day. Bed rest is most often prescribed to control preterm labor and complications, like IUGR or too little amniotic fluid, that threaten the health of a baby and the overall well-being of a pregnancy.

Recent studies, however, have shown that in the case of preterm labor, *strict* bed rest (when you can't get out of bed) doesn't necessarily prevent it, and the costs associated with bed rest—physical, emotional, and financial—can be quite high. While on strict bed rest, women can become weak, and they may find it difficult to care for their children once they're born. They can become depressed; and they may have to pay for extra help with other children and/or take a (possibly unpaid) leave from work.

Do these new studies mean that bed rest is never useful? No. In certain circumstances, strict or moderate bed rest is appropriate and will help a pregnant woman get closer to term. Some women find that bed rest decreases uterine activity and helps them maintain the pregnancy longer. Bed rest can help promote the growth of babies with IUGR and low amniotic fluid. Should prenatal health care providers think twice before prescribing bed rest? Absolutely. Bed rest can't be used indiscriminately. But, prescribed prudently, it's an effective and important tool.

baby, which could lead to a smaller baby. Placenta previa is reported in about 0.5 percent of live births (one in two hundred).

• *Causes:* Placenta previa occurs more frequently in women over thirty-five, typically those who have already given birth to several children, and in African-American women. Another risk factor is previous uterine surgery (like a C-section), when the placenta can implant over the scar.

• *Symptoms:* Painless, bright red bleeding in the second or the third trimester is the classic symptom of a previa. (If the bleeding is severe, which is relatively uncommon, delivery will have to take place immediately.) Sometimes, however, a previa doesn't bleed at all.

• *Diagnosis:* If you start to bleed bright red (new) blood, you'll have an ultrasound to determine if you have placenta previa. Alternatively, a previa may be detected in the second trimester during a level 2 ultrasound, given between weeks eighteen and twenty (see "Ultrasound—Level 2" on page 303). If a previa is spotted, your care provider may follow up with ultrasounds at twenty-four, twenty-eight, and thirty-seven weeks, or some combination thereof. Keep in mind, though, that a previa diagnosed early (at eighteen to twenty weeks) might not be present at your due date. Here's why. In an ultrasound, the placenta may appear to cover the cervix. As the uterus expands, the placenta, which is in a fixed position, can move farther away relative to the cervix. (Think of a balloon with a spot on it near the opening. As it fills up with air, the spot moves farther and farther up the side of the balloon.) By thirty-seven weeks, more than 90 percent of women diagnosed with placenta previa at eighteen to twenty weeks will no longer have the condition. A diagnosis of placenta previa is more worrisome after thirty-two weeks, when it's less likely that the relative position of the placenta will change significantly.

• *Follow-up:* If the placenta previa is still present at thirty-two weeks, you may start to have biophysical profiles and/or non-stress tests (see pages 288 and 299) to assess the baby's well-being, as well as ultrasound growth scans. The timing and prescribing of these tests will vary, and you should talk to your care provider about what tests she feels would be best for you.

• *Birthing options:* Birthing options must be evaluated individually based on the location of the placenta. For example, if the placenta completely covers the opening of the cervix, a C-section will be necessary. (Since the baby's blood supply comes from the placenta, and the cervix must open for the baby to be born, during a vaginal delivery with a previa, the baby could bleed to death and/or the mother could hemorrhage severely. This risk is significant.) If a very small portion of the placenta overlaps with the cervix, you may be able to try a vaginal delivery. Discuss with your care provider the possibility and safety of a vaginal delivery in your situation.

Note: If you're diagnosed with placenta previa, your caregiver may ask you to abstain from intercourse and possibly to avoid having an orgasm. Also, you may be put on bed rest, but that depends on where exactly the placenta is, how much bleeding you've had, and how far along you are.

Coping with Bed Rest

✦ *Let go of control and work with your partner:* Among my patients, one consistent challenge that bed rest brings is giving up control of their homes. A prescription for even limited bed rest often means negotiations with a partner about when and how chores get done. For example, your partner may do the laundry very differently from how you do it. This kind of thing can be aggravating at first—but liberating to let go of! Also, keep in mind that bed rest, while difficult and challenging for you, can put a lot of pressure on your partner, who might be working while caring for you and your other children (if you have them), and picking up additional responsibilities at home. All in all, stress and frustration between partners can build up quickly when you're on bed rest, and one way to defuse it is to talk directly about the situation. (This sounds simple but often isn't.)

Before you start the conversation, identify what's most important to each of you, what needs to get done in the house and what can wait, and then together decide when it's time to ask for help from a friend or family member or to look into hiring help. Sometimes, women find the process of evaluating their needs, talking to their partners about even the most mundane details of housekeeping, and letting go of a certain kind of control to be enormously and surprisingly cathartic. After sorting out the particulars, my patients talk about having more energy to concentrate on connecting with their babies or to work through anxiety they may have about the baby's health, their own health, and the upcoming birth.

• *Stress relief and visualizations:* I encourage women on bed rest, and those with any complication, to practice stress reduction exercises such as belly breathing (see page 63) and to adapt visualization exercises to help them connect with their children emotionally and energetically. For example, you might dedicate anywhere from five to fifteen minutes each day to visualizing your healthy baby, surrounded by water and warm light, safely tucked into your womb. You could imagine the placenta and umbilical cord, the physical connection between the two of you, pulsing not only with blood and nutrients, but also with love and joy. (See "Cultivating the Positive," page 355.)

• *Use your time:* No matter what, the hours on bed rest can get long. Friends and family can be an enormous source of support, but a project—like knitting a sweater, organizing family photos, reading parenting books or one of those books you never seem to have the time for—can really help. Some women find it useful to create a loose schedule; they set aside two-hour chunks for a project (organizing photos, a craft), reading, or watching a movie or a favorite TV show. A routine can be reassuring when everything feels out of control because you're consigned to the couch.

• *Stretching exercises:* Every day, practice simple stretching exercises. For example, lying on your back with a pillow under your hip to prop your left side up to a fifteen-degree angle, stretch your right leg out to the right side (you may want to loop an old tie or belt around your foot to get a deeper stretch), then switch sides (you can move the pillow if that's more comfortable for you). Next, again propped up on a pillow, bend your left knee and bring your left foot to the outside of your left hip (as in a "runner's stretch" or half of the yoga pose *supta virasana,* page 264), then switch sides. Roll your ankles and wrists to one side, then the other. Stretch your arms and shoulders by reaching your right arm up and bending it at the elbow so your right hand touches your left shoulder. Bring your left hand to your right arm just above your bent elbow and gently apply pressure. Switch sides. Don't lie flat on your back at any time on bed rest. If you're going to lie on one side without a pillow under your hip, choose your left side; it's better for circulation because of the location of major blood vessels.

• *Eating:* While on bed rest, you should still consume about the same number of calories per day as you normally would at your stage of pregnancy (see page 241). But because you can't move around, it's more important to eat nutritious foods like whole grains, fruits, vegetables, and low-fat proteins (chicken, fish, beans, nuts, nut butters), as opposed to foods with empty calories like candy, cookies, chips, and ice cream. That doesn't mean you have to avoid treats altogether, but it does mean you should try to be more moderate in eating them—both in portion and in frequency.

Have a frank discussion with your care provider about your diet while on bed rest. There are certain situations (such as managing preterm labor) where long-term bed rest does mean slightly reducing caloric intake, but there are others (such as IUGR) where it's important to maintain the normal number of calories recommended in pregnancy.

REAL VOICES

I was very distracted even before I went on bed rest with my twins. I mean, all I wanted in the whole world was to have these little children. I'm a big reader, but I found that I couldn't concentrate on reading or TV because I was so stressed about doing whatever I could to have healthy children. Then

Cultivating the Positive . . . Even on Bed Rest

✦ Bed rest can be extremely challenging physically and emotionally. I often ask the women for whom I prescribe it to have a phone session or two with Tullia Forlani Kidde, MSC, NCACII, NBCCH, a psychotherapist, spiritual counselor, and hypnotherapist with whom I work closely.

Q: What's important for women to know about bed rest?

Tullia F. Kidde: The first thing to understand about bed rest is that it inspires fear. This is normal, because the future is uncertain and you're worried about the health of the baby. But what's important is to learn how to overcome fear and then how to relax into a sense of trust that all will be well for you and your baby.

Q: How do you do that?

TFK: You start by identifying the positive aspects of the experience. Pregnancy is a very special time in life; it's a time of love and dedication to the task of nurturing a new life—there's sacredness to that work. So when you're in bed, consider the time as something of a gift, time that you can use to connect with the baby and work through your anxiety, which you can do primarily by breathing. All you have to do is breathe consciously, bringing slow, rhythmic breaths into the abdomen. You can set aside a specific time to do this each day, or simply start to breathe whenever the mood strikes you. Every time you feel fear or dark thoughts coming over you, breathe through them. If you're feeling bored or restless, slow down your breath and imagine it filling your womb with energy, hope, and love. Really immerse yourself in your breath, swim in it, and let it relax you, as it does naturally. But if breathing becomes boring or your attention is wandering, don't try to focus on it and return to normal.

Affirmations also help women learn to relax and develop a sense of trust. You can repeat an affirmation such as:

- I am peaceful and serene. I am well.
- My baby is growing well and is strong. I trust in the best outcome.
- I let go of fear and doubt. I am peaceful and serene.

Create an affirmation that suits you.

When you use an affirmation in a situation like bed rest, repeat it so only these words fill your mind and nothing else can penetrate. That way, the feeling behind the words is absorbed into your subconscious. As with breathing, you can practice repeating an affirmation at any time in the day when you have five minutes during which you know you won't be disturbed. Also, repeat the affirmation before going to sleep, because our subconscious mind will respond to the last thing it's aware of before drifting off to sleep.

Q: What practical strategies do you recommend to women on bed rest?

TFK: Well, I don't think it's constructive to spend a lot of time on the phone talking about how boring bed rest is or how anxious you are—especially if you're telling this to a very emotional person who will egg you on. While it's important to give yourself the space to feel and express your anxiety, discomfort, boredom, etc., it's most useful to do so with someone who can be objective, someone who won't feed your fears and will help you move from a negative space to a more positive one. This can be a therapist or a friend whom you know to be level-headed.

Also, have some fresh flowers or a plant in the room. Even if it's only one bud, a flower can remind you of the natural world and your place in it as someone nurturing new life.

Spend time doing something you love to do right now—reading, a craft, listening intently to music—whatever it is.

Finally, find ways to bring in joy and humor. Watch good movies, read books you've always wanted to, look at pictures of joyous moments of your life, read a favorite story to your baby, which will enrich your relationship from the start.

Try to remember that this isn't a time for gloom and doom, and that with good prenatal care the odds are very good that everything will be fine.

While you're on bed rest, it can feel like a big risk to fall further in love with your baby. But life, and love, take courage. We can choose to spend our time protecting ourselves or trying to open our hearts and spirits as much as we can.

somebody gave me the great advice that I should teach myself a skill, and so I taught myself to quilt. Before I went on bed rest, I managed to pick fabric and take a couple of classes. I had my husband do the cutting and measuring, and lying down, I made this crazy quilt that I'm still so proud of. By the end, I had such bad carpal tunnel that I couldn't move the needle unless I held it with a pliers! But I did that because I was determined to finish that quilt. I finished it on April 7 and they were born on April 10.

Katherine, mom of two

Preeclampsia

Preeclampsia is a mysterious and potentially dangerous syndrome that affects 3 to 7 percent of pregnancies. (Some estimate that it affects as many as 10 percent of pregnancies.) Once called toxemia, preeclampsia can range from mild to severe. It usually appears in the second half of pregnancy, most often in the third trimester. The earlier it appears, the more severe it's likely to be. It most often affects first pregnancies.

Left unchecked, preeclampsia can limit blood flow to the baby, putting him at risk for IUGR and, in severe cases, stillbirth. In the mother, untreated preeclampsia can lead to a stroke, hemorrhage, seizures, and even death.

No one knows what causes preeclampsia, but the body has a complex reaction when the syndrome strikes. It seems that some women have a particular response to a chemical in the blood that's unique to pregnancy. The chemical triggers a narrowing of the blood vessels, which constricts blood flow and raises blood pressure. Higher blood pressure can cause lesions to form in the kidneys, which then don't work normally and leak protein into urine. (Protein in urine is an early sign of preeclampsia, and it's one of the reasons you give a urine sample at every prenatal visit.) Extra protein in the urine means there's not as much protein in the blood, which makes the blood thinner. Because the blood is more dilute, water leaches out of it in order to establish a balance between the fluids outside the blood vessels and the blood within. (This follows a basic principle of chemistry that water likes to create equal concentrations in neighboring environments.) This leads to swelling, also called edema, often in the face. (Ironically, a woman with swelling from preeclampsia sometimes needs to be given fluids to replace those lost from her blood.) Other symptoms of preeclampsia include blurry vision, pain around the liver (in the right upper quadrant of the torso), and, in severe cases, an inability to stop bleeding (see *Symptoms*, below).

• *Symptoms:* These symptoms can appear individually or in clusters of two or more. Call your caregiver if you feel you have any or several of these symptoms, or if you simply don't feel right:

— *Pain around the liver* (in the right upper quadrant of the torso)
— *Blurry or double vision or seeing stars*
— *Persistent headache:* Either a headache that you'd describe as "usual" or "mild" that lasts at least two days or a very severe headache no matter the

duration (it deserves evaluation even if it lasts only an hour). Either a short or long headache would be more worrisome if it didn't improve after taking acetaminophen (Tylenol).

— *Dizziness*

— *Swelling (edema):* Normal, pregnancy-related swelling is affected by gravity; it gets worse later in the day and is mostly in your hands, legs, and feet. By comparison, gravity doesn't affect swelling from preeclampsia. This swelling is severe throughout the day (though it may be better in the morning), and it's especially noticeable in the face, specifically around the nose.

— *Sudden weight gain due to swelling*

— *Bleeding that can't be stopped* (from the gums or nose, for example)

— *High blood pressure*

— *Protein in urine*

Note: Nausea and vomiting, rapid heartbeat or a racing pulse, stomach pain, or right shoulder pain are less common symptoms of preeclampsia.

Caution: Contact your care provider right away, day or night, if you have blurry vision, sudden pain in the right upper quadrant of your torso, or a severe headache that doesn't get better after taking acetaminophen.

• *Diagnosis:* Because preeclampsia can appear through a range of symptoms, it can be difficult to diagnose. If a woman displays any one of the classic symptoms (headache, blurry vision, right upper quadrant pain), her blood pressure will be taken, and blood and urine tests collected when she goes to her caregiver's office or an emergency room. Taken together, the results of these tests contribute to a diagnosis of preeclampsia. If a woman is diagnosed with the condition, she'll be followed closely with biophysical profiles and possibly non-stress tests (see pages 288 and 299 for a description of these tests), and delivery may be considered.

• *Treatment:* How preeclampsia is treated depends on its severity. Since there's no known cure—besides giving birth—the goal of treatment is to keep the syndrome under control for as long as possible, so a woman can get as close to her due date as possible. In very mild cases, a woman may be asked to limit her activities, stop exercising, and generally take it easy. In moderate but still relatively mild cases, modified bed rest, which helps keep blood pressure low and improves blood flow to the kidneys, may be prescribed. Medication and/or hospitalized bed rest may be necessary in more severe cases. In the most extreme cases, the baby must be delivered, no matter how early in the pregnancy it is.

Stress Relief Exercises for Preeclampsia

✦ Any mind-body exercise that you're comfortable with can be adapted to preeclampsia. You can adapt a visualization exercise to the specifics of your condition or meditate daily to help clarify your feelings about the syndrome and manage its symptoms. Here are two examples:

• *Visualization (for high blood pressure):* Begin by practicing belly breathing for a few minutes. (For a complete description, see page 63.) Slowly inhale and exhale, focusing exclusively on your breath. Say the word "soft" on the inhale and "belly" on the exhale. Once you're relaxed, begin to imagine your blood vessels and your heart. Don't worry about being scientifically accurate, simply call to mind an image that makes sense to you right now. Since your blood pressure is high and your whole cardiovascular system is working hard, imagine your heart and blood vessels working together in a relaxed and easy fashion. See your blood move smoothly through your blood vessels, which contract just enough to maintain a healthy flow. The blood moves easily, carrying with it calm, soothing, nourishing energy that reaches into every corner of your body and brings your baby nutrients, warmth, and love. Let your senses quiet down as you stay with the image for several minutes allowing yourself to experience the healthy, easy flow of blood and the serenity you have within you. When you feel ready, slowly draw your focus away from the image you've been holding and bring it back to your breath. Begin to practice belly breathing once again, and gently reenter your day.

• *Meditation:* If you're on bed rest or you're modifying your activity, it can be challenging to practice a meditation based solely on your breath (see page 63). But meditation can have enormous benefits when you're trying to manage preeclampsia (or any type of high blood pressure), so it's worth trying even once to see if it helps you. If it does, try to meditate regularly. If you already meditate regularly, by all means continue to do so. One technique that can be helpful if you're new to meditation and have preeclampsia is a concentrating meditation using a candle. (For a description of different types of meditation, see page 67.)

Begin by setting up a candle where you can see it easily and comfortably. Light the candle and focus on its flame by gently narrowing your eyes so that the light from the flame appears to expand in many directions. Continue to focus your attention on the flame, paying close attention to its dancing movements. When you feel your gaze is fully on the flame, relax your eyes and slow your breathing. Let your mind and senses quiet as you concentrate on the flame. As you sit for five to fifteen minutes, or until you feel satisfied, let your mind be empty, free of thoughts or worries. Just let yourself be, and breathe with the flame. When you feel complete, blow out the candle, continue to breathe quietly and steadily for a minute or two, and then slowly return to your day.

• *Nutritional/supplement recommendations:* In cases of mild preeclampsia, I recommend taking:
  – 400–600 mgs of magnesium daily to help lower blood pressure
  – 400 IUs of vitamin E daily (in addition to the 30–40 IUs in your prenatal vitamin) as an antioxidant (do not exceed 800 IUs total)
  – 1,000 mg of vitamin C daily (in addition to what's in your prenatal vitamin) as an antioxidant
  – Up to ten three-ounce servings of brightly colored fruits and vegetables per day for a whole food source of antioxidants (Ten servings sounds like a lot, but three ounces is less than half a cup, and at that size, servings add up fast.)
  – 3 mg of folic acid daily (in addition to what's in your prenatal vitamin); you may need up to 5 mg, depending on your homocysteine levels (see note, pages 361–362)

These recommendations are based on promising new research documenting low levels of antioxidants in women with preeclampsia. Low calcium levels have also been shown to have a relationship to preeclampsia, so it's very important to make sure that you're getting 1,500 mg of calcium per day, either through supplements, food, or some combination thereof. (For more on calcium in pregnancy and calcium-rich foods, see page 220. Do not take more than 2,500 mg of calcium per day.)

In all cases of preeclampsia, mild and more severe, I recommend taking 3,000 mg a day of omega-3 essential fatty acid (fish oil) supplements (equal parts EPA and DHA). Omega-3 essential fatty acids are considered a promising, if not yet thoroughly studied, nutritional intervention for managing preeclampsia. They've got many additional benefits for pregnancy (see page 227), they certainly won't make the preeclampsia worse, and they may even help improve things. *Only take a supplement that guarantees it's free of PCBs and heavy metals.* (See "Resources," page 522, for recommendations.)

> ## Preeclampsia—Related Syndromes
>
> ✦ *HELLP syndrome:* A severe form of preeclampsia, HELLP stands for hemolysis (when the body breaks down its own red blood cells), elevated liver enzymes, and lowered platelets. It's diagnosed through blood tests and occurs in 2 to 12 percent of women who develop preeclampsia. Women with HELLP don't necessarily have high blood pressure or protein in their urine; instead, they have stomach or right shoulder pain, nausea or vomiting, or flulike symptoms. In fact, HELLP can be mistaken for the flu or a gallbladder problem. Management and treatment—including bed rest, medication, and delivery—is the same as for preeclampsia.
>
> • *Eclampsia:* Eclampsia is an extremely rare form of severe preeclampsia marked by seizures and the temporary loss of consciousness. Magnesium sulfate, as well as delivering the baby, is the standard medical treatment for eclampsia.

Note: These recommendations for using nutritional supplements to manage preeclampsia are not generally accepted in the conventional medical community. They are based on the latest scientific literature as well as my collaboration with Magdy S. Mikhail, MD, a colleague at Albert Einstein College of Medicine, who has researched and published in the area of antioxidants and preeclampsia.

- *Risk factors for preeclampsia:*
  - First-time pregnancy
  - If a mother is over forty or under eighteen
  - Previous case of preeclampsia
  - Family history of preeclampsia
  - Obesity
  - Pregnant with multiples
  - A history of chronic high blood pressure, diabetes, or a kidney disorder
  - Being African-American

Note: It's long been known that African-American women have a higher risk of developing more severe preeclampsia earlier in pregnancy. Why this is remains a mystery, but one recent study sheds some light. In a small sample of white and

African-American women, researchers found that the African-American women who developed preeclampsia had higher levels of an amino acid called homocysteine and lower levels of folic acid than the white women in the study. The study opens the door for further research into the role of folic acid in preeclampsia. In the meantime, it may be worthwhile for African-American women with elevated homocysteine levels to take an extra 3 mg a day of folic acid (or as little as 1 mg and as much as 5, depending on their individual homocysteine levels, the type of folic acid they take, and their care providers' recommendations).

In addition, I would recommend that all women with, or at risk for, preeclampsia have their homocysteine levels checked and take enough folic acid and B vitamins to keep them in the normal range. This is not a standard test or treatment, but if you're concerned about preeclampsia, discuss these recommendations with your care provider.

REAL VOICES:
When I had my first baby, most of the pregnancy was normal, but I started to retain a lot of water at about thirty-six weeks. At that point there was no definitive diagnosis of preeclampsia, but the doctor I saw that visit was concerned and had me come in once a week or so for blood pressure checks and to make sure that everything was staying on track. At about thirty-eight weeks my blood pressure went up, but they didn't start talking about taking the baby out, they just kept monitoring me. Right around the baby's due date they said, "You have preeclampsia, we're not going to induce yet. We're going to watch your blood pressure and make sure that you don't fall apart. Let's see if the baby comes out on his own, but take it easy." But, again, it was really mild. It wasn't what I had always heard about preeclampsia, you know, "Must induce immediately!" None of that. Instead, I took it easy, and they checked my blood pressure every day. Six days after that—I probably wasn't taking it easy enough—I was walking around the San Francisco Museum of Modern Art with my mom because I was desperate to get out of the house. I started to get really dizzy, I got a really bad headache, and my hands swelled up. I mean, I had ditched my rings and most of my shoes weeks before, but now my hands started swelling up so badly that I had to hold them up in the air. It was really scary. A midwife who I saw a lot of the time (I went to a combined MD-midwife practice) had me come in right away. Then she sent me to neonatal testing, and they said, "We're going to induce tomorrow. You're done." After twenty-four hours of labor, I ended up having a C-section. . . . For me, the preeclampsia wasn't that bad, but it was a really good reminder

that stuff can happen, that this is why you get all the medical care you do, this is why you need to watch out for things.

Jill, mom of two

Preterm Labor

Preterm, or premature, labor is defined as labor that begins before thirty-seven weeks. Preterm labor occurs in about 12 percent of pregnancies, and it can be spontaneous or planned. The latter is labor that's induced in response to a health problem with the mother or baby, such as preeclampsia, low amniotic fluid, or IUGR.

Spontaneous premature labor can occur for a number of reasons, including infection, too much amniotic fluid, multiples, an anatomical problem with the uterus, in reaction to a trauma such as a fall or a car accident, or, as is most often the case, for unknown reasons. It can be mild—for example, you can have contractions that are controllable with moderate bed rest and don't progress to full-blown labor—or it can be more severe and contractions will progress relatively rapidly into labor. Depending on when and how labor begins, medication may be used to stave off delivery for several days.

• *Symptoms:* Premature labor doesn't necessarily feel like regular labor (or how you'd imagine regular labor to feel). A woman might feel pressure in her pelvis; she could have a backache, increased vaginal discharge (it would be watery, mucuslike, pink, or bloody), spotting or bleeding, menstrual-like cramps, and contractions that may or may not be painful. While these are typical pregnancy symptoms, if you have one of them and it's more noticeable than usual, you should call your caregiver that day. If you have more than one of these symptoms, call your caregiver immediately. (See sidebar for a complete list of symptoms.)

• *The risks:* Preterm labor can pose serious risks to the baby—how serious a risk depends on how early the baby is born. Babies born between thirty-four and thirty-seven weeks are typically healthy. While they might have to spend some extra time in the hospital, they generally don't experience serious health complications.

Babies born between thirty and thirty-four weeks most often come home from the hospital in good health, but they are at risk for neurological, digestive, or breathing problems. Later in life, some of these children *may* have developmental issues such as learning problems.

SYMPTOMS OF PRETERM LABOR:

Contact your care provider immediately if you experience any combination of these symptoms:

- Increased vaginal discharge that's watery, mucuslike, pink, or bloody
- Vaginal bleeding or spotting (It's usually dark in color.)
- Lower back pain (It's typically dull.)
- Pressure in the pelvis
- Contractions: more than four in an hour for two hours
- Menstrual-like cramps
- Abdominal cramps with or without diarrhea

Twenty-eight weeks has long been considered the benchmark for "viability"; that is, the chances that a baby born at twenty-eight weeks will survive are extremely good. How good depends on the particulars of the situation (the baby, access to sophisticated and experienced care, etc.).

Babies born before twenty-six weeks face the grave risk of death in the first few days and weeks of life. Once stable (because of advances in medical care, many babies can be stabilized even at this early gestational age), they generally stay in the hospital until close to their due date (although sometimes they're released weeks sooner), and they're followed closely after being discharged.

If you're currently being treated for preterm labor, I strongly recommend talking with your provider about the risks to your baby if he were to be born prematurely. Depending on how far along you are in your pregnancy (and certainly if you are thirty-three weeks or less), you might want to include a specialist in the care of newborns (neonatologist) in the discussion.

• *Diagnosis:* If you and your care provider suspect preterm labor, you'll go into the office for an examination. Your care provider will assess your cervix to see if it's at all dilated (open) and/or effaced (thinned). You'll probably be put on a monitor to see if you're actually having contractions. If so, you might be given IV fluids since dehydration is associated with contractions (including Braxton Hicks, see page 193) and preterm labor. If the contractions stop after you receive fluids, you'll be allowed to go home, with the instructions to stay hydrated and take it easy.

Depending on your symptoms, your caregiver may recommend giving a fetal fibronectin test (see page 302). Fetal fibronectin is a protein that's not normally found in the vagina or cervix after twenty-two weeks. If it's there, labor may begin within the next two weeks. You might also have a transvaginal ultrasound to measure cervical length, because a shortened cervix puts you at risk for preterm labor. If your cervix is short, your caregiver may suggest follow-up sonograms every week or even every few days.

- *Risk factors:*
    - Having already delivered a preterm baby (the earlier the previous delivery, the greater the risk in the next pregnancy)
    - Pregnant with twins or higher-order multiples, particularly if you conceived using artificial reproductive technology
    - A uterine or cervical anatomical abnormality
    - Fibroid(s), particularly a large fibroid
    - Too much amniotic fluid
    - Being African-American (17.4 percent of African-American babies are born prematurely)
    - Low pre-pregnancy weight (a BMI of under 19.5; see appendix 4)
    - Low weight gain during pregnancy
    - Being younger than eighteen or older than forty
    - Conceiving within six to nine months of giving birth
    - Continuous high stress levels or standing during work more than forty hours a week
    - Smoking, alcohol, or illegal drug use (especially cocaine) during pregnancy

- *Treatment:* Unless the baby shows signs of distress (as determined by a biophysical profile or a non-stress test, see pages 288 and 299), the goal of treatment for preterm labor is to delay birth for as long as possible. The best way to do this depends entirely on the situation. For example, if you go into labor before thirty-four weeks, your water hasn't broken (in other words, your membranes are intact), and the baby's heart rate doesn't show signs of distress, you may be hospitalized and given IV fluids and possibly antibiotics (in case you have group B strep or another infection). You could also be given medication to stop the contractions and steroids to speed the development of the baby's lungs and other organs. (Magnesium sulfate and terbutaline are two drugs that are commonly given to control preterm labor.) Studies have shown that drugs don't stop labor for long periods, but they can give you enough time to take other medications, like steroids, that help mature the baby's lungs before birth.

If your water has broken, your care provider will have to balance the risk of delivery with the risk of developing an infection. (Once the membranes break, there's nothing keeping infection-causing bacteria out of the uterus.)

Sometimes, simply increasing your fluid intake and resting may control preterm labor. Or the labor may simply go away on its own after a limited hospital stay.

Note: While bed rest is often prescribed for preterm labor and in my experience often helps control it, there's no evidence from in-depth clinical studies that it actually helps limit or stop it. That said, if you go into preterm labor, it makes sense to take things easy and to stop exercise and sexual activity until the situation improves.

• *Herbal medicine for preterm labor:* When preterm labor is mild—that is, when contractions are persistent enough to warrant continued observation, examination, and reduced activity but not strong enough to require medication—blackhaw (*Viburnum prunifolium*) may be used to try to control uterine activity. This shrub is native to the northeastern United States and is closely related to the European shrub known as cramp bark (*Viburnum opulus*). In fact, both herbs are gentle and effective in slowing muscle spasms. While cramp bark may be used, blackhaw has a longer history and there's more evidence of its effectiveness.

Dose: For tea, add one teaspoon of recently dried inner bark to eight ounces hot water, steep for ten minutes, and drink up to three cups a day. Blackhaw may be combined with red raspberry leaf; the latter herb has a toning effect on the uterus. (See "Resources" for herb recommendations on page 523.)

Note: The medical material in this chapter was reviewed by Dr. Cynthia Chazotte, professor of clinical obstetrics and gynecology and women's health, and director of obstetrics and perinatology, Weiler Hospital of the Albert Einstein College of Medicine/Montefiore Medical Center.

18

Pregnancy Loss

Unfortunately, first-trimester miscarriages are not uncommon in the reproductive lives of many women. However, a loss between twelve and twenty weeks is rare, and stillbirth is even more unusual. (Helping my patients cope with stillbirth while performing the necessary medical care has presented one of the greatest challenges I've had as a doctor and a human being.) In this chapter, I discuss the signs, symptoms, and causes of losses at different stages of pregnancy and share some of what I've learned from my patients about coping with miscarriage. This topic is always difficult to discuss, but it is my sincere hope that the material I present here will be helpful.

❖   ❖   ❖

In this chapter you'll find:

- Early Miscarriage
- Recurrent Miscarriage
- Late Miscarriage and Stillbirth

Early Miscarriage

When a woman miscarries before week 12, it's considered an "early miscarriage." These losses most often occur by week 8. When a woman miscarries between nine and twelve weeks, the loss often appears to have taken place weeks before the symptoms of the miscarriage—primarily bleeding—begin. Estimates of the frequency of (first-trimester miscarriage) vary (some are as high as 35 percent), but it's widely accepted that 15 to 20 percent of pregnant women miscarry in the first trimester.

Miscarriage rates in general have gone up in recent years, partly because we're now able to diagnose a pregnancy much earlier, in some cases even before a missed period. Therefore, more women today know they've miscarried while, twenty years ago, they might've just assumed their periods were a little later and heavier than usual.

• *Symptoms of early miscarriage:* The intensity of the miscarriage symptoms is related to how soon the pregnancy stopped developing. For example, women who miscarry very early (before week 6) may have no symptoms other than a period that's late and slightly heavier than usual. Women who miscarry later will have more significant symptoms:

— *Bleeding:* The most typical symptom of a miscarriage, it can be bright red (if the loss is very recent) or dark brown (if the loss is older). Keep in mind that 10 to 20 percent of all pregnant women experience some spotting or bleeding over the course of their pregnancies. Just because you bleed, even if you bleed fairly heavily, it doesn't necessarily mean you're miscarrying.

That said, *any* spotting or bleeding *always* warrants a call to your caregiver—the urgency of the call depends on the nature of the bleeding. For example: Light spotting, for which you only need a panty liner, warrants a call to your care provider during the day but not necessarily in the middle of the night (unless you have some other symptoms, such as pain on one side, see note, page 369). If your care provider doesn't feel you need to come to the office, but you think you do, ask for an appointment anyway.

Continuous or heavy bleeding that requires changing a pad every hour or so means you should call your care provider immediately or go to the nearest emergency room. If you notice any clots or tissue (tissue would be pink, white, or grayish), try to collect it in a plastic bag or jar and put the bag or jar in an ice-filled container to keep the contents cool. Or if there are clots on your sanitary pads that look to you like they might contain pregnancy tissue, you could bring the pads into your caregiver's office. You and your caregiver can then decide if the tissue or clots should be tested to determine if the loss was caused by a chromosomal (genetic) abnormality.

What Your Caregiver Will Ask When You Call

✦ No matter how heavy the bleeding, there are standard questions your caregiver will have for you about the nature of your symptoms. Your answers will give her some idea of what's going on. These questions include:

- How long have you been bleeding?
- What color is the blood?
- Are there any clots or have you seen any tissue (pink, white, or grayish in color)?
- Do you have pain? What's it like? Is it located in a particular area? Is it like you're having a bad period?
- Are you at all dizzy or do you have shoulder pain? (Shoulder pain is a sign that an ectopic pregnancy has burst and is causing internal bleeding. This is a life-threatening emergency. If, early in pregnancy you have pelvic pain, vaginal bleeding or spotting, or shoulder pain, then call your caregiver and go to the nearest emergency room *immediately*.)

— *Cramping and pain* similar to that of a heavy period may also occur when you miscarry.

Note: If you have any bleeding accompanied by pain on one side, shoulder pain, or dizziness, you need to be checked for an ectopic pregnancy as quickly as possible. (For more on ectopic pregnancies, see page 125.) If you experience any combination of these symptoms, or just have severe pain in your shoulder, side, or pelvis, call your caregiver immediately, day or night, even if you're only spotting lightly.

• *Diagnosing and treating an early miscarriage:* After talking with your provider about the spotting or bleeding, you'll be asked to go to her office that day or the next, or to an emergency room, depending on your symptoms. You'll probably have an ultrasound to see if there's a fetal heartbeat and to check on the placenta. If there's no heartbeat, you've had a miscarriage. (Only an ultrasound can diagnose a miscarriage before any tissue has passed. After twelve weeks, the failure to hear a fetal heartbeat with a Doppler on the abdomen raises the suspicion of a miscarriage, but an ultrasound exam is necessary to confirm a loss. As a clinician, I find it's impossible to predict what an ultrasound will show: I've had women come to the office with

WHAT CAUSES SPOTTING OR BLEEDING IN THE FIRST TRIMESTER?

There are several causes of bleeding in the first trimester, most of which can be diagnosed by ultrasound:

• *Menstruation* (typically between weeks 4 and 5): While pregnancy hormones usually shut down the mechanisms that trigger menstruation, every so often they fail to do so completely. When this happens, you could have what seems like a very light period and still be pregnant.

• *Implantation* (typically between weeks 6 and 12): As the embryo burrows into the lining of the uterus and the placenta establishes its connection to the mother's blood vessels, a slight leak can develop, resulting in some bleeding.

• *Separation of placenta* (typically between weeks 8 and 12): The placenta, once established inside the uterus, can separate slightly. This can cause bleeding, which can sometimes be heavy. (See "Placental Abruption" on page 349.)

light spotting and an ultrasound showed there was no heartbeat, and women who've come in with heavy bleeding when I was very concerned something was wrong and we've found a healthy heartbeat.)

Once a loss is confirmed, you will have a pelvic exam so a care provider can see if your cervix is open or closed. At that point, she can assess whether or not, in her opinion, all of the tissue has passed. If the cervix is still open, or if there appears to be some tissue around it, a care provider will know that all the tissue hasn't passed, and can recommend the surgical procedure known as a D&C, which stands for *dilation and curettage*. During this procedure, the cervix is opened (dilated) to allow the doctor to remove the remaining tissue. If left in the uterus, the tissue could cause a serious infection. A D&C may be done in a hospital or a doctor's office, depending on the anesthesia used: local (an injection is given around the cervix), "twilight" (drugs are given that induce a sleepy, "dreamlike" state), or general ("going under"). General and twilight anesthesia are typically administered in a hospital; a doctor may use a local anesthesia in his office.

You don't necessarily have to have a D&C after a diagnosed miscarriage; if you choose to forgo the procedure, you may have to wait several days or weeks for the tissue to pass, you may experience prolonged bleeding when it does, and you have an increased risk of infection.

• *Follow-up:* After a D&C, there's the possibility of an infection developing, symptoms of which are pain in your lower abdomen, greenish or yellow discharge, and fever. I typically prescribe an antibiotic after performing a D&C. As always, whenever I prescribe an antibiotic, I recommend taking the probiotic acidophilus, two capsules a day of a reputable brand that guarantees between 2.5 and 5 billion live bacteria per capsule up through the expiration date. This helps maintain good bacteria in the gut, which antibiotics may break down. The only other testing routinely recommended is a blood test for Rh compatibility after a miscarriage if you haven't already had it done (see page 93).

Note: Medical professionals sometimes refer to miscarriages as abortions. This is the term medical textbooks use, but it can be painful to hear. If your caregiver uses "abortion" instead of "miscarriage" with you and you find it upsetting, let her know that you need her to be more sensitive about the language she chooses with you.

• *Using acupuncture and Chinese herbs after a loss:* If a miscarriage has been confirmed by ultrasound but the tissue or embryo sac has yet to pass, an experienced acupuncturist/Chinese herbalist can provide you with powerful Chinese herbs that are designed to make the uterus empty itself in the hope of avoiding a D&C. If you choose this option, you can avoid a surgical procedure, but the downside is you face possibly prolonged bleeding and the risk of infection. The herbs can't be used in certain circumstances—if you have fibroids, for example—which is why they should only be used under the supervision of a qualified herbalist. Discuss these issues with your practitioner and caregiver.

If you've had a D&C, a combination of Chinese herbs and acupuncture may be used to help you rebuild your energy and mend any slight internal bleeding that remains. In my own practice, acupuncture and Chinese herbs have been quite helpful in this regard.

REAL VOICES
We'd only been trying for a few months, but I was so excited to get pregnant! I'm such an inveterate reader that I was fairly circumspect and knew how common miscarriage was. But this was at eleven or twelve weeks, and I'd had an eight-week ultrasound and seen the heartbeat. I'd talked to my midwife about traveling, which she said was fine. The morning we were scheduled to leave for a two-week vacation in Morocco, I started bleeding. I called my midwife, and I was so relieved because she said it could just be spotting, but to keep an eye on it. Over the course of the morning, the bleeding just got heavier, and I realized that I was losing the baby—and I wasn't going on vacation. At some point my midwife told me she was sending the doctor to

meet me at the emergency room. I have generally negative feelings about doctors, and I very consciously chose a midwifery practice that had a couple of doctors associated with it, but I have to say that for a horrible experience the doctor was like a textbook example of how to be humane and sympathetic. She was amazing. She met me at the emergency room and got me a little cube. While I was there I felt the tissue pass. Then she did an exam and said it looked like there might still possibly be something left so I had to have a D&C. She was really sympathetic about it. I had been crying my eyes out all day when it became clear that this pregnancy was over. But, thanks to drugs, I woke up after the procedure feeling much better. Afterwards, I think I was okay for a couple of months. I was just like, "We'll get back on the horse, we'll do it again." And it wasn't until three or four months later that I realized that I was *really* upset.

In retrospect, trying again was hard. Every month I wasn't pregnant, I felt worse. But I have a friend who'd delivered a stillborn baby, and compared to that? "Good Lord!" I thought, "I have no right to be so worked up about this." On the one hand, I thought I was being a drama queen, but on the other, I still felt miserable. At the time, I hated my job, so I quit and went back to freelance writing. And I started therapy, which was really important for me because I could just talk about what I was feeling without worrying about anyone else. I also read two books that really helped: *Miscarriage: Women Sharing from the Heart* and *Our Stories of Miscarriage*.

Marjorie, mom of one, pregnant

• *Recurrence:* Once you've miscarried, the fear of a second loss can be profound. Because the statistics that describe the risk of pregnancy loss include the full range of causes, including those related to age, if you've miscarried once, *statistically* speaking your risk of a second loss goes up *slightly*. But your own risk of another loss depends on the cause of the first loss. For example, if you've miscarried because of a chromosomal abnormality (a spontaneous event that's the most common cause of early pregnancy loss, see "Causes," page 373), your risk of a second loss doesn't go up (except when age is a factor).

The most important statistics to keep in mind are these: *At least* 85 percent of couples who've experienced one loss go on to have a healthy pregnancy the next time. *At least* 75 percent of those who've had two or three losses do the same. In the midst of all the negative feelings around a loss, I've found that it's often useful to remember these statistics because they reflect the *extremely* good odds that a woman who's miscarried will go on to have a healthy pregnancy.

• *Causes:* I don't want to sound preachy, but when considering the causes of a miscarriage, remember this important point: You can't cause a miscarriage. Not by going on an airplane, not by exercising, not by having sex. Even if you had a few drinks or a couple of cigarettes before you learned you were pregnant, it would have no impact on whether or not you miscarry. (If, however, after you learn you're pregnant, you continue to drink heavily, smoke heavily, or use illegal drugs, you do increase your risk of a miscarriage.)

That said, these are the basic medical causes of miscarriage:

— *Chromosomal abnormalities:* More than 50 percent of miscarriages can be traced to a chromosomal abnormality. A sperm and egg each contain 23 individual chromosomes. When they come together, the embryo that develops should have 46 chromosomes or 23 pairs (22 plus the pair that determines sex). However, the cell division that takes place in the first hours after conception is extremely complex, and mistakes can occur that result in, for example, an embryo having three copies of a particular chromosome instead of two. (The word "trisomy" refers to this phenomenon; "trisomy 21" means an embryo has three copies of the twenty-first chromosome. Trisomy 21 is also known as Down syndrome, and it's one of the few chromosomal trisomy errors that an embryo can survive.)

Whether or not a woman has an increased risk for a second loss due to a chromosomal problem depends on her age. The risk of a spontaneous chromosomal abnormality increases as a woman gets older. Risk increases significantly over thirty-five, but it's not confined to women over thirty-five. (Women who experience repeat miscarriages due to chromosomal abnormalities and/or those who are older may be candidates for pre-implantation genetic diagnosis (PGD). (See page 16.)

Diagnosis: A chromosomal abnormality can only be diagnosed by analyzing embryonic tissue that a woman has passed or that's collected from a D&C. This is why caregivers recommend saving any tissue that might be passed while bleeding.

— *Blighted ovum:* After conception, cells divide into those that will become the pregnancy sac and those that will become the embryo. With a blighted ovum, the pregnancy sac develops, but an embryo never does. A problem with the chromosomes of either the sperm or the egg is thought to be the cause, and it's more common among older couples (when the woman will be thirty-five or older at her due date; there are conflicting data on the effects of the father's age). The medical literature often makes a distinction between a blighted ovum and a miscarriage. But in both instances a pregnancy ends, so emotionally the distinction has always struck me as unnecessary.

Diagnosis: A blighted ovum may not be diagnosed until an ultrasound or Doppler exam at an eight- or twelve-week visit fails to find a heartbeat. An ultrasound exam can confirm a blighted ovum.

— *Progesterone deficiency:* When a woman doesn't produce enough progesterone in the second half of her menstrual cycle or after she conceives, her risk of miscarriage goes up significantly. This is sometimes called a luteal phase defect (see page 54). Using progesterone supplements in the form of pills or suppositories from when you learn you're pregnant through weeks 11 to 12, when the placenta takes over hormone production, can significantly improve your chances of carrying to term. Hormonal imbalances are thought to cause between 5 and 40 percent of miscarriages that occur before week 10.

Diagnosis: To diagnose a progesterone deficiency, a woman would have a blood test on day 21 of a (non-pregnant) cycle and/or an endometrial biopsy, in which a piece of the uterine lining (endometrium) is taken and analyzed. Because low levels of progesterone are a relatively common cause of miscarriage, your caregiver may recommend bloodwork after a first early miscarriage.

REAL VOICES

I miscarried the first time I got pregnant and found out afterwards that I had low progesterone. So in my next two pregnancies, I had to have these vaginal suppository things. That was a little scary because I had to take them until eleven or twelve weeks, and I had to have my blood taken every week, and then finally after twelve weeks I was in that period where I was like, "Okay, the baby's fine."

Shawn, mom of two

• *Miscarriage prevention:* I want to repeat that according to all the data, there's nothing *you* can do to prevent a first-trimester miscarriage once you're pregnant.

Even if your caregiver suspects a problem with the pregnancy or you start bleeding, a situation technically known as a "threatened abortion," there's no known intervention, except for maintaining normal progesterone levels, that can stop a loss from occurring—although taking it easy in this situation isn't a bad idea.

If, however, you've experienced more than one or two miscarriages, you can be tested for the potential causes discussed on page 373 and above and treated in any way that's appropriate.

• *Steps toward better health:* Given that for most women and couples there are no concrete medical steps to take after a miscarriage and before your next pregnancy, once you decide you're ready to try again, I would recommend taking steps toward improving your general emotional and physical well-being before becoming pregnant again.

Unless you have a preexisting medical condition that should be controlled before you conceive, improving your health before conceiving won't necessarily affect your risk of miscarrying, but it will improve your overall health in your next pregnancy. This doesn't mean that you have to be in tip-top shape or eat a perfectly healthy diet before you conceive again. From a medical perspective, none of that would make a difference when it comes to maintaining your next pregnancy. But from a commonsense perspec-

---

RISK FACTORS FOR MISCARRIAGE

Even though you can't prevent a miscarriage, certain factors may increase your risk of miscarrying. These include:

- Uncontrolled diabetes or high blood pressure
- An autoimmune disorder such as lupus or MS
- Anatomical problems in the uterus: fibroids, depending on their location, or uterine polyps or a structural anomaly of the uterus (see "Uterine Abnormalities" on page 381)
- Inadequate progesterone production in the second half of the menstrual cycle
- A previous miscarriage (see "Recurrent Miscarriage," page 378)
- When the mother is over thirty-five
- Smoking, drinking, or recreational drug use

---

tive, if you're feeling emotionally and/or physically worn out, it's reasonable to take steps to restore yourself in ways that are most important to *you* before embarking on the potentially demanding physical and emotional journey of trying to conceive and pregnancy. Simple steps that you might consider to encourage overall well-being include:

— Eating a clean diet (see page 28)

— Spending time outdoors walking, gardening, biking, or simply sitting and breathing

— Setting aside time to move your body each day, for example by exercising and/or dancing around your living room

— Seeking out a therapist or spiritual counselor

— Trying a complementary therapy that can help your body restore its energy,

From My Office: Making Sense of the Loss

✦ Whether or not you can pinpoint an identifiable cause for a miscarriage, like a chromosomal abnormality or a progesterone deficiency, I've found that some women are comforted when they find some kind of purpose for their loss. This doesn't help everyone, but for some it helps a deeper level of healing emerge.

I'll never forget the first time a patient who had been grieving a miscarriage described a loss in terms of a bigger purpose. Maggie had miscarried at eight weeks; it was her first pregnancy. At a follow-up appointment after the loss, I asked how she was feeling, and she began to describe how she felt a soul had been alive in her, very briefly, for a reason. She said, "Dr. Evans, I have to tell you, I had this very weird dream the other night. I dreamed that this very old soul was talking to me. She was a woman, and she said that she had wanted to figure out if she should take on a physical form again in order to progress further in her own growth. My pregnancy had allowed her to have the 'taste' of physical life that she needed to continue her own evolution. She was filled with gratitude towards me for allowing her to have that experience. I don't know why, but for some reason, I knew this old woman, this old soul, was my baby. And I feel much better knowing that I was able to help her."

After that conversation, I asked other women how they made sense of what had happened, and I was surprised at the range of responses.

Many more than I would have thought felt like Maggie did—that their baby had a soul that had been with them for a reason and their pregnancies had been a vehicle for something separate from themselves. Others felt that after the miscarriage they had greater insight into their own lives, particularly in areas of conflict, for example if a marriage was troubled or if a woman was very ambivalent about parenthood. Still others felt that their loss was heartbreaking, but without a greater spiritual or psychological purpose.

The point is there's no right or wrong way to understand a pregnancy loss, but every woman should take the time to make sense of her experience, grieve, and recover in her own way.

such as acupuncture, reflexology, or chiropractic. (For descriptions of each, see the CAM glossary in appendix 2.) I typically recommend pursuing the type of energy/body work that appeals to you. (For a discussion of preconception physical and emotional health, please turn to chapter 2.)

• *Lifestyle and emotional issues:* Because there's no scientific evidence to support recommending a particular lifestyle change or addressing an emotional need before trying to conceive again, many medical professionals don't raise these issues with their patients after a miscarriage.

I take a different approach simply because I trust the power of personal intuition to explain medically unexplainable events. I like to explore with a woman whether she believes, in her gut, that something she did contributed to her loss. If *she* thinks something in her life was a factor in her miscarriage, then I work with that belief and help her, if I can, confront and overcome any guilt she may feel. For example, I've had many women ask me if I thought the fact that they worked very long hours contributed to their miscarriages. My answer is always the same: "Do *you* think it affected you?" If a woman says yes, I explain that there's nothing in the medical literature to suggest that long hours would contribute to a miscarriage, but if she strongly feels that her workload influenced her loss, we'll talk about how she might be able to modify her work habits before she conceives again.

Whatever the issue is, and there are many that come up besides work (for example, problems in a marriage, emotional exhaustion from family stress), I've found it helpful for many of the women I've worked with to spend time exploring not only the emotions of grief and loss, but what the experience of the miscarriage exposed about their lives, relationships, and inner world. This is certainly not to say that working long hours, a shaky relationship, or ambivalence could cause a miscarriage, only that the process of grieving for the loss can sometimes bring unexpected clarity to a range of difficult life issues.

• *When is it safe to try again?* Physically, I recommend waiting until you've had two menstrual cycles before trying to conceive again.

It's hard to predict when you'll first menstruate after a miscarriage—it can happen in two weeks or three to four months. Most women will menstruate within three months. If you don't have a menstrual period within four to six months of a miscarriage, let your caregiver know—it's likely he'll give you medication to induce your period and run some tests to investigate reasons for the delay.

The emotional recovery from miscarriage, however, is as important as the physical, and for that there's no set time frame. Pregnancies begin in so many different ways—soon after starting to try, after months of trying, after fertility treatment, accidentally—that it's almost impossible to predict the impact a loss will have on a woman or couple who are trying to have a child, and what it means to be "ready" to try again. Each woman, and each couple, must come to their own decision about when the time is right.

REAL VOICES

Shortly after I got pregnant again after miscarrying, I was at a spa in Sedona for work. I was getting Reiki, which is the most *woo-woo* treatment in the world, and I was really hoping to have some kind of revelation. It was like I wanted to know somehow that the spirit of the miscarried baby was blessing the spirit of the new baby, or I just wanted some kind of sign that everything was going to be okay.

I was lying on the massage table and the woman's hands were, like, waving over my body in the bizarre way of Reiki, and I was waiting for something to happen but nothing did. Then all of a sudden a Samoyed came into the room—a big, white fluffy dog—and it lay down next to the massage table. I thought, "That is so cool, that this spa is so chill that they have these beautiful animals that can come in and it doesn't bother anybody." And the dog just went to sleep next to the table. And then I thought, "Okay. Wait. My eyes are closed." And I actually opened my eyes and looked, and there wasn't a dog there. But there was this feeling of "That's so nice." I just felt really calm and not worried. It didn't tell me this baby was going to be fine, but it told me *I* was going to be fine. I'm a little teary just thinking about it. It was this moment when I knew that I was going to survive, no matter what.

Marjorie, mom of one, pregnant

Recurrent Miscarriage

Your doctor or midwife may not recommend any testing beyond chromosomal testing of fetal tissue after one first-trimester loss. Traditionally, testing is recommended after three first-trimester miscarriages, at which point a woman is diagnosed with "recurrent miscarriages." But, depending on your situation (e.g., your age, how easily you've conceived, your general health, your feelings about medical testing), you may want to pursue testing after a second miscarriage. Talk with your caregiver about what kind of testing options are available, and decide what makes the most sense for you.

Causes of repeat miscarriage include the following (in alphabetical order):

• *Advanced maternal age:* Technically, this term applies to a woman who'll be thirty-five or older when she gives birth. Age is a risk factor for miscarriage because, as a woman ages, her egg supply does, too. It appears that when older eggs are fertilized, they're more likely to develop chromosomal abnormalities, such as Down syndrome.

Diagnosis: Doctors evaluate egg quality by testing the level of follicle-stimulating hormone (FSH) in a blood sample. A test known as the clomid challenge test could also be used to evaluate FSH levels and egg quality. (See page 53 for more on elevated FSH.)

Note: In my practice, we've found acupuncture/traditional Chinese medicine to be very helpful in treating women with diagnosed elevated FSH levels.

• *Chromosomal translocation in either parent:* If specific chromosomal abnormalities appear in the genetic test results of the pregnancy tissue, your caregiver might recommend that you and the baby's father be tested for what's called a chromosomal translocation. When someone has a chromosomal translocation, pairs of chromosomes are mismatched. In a typical set of chromosomes, the chromosome pairs, which scientists number, are matched—for example the eighteenth chromosome from the sperm is paired with a second eighteenth chromosome from the egg. But if someone, let's say the man in a couple, has a translocation, part of his chromosome 18 might be attached to his chromosome 21 and vice versa. Because all of the genetic material is present, the man is totally normal. However, since his sperm carry one copy of his chromosomes, there's a good chance it would include one of the flipped pairs. When a sperm with a translocation fertilizes an egg that has a normal set of chromosomes, the embryo will have abnormal chromosomes and a miscarriage will result.

Approximately 5 percent of couples struggling with repeat miscarriage have this problem. It can be diagnosed, but there's no treatment. (However, pre-implantation genetic diagnosis combined with in vitro fertilization offers couples with certain translocations a viable treatment option; see page 16.)

Diagnosis: A translocation is diagnosed by a simple blood test that analyzes all the chromosomes (karyotype). The test can be expensive, but most often it's covered by insurance.

• *Immune system problems:* Problems with a woman's immune system that contribute to first-trimester losses fall into two categories:

1. For unknown reasons, the body sometimes produces antibodies, known as auto-antibodies, that attack the body itself. (This is what happens in autoimmune diseases like lupus and MS.) Certain auto-antibodies, particularly

antiphospholipid antibodies and anticardiolipin antibodies, attack the surface of blood cells and cause excessive clotting. The clotting restricts blood flow to the embryo, denying the embryo needed nutrients and making miscarriage likely. When this is diagnosed, treatment with baby aspirin or heparin (the latter is taken by injection), both used to thin the blood, can help a woman avoid another miscarriage.

Natural supplements that have a very mild blood thinning effect include omega-3 essential fatty acids (found in fish oil), garlic, and vitamin E. If you test positive for one of these auto-antibodies and your doctor recommends medication, I personally would follow that recommendation. If, however, you don't want to take the medication, then these supplements in the doses listed below can serve as an alternative.

If your doctor doesn't recommend taking the blood thinners, or you don't want to be tested for the antibodies but you want to do all you can to prevent miscarriage, then you could follow the regimen of supplements described here, but halve the doses of EPA/DHA and vitamin E. Taken in the proper amounts, the supplements will not harm you or your baby, and they may serve as a natural way to help prevent a miscarriage caused by excessive blood clotting.

Dose:

○ *Omega-3 essential fatty acids:* 3 grams daily of combined EPA and DHA
○ *Vitamin E:* 800 IUs of natural tocopherols
○ *Garlic:* one capsule containing 6,000 mcg of allicin

Caution: Do *not* take these supplements together with baby aspirin or heparin without the approval of your doctor.

Note: Only take an omega-3 essential fatty acid supplement that guarantees it is free of heavy metals and PCBs. (See page 521 for resources.)

2. When a woman conceives, her immune system, which typically attacks foreign entities, theoretically should treat the embryo as foreign because it contains genetic material from the father. (Think of organ transplant recipients; they have to take strong medications throughout their lives to prevent their bodies from rejecting the foreign transplanted organ.) In a typical pregnancy, however, the immune system turns off its attack mechanism—how this happens is one of the great mysteries of biology.

Very rarely, a woman's immune system fails to shut off the attack mechanism, and so it treats the embryo as if it were foreign, attacking it and causing a miscarriage. Currently the treatment for this is to immunize the woman with white blood cells either from her husband or from blood product from the general population with what's known as intravenous immune globulin, or IVIG. The benefits of this treatment are uncertain and its use is highly controversial. It can only be given at specialized medical centers, and it can be expensive.

Diagnosis: Blood tests performed at several specialized labs around the U.S. can diagnose the presence of auto-antibodies and an immune system that identifies an embryo as foreign.

Nutritional strategies: If you've been diagnosed with this immune problem, you may want to consider dietary changes that would keep your immune system from being "turned on" (as pollen "turns on" an allergic response in someone with hay fever), especially if you already have symptoms of an overactive immune system such as a known food allergy, joint pain, headaches, rashes, or eczema.

In addition to the immune testing you've had, I'd recommend getting tested for food allergies and cutting out any foods that are found to trigger an allergic response. I'd also follow an anti-inflammatory diet (see page 52) and take 2 grams of an omega-3 essential fatty acid supplement that contains at least 2 grams (or 2,000 mg) of EPA twice a day. Whether these dietary interventions will help you maintain a pregnancy is untested, but if your immune system is "turned on," they certainly won't hurt you, and your overall health may improve.

Note: One other clotting problem may cause miscarriage. There's a genetic mutation of the blood called the factor V Leiden mutation. A woman may have one or two chromosomes with this mutation—if she has two, her risk of miscarriage, and preeclampsia, goes up; having one such chromosome is considered less of a risk factor. (The mutation is relatively common among Jews of Eastern European descent.) Factor V Leiden mutation may be diagnosed by blood test, and, especially if you have two copies of the chromosome, it may be treated with baby aspirin or heparin. If you have one copy of the chromosome, you may consider following the regimen of natural blood thinners described on page 380, halving the doses of omega-3 essential fatty acids and vitamin E.

• *Uterine abnormalities:* One of these uterine issues affects 10 to 15 percent of couples coping with repeat miscarriages in the first or second trimester (see "Late Miscarriage," page 382):

  1. An anatomical issue with the uterus—it might be small, misshapen, or partially or completely split down the middle (bicornate)
  2. Fibroids that interfere with implantation or an embryo's growth because of where they have attached to the uterus

3. An "incompetent" cervix

Depending on your situation, particularly with fibroids, surgery for these conditions can improve your chances of conceiving and carrying a pregnancy to term. In the case of an incompetent cervix, close monitoring of the cervix with ultrasound and/or surgically stitching the cervix is the standard treatment. (For more on an incompetent cervix and its treatment, see page 343.)

Diagnosis: Either a hysterosonogram, an ultrasound done after saline is injected into the uterus, or a hysterosalpingogram, a fluoroscopy (a sophisticated X-ray) done after dye is injected into the uterus and fallopian tubes (see page 49), is used to diagnose these uterine abnormalities.

Late Miscarriage and Stillbirth

- *Late miscarriage:* A miscarriage that occurs between twelve and twenty weeks is sometimes called a late miscarriage. It's not at all common. In fact, according to medical textbooks, once an ultrasound confirms a viable pregnancy at sixteen weeks, the future loss rate is just 1 percent. The causes of a spontaneous late miscarriage include:
  - *Anatomical:* if the uterus is small or misshapen or a woman has a weak (incompetent) cervix (see page 343 for more on an incompetent cervix)
  - *Infections:* listeria (page 246), toxoplasmosis (page 321), rubella (page 15), fifth disease (page 328)
  - A *blood group incompatibility:* for example, an Rh-negative mother carrying an Rh-positive fetus (page 93).
  - A *chromosomal abnormality:* Rarely, a chromosomal abnormality isn't apparent until the second trimester, when swelling or a severe anatomical problem may cause fetal death.
- *Anatomical problem:* A first-time loss because of an anatomical problem such as an incompetent cervix can't be predicted but also can't be missed: The symptoms develop quite quickly. Suddenly a woman might feel a bulge in her vagina or a gush of water, and she'll deliver shortly thereafter. She may feel some mild cramping but no significant labor pains. After one such loss, a woman will be followed very closely in her next pregnancy and possibly treated by putting a stitch in her cervix to help her hold onto the pregnancy. (See page 343 for a discussion of an incompetent cervix and its treatment.)
- *Viral infection:* A loss that's the result of a viral infection is usually accompanied

by flulike symptoms and possibly a rash. If you've had contact with any of the viruses listed on page 382, let your caregiver know as soon as you can. If you've had contact *and* develop a fever above 100.4 accompanied by *any* other flulike symptoms, contact your caregiver immediately.

• *Rh incompatibility, blood group incompatibility, or chromosomal abnormality:* If a miscarriage is caused by a blood group incompatibility or chromosomal abnormality, you may not know it until a routine office visit or a level 2 ultrasound reveals a problem. If you're tested for Rh incompatibility early in pregnancy, as almost all women are, you'll know if this is an issue for you. If you have been "Rh sensitized" from a previous pregnancy, meaning your Rh-negative blood mixed with the Rh-positive blood of the baby or the baby's father (which could happen during labor, a miscarriage, or a termination), this pregnancy will

> ### LOSS AND MULTIPLES
>
> It's highly unusual to lose one fetus in a multiple pregnancy, but it does happen. The most common reason for it is a condition known as twin-twin transfusion syndrome, which only occurs in identical twins that share a placenta (known as monozygotic, monochorionic twins).
>
> If there's a problem with the placenta, then one twin can get more blood and nutrients than the other. The twin that gets more blood can develop problems in her heart and circulatory system, and the twin that doesn't get enough blood can develop severe anemia—either twin can die from these complications.
>
> Twin-twin transfusion syndrome can be diagnosed during the monthly growth scans that are routine for women carrying multiples. Once it's identified or suspected, a high-risk specialist (perinatologist) will usually take over managing the pregnancy to try to prevent a stillbirth.

be watched closely, and your baby may require an intrauterine blood transfusion or early delivery before any complications develop. (For more on Rh incompatibility, see page 93.)

Note: Rh incompatibility creates problems when your Rh-negative blood mixes with Rh-positive blood from the father or baby. It cannot cause problems in a first pregnancy. Only women who had an Rh problem from a *previous* pregnancy can miscarry because of Rh incompatibility.

• *Stillbirth:* After twenty weeks, a loss is defined as a stillbirth (the term "stillbirth" has legal implications that vary from state to state). While rare, a stillbirth is absolutely devastating, and much of prenatal care, especially at the end of a pregnancy,

PRENATAL TESTS TO MONITOR FETAL WELL-BEING

- Biophysical profile
- Contraction stress test
- Doppler blood flow measurement
- Non-stress test

For descriptions of all of these tests, see chapter 15.

is designed to help doctors and midwives confirm that a baby is doing well in the womb in order to prevent a loss.

- *Symptoms:* Bleeding—anything from spotting to heavier bleeding—and detecting a change in, or stopping of, fetal movements are the most important symptoms of a stillbirth. If you pick up any deviation in your baby's movement pattern after twenty-eight weeks, call your care provider; if there are less than six to ten movements per hour for two hours, call immediately, no matter what time of day or night. (For counting fetal movements, see page 347.)

- *Common causes of stillbirth:*
  - *Cord accidents:* The umbilical cord measures, on average, twenty-two inches. It's coated (in utero) with a substance known as "Wharton's Jelly" which protects blood flow to the baby when the cord has a knot in it or is wrapped around the baby's neck. As a result, in the great majority of births, the cord doesn't pose a danger, even if it's wrapped around the baby's neck (its position in almost one out of four births). It's only in extremely rare cases that the cord is knotted or wrapped around the baby's neck so tightly that it cuts off oxygen and causes a stillbirth.
  - *Infection:* Listeria (see page 246), toxoplasmosis (see page 321), fifth disease (see page 328), and rubella (see page 15) can cause fetal death.
  - *Intrauterine growth restriction (IUGR):* In this condition, the baby's growth is hindered because, for some reason, he's not getting enough nutrients. Left untreated, this can lead to a stillbirth. (See page 345.)
  - *Placental abruption:* If the placenta separates—entirely or partially—from the uterine wall, it's known as a placental abruption, which causes bleeding because the blood vessels that connect the uterus and placenta tear. In severe cases, an abruption can cause so much bleeding it threatens the life of the baby and possibly the mother. (See page 349.)
  - *Placenta previa:* If the placenta attaches over the cervix, two problems may develop: (1) The baby may not be able to get enough nutrients, and IUGR

may develop; and (2) the placenta could cause excessive bleeding during childbirth, which could create a life-threatening emergency for the baby and mother. (See page 350.)

— *Preeclampsia:* Because this condition can cause the mother's blood vessels to constrict, blood flow to the baby may be limited. In severe cases, this limited blood flow can cause fetal death. (See page 357.)

— *Uncontrolled diabetes:* If maternal blood sugar can't be controlled, the baby is at risk for a range of metabolic problems that can lead to stillbirth. In addition, high blood sugar very early in a pregnancy, due to either juvenile diabetes or adult diabetes that has never been diagnosed, can cause major malformations that can result in stillbirth later in pregnancy.

— *Unexplained:* Sometimes stillbirth is unexplained; we never find a reason for it.

— *Unexplained elevated AFP:* There's a relationship between stillbirth and an unexplained elevated AFP level (alpha-fetoprotein; see page 281). No one knows why. So close monitoring through non-stress tests and biophysical profiles (see pages 299 and 288) are recommended to a woman with unexplained elevated AFP in order to prevent a stillbirth.

— *Vasa previa:* A rare condition that occurs in approximately one in three thousand pregnancies, vasa previa is an abnormality of the umbilical cord. Typically, the cord attaches in the middle of the placenta, but with vasa previa, the cord attaches to the fetal membranes (the "bag of waters"). Sometimes when this happens, fetal blood vessels, which are usually protected by the umbilical cord, run through the membrane and into the cervix. If this is the case, the blood vessels will rupture when the membranes rupture ("breaking the water") before or during labor, and the blood loss from the broken blood vessels will create a severe threat to the infant's life. When detected through ultrasound, serious complications during labor from vasa previa can be prevented by scheduling a C-section as soon as the baby's lungs are mature (typically around thirty-seven weeks; an amniocentesis can determine lung maturity, see page 287) and before he is full term.

Note: When a woman hasn't delivered by forty-two weeks, her risk of stillbirth goes up because the placenta no longer functions as well as it should.

Detecting a problem: If your caregiver suspects a problem either after a test or a prenatal exam, she might suggest either monitoring the fetal heart rate or taking a Doppler blood flow measurement (see page 129) to assess the blood flow to the placenta. Both of these tests should be available at the nearest hospital.

• *What happens next?* If tests show that a baby has died, a mother has to deliver the baby. This most often involves inducing labor; only rarely is a C-section necessary. If a woman doesn't elect to induce, she will probably go into labor spontaneously within two weeks. While there's no medical reason to induce right away, most of the women I've worked with considered the strain of continuing the pregnancy too emotionally overwhelming. (Also, blood clotting problems may develop if a woman doesn't deliver the baby within two to four weeks.)

As a physician, my role is to support the mother and her partner in whatever way I can. Personally, I recommend pain medication for these deliveries, and a woman can choose to have as much of it as she wants. (Usually pain medication is managed to minimize its effect on the baby; see page 461.)

After the delivery, the medical team typically cleans and swaddles the baby, even putting on a little hat as they would with any newborn. Most hospitals take a photograph of the baby and offer it to the parents. Sometimes they don't want the photo, but a caregiver or the hospital should be able to keep it in the patient's file in case she changes her mind.

Parents are then offered time alone with their baby. If a couple declines, I gently recommend that they reconsider. In my own experience and in the medical and psychology literature on the subject, time with the baby has been found to be extremely important for the mourning process. This baby has been an intimate part of a couple's world and imagination for a long time, and it helps many to spend time simply holding their child.

• *Trying again:* From a purely physical perspective, I recommend women wait for at least four menstrual cycles before trying to conceive again. This gives the body some time to restore itself. But more than physical readiness, emotional healing is crucial before a woman or couple tries to have another child. No one can say how to mourn and recover. For some women it's prayer, for others therapy. Mind-body exercises work for some, and even a craft or volunteer activity can bring a particular kind of relief. Sometimes professional help, either from a therapist or clergy, becomes an important part of the mourning process. Once a woman and her partner find a medium of healing that gives them insight into their experience and creates some sense of peace, I recommend continuing its practice, with any modifications that feel right, during their next pregnancy.

• *Recurrence rate:* The recurrence rate for stillbirth is anywhere from 0 to 8 percent, depending on the cause and the population of women. And the prenatal care a woman receives will be different if she chooses to get pregnant again. For example, if she had an unexplained loss at forty weeks, her caregiver might recommend inducing at thirty-eight weeks. If there were any genetic causes, she and her partner would be tested for chromosomal translocations (see page 379) before she conceived. No matter the cause, though, the medical professionals she works with would closely monitor her next pregnancy and do everything possible to prevent a second tragedy.

Note: The medical material in this chapter was reviewed by Dr. Cynthia Chazotte, professor of clinical obstetrics and gynecology and women's health, and director of obstetrics and perinatology, Weiler Hospital of the Albert Einstein College of Medicine/Montefiore Medical Center.

Preparing for Labor and Birth

No two women will want or need the same things from either their preparation for birth or from the experience itself. So when you talk to other people about labor—your friends, care provider, doula, childbirth educator—try to pay attention to your own instincts and listen to your own inner voice.

In this chapter, I describe how you can identify what you want in labor and birth in order to prepare emotionally for the experience. I also discuss some of the practical aspects of childbirth preparation, such as your childbirth education options, where you want to give birth, and basic pelvic exercises.

✦ ✦ ✦

In this chapter you'll find:

- Preparing for Birth
  - "Seeing" your labor and birth
- Creating a Birthing Team
- Connecting with Your Baby Before Birth
- Childbirth Classes
- A Birth Plan
- Preparing the Pelvis: Kegels and Perineal Massage
- Birthing Locations

Preparing for Birth

Preparing for both the emotional and practical aspects of birth means walking a fine line between the present and future. When you start to figure out how you feel about birth, it's easy to become overwhelmed by medical facts and lost in an imaginary world of details. Many of the pregnant women I work with spend so much time during their prenatal visits asking about particular hospital procedures for labor and birth that it sometimes feels like we get lost in a swamp of "what ifs," when we really should be talking about "right now."

For example, if a first-time mother who's around thirty weeks pregnant has a lot of questions about being induced—what medications are given, why she would be induced, would she be more likely to have a Cesarean delivery—I answer them, and it's obviously important information for her to have. But at the same time I might wonder why she's spending so much energy *now* thinking about being induced. Is she afraid of it? Was a friend induced and had a bad experience? Would she prefer to be induced for some reason? If so, why? The emotional questions that lie behind the medical questions are really the ones that can help you tap into your feelings about birth—your fears, excitement, attachments.

When you think about what you hope for and need in labor and childbirth, open yourself up to the future event while being conscious of the present moment. Is there something happening right now that's driving a particular concern? Let your ideas and emotions evolve as your daily experience of being pregnant changes.

By giving yourself room to explore your feelings about labor and childbirth, learning the facts of the process *and* living in the present moment, you can work—alone and together with your care provider and partner/coach—toward the best outcome for childbirth: a healthy mom, a healthy baby, and a satisfying birth experience.

"Seeing" your labor and birth

There's no right way or wrong way to start thinking about your labor and birth experience. If you're more comfortable finding out about the facts of labor, for example, how it generally progresses and standard medical procedures that may be used, then I suggest turning to chapters 21 and 22. If you want to start preparing by investigating your own assumptions and ideas about labor and birth, regardless of whether or not they're based in "facts," then the following exercise is a useful place to begin.

It will help you envision your experience and, to some degree, express your hopes, expectations, and concerns.

I usually recommend this exercise when you're between twenty and twenty-four weeks, because by then you've completed any prenatal testing you're planning to have. Any concerns you've had about your baby's health have been resolved, and you're feeling relatively comfortable and confident in your pregnancy. Also, you'll have plenty of time to think about what you find out in the exercise and apply it to your birth preparation. But, in the end, there's no right or wrong time to do this exercise. *Whenever* the time is right for you—at fifteen, twenty-two, twenty-eight, or thirty-eight weeks—this exercise can help you articulate a range of feelings about childbirth.

Note: This exercise takes between ten and twenty minutes to complete. If you don't wish to do this exercise now, then I *strongly* recommend skipping over this section until you're ready to do it. If you read the description without the intention of doing the exercise right away, it will be far less effective when you do it.

- *What you'll need:* a box of 64 crayons, a pen or pencil, 2 blank pieces of paper
- *Optional:* candle, relaxing music
- *How long it will take:* 10–20 minutes

- *Instructions:* Clear a space at a table or desk and place the crayons and paper in front of you. If you like, light a candle and play some music you find relaxing. You're going to draw two pictures; each should take five to ten minutes to complete.

To begin, focus on your breathing for a few minutes. Sit quietly and notice your breath as you inhale deeply and exhale gently. If you've lit a candle, focus on the flame for a minute or two as you breathe, which will help you quiet your mind.

When you feel centered, bring your attention to the paper, take the pen or pencil, and write "How I see my labor and childbirth" across the bottom of the page.

Then close your eyes and let yourself start to imagine your labor and childbirth. Focus on any aspect of it you like. Notice whatever images come naturally to you— it could be where you're laboring, the people with you in labor, you holding your baby, you giving birth in any position (including if you imagine a Cesarean), or even an abstract image of a feeling—like pain or love or joy. Don't try to manage the images or change them. Draw as much as you can of what you see in your mind's eye. Use whatever colors move you, and don't worry about how good or bad the drawing is. It doesn't really matter if it's anatomically or factually correct. What matters is taking the image in your head and moving it onto the paper.

When you're done with the first drawing, take a few moments to quiet your mind again. Breathe deeply and focus on the candle, if you find that helpful. When you feel centered, bring your attention to the second blank sheet of paper. On the bottom of it write: "How I *want* my labor and birth to be." And ask yourself: In your heart of hearts, what do you want your birth experience to be like? Then let the images come to you. Try not to edit what you're drawing—let whatever pops into your mind by way of your heart find its way to the paper. No one will be judging this or you.

When you've finished the second drawing, put away the crayons, sit quietly, and breathe for a little while longer. Again, if the candle helps you focus, use it to bring you back to your center.

Now you can choose what to do next—either look at the drawings right away or set aside a time later today or tomorrow to do so. Whichever you choose, take a few minutes to breathe deeply before returning to your day.

When you're ready to look at what you've drawn, first clear your mind just as you did before drawing the pictures. Then, begin to note the details of each picture. Can you tell if it is day or night? (This sometimes is a clue to when you will give birth.) Who's in the room in each picture? Where are they in relation to you? Is everyone happy? What colors have you used? What do the colors mean to you, if anything? Notice the differences between the drawings of what you believe your birth experience will be and what you want it to be. As you do this, you can jot down a few words (about five) that pop into your head when you look at each of the two pictures. Or you can note the different details that really jump out at you. There are no right questions or right answers. Let your mind and heart lead you to whatever insights the pictures offer.

If the pictures are very similar and you feel good about what you see, then you can build on those positive feelings about childbirth and embrace their potential to become a reality. For example, you can use the words that you used to describe the drawings to prepare. Repeat them when you feel like talking to your baby ("I imagine your birth will be like . . .") or when you get nervous or anxious about something related to the birth ("My inner self believes labor will be filled with . . . and I trust in that feeling.").

If the pictures are different, and you're not comfortable with the differences, ask yourself, "What would it take to make the labor and birth I *believe* I will have more like the labor and birth I *want* to have?" Are there steps you can take to bridge the gap? The idea is to help you get to a place where you can approach childbirth with

From My Office: Putting a
Drawing to Work in the Delivery Room

✦ A few years ago, a patient named Amy, who was pregnant with her first baby, drew her birth pictures as cartoons in a series of frames. In the birth she thought she'd have, there was a frame or two about labor, and then a frame of the actual birth. Her husband was in each frame, and I was in the frame of the birth. In it, I was using enormous forceps to deliver the baby. In the final frame, she was holding her son, her husband had his arm around her, and all three were smiling. I was also in the drawing of the birth she wanted to have, but I wasn't using forceps. Over the next few months, I talked at length about forceps, why and when they're used, and that she probably wouldn't need them. But she never let go of the idea that forceps were inevitable for her. She was a small person, and she felt that she wouldn't be able to push the baby all the way out on her own. There was no medical reason for this, but Amy was convinced, and nothing would shake her belief. (Forceps are typically used when the baby gets "stuck," or stops progressing, relatively low in the birth canal; see page 473.)

I was there when Amy gave birth. And wouldn't you know it? The baby stopped progressing downward through the birth canal, and unfortunately, he stopped moving in a funny spot. It was low enough to potentially make a Cesarean difficult, but high enough that forceps might be challenging as well. The baby was truly in a place where the two options, a Cesarean or forceps, were equally medically acceptable. I had to make a quick decision about what to recommend. I took a few deep breaths to focus, and Amy's drawing popped into my head. I saw the image of me holding the forceps, and I saw the final frame of Amy, her baby, and her husband all healthy and happy. I decided to recommend the forceps, Amy agreed, and it turned out to be one of the smoothest forceps deliveries I've ever done. Amy's son slid out with the next contraction, and soon after, her new family was together and happy—just like in the final frame of her drawings.

excitement. It may be helpful to write up a list of the differences between the two pictures and share it with people connected to your pregnancy—a doctor or midwife, a doula, a close friend, your partner, or a therapist—someone who can help you work toward the birth you want to have. Alternatively, you could explore in a journal the feelings the exercise sparked, or continue to do the exercise every few weeks as your pregnancy progresses, to see how your vision of birth evolves.

Nobody can control what will happen in labor and birth, and this exercise can't guarantee anything about your labor and childbirth experience. But by imagining the experience, you can identify what you want and what you might fear and open yourself up to the complexity and mystery of childbirth.

• *Patterns in drawings:* Here are a few patterns that have emerged among the pregnant women I've worked with when we've looked at their two drawings.

— *Who's the care provider?* Often, there will be a different care provider in each picture. In any group practice (of doctors or midwives), it's impossible to predict who's going to be on call when you go into labor. (This is true even with a solo practitioner if your due date falls around his vacation.) The question is: Does this uncertainty make you anxious? Is there something you can do to become more comfortable with the other doctor(s)/midwives? What is it about one caregiver that makes you uncomfortable? Does it feel right to talk about it with the caregiver you like, or the one you don't? Do you feel comfortable sharing your birth plan and general preferences with a caregiver you don't like? (See "A Birth Plan" on page 411.)

— *Will you have a C-section?* Some women are convinced they'll have a Cesarean delivery when they truly want a vaginal birth. They draw the labor and birth they think they'll have in an operating room, and the labor and birth they want to have in a birthing room.

In some cases, the conviction that a C-section is inevitable or highly likely is based on a medical fact, for example, if a woman has a large fibroid located in a place that would make a vaginal delivery dangerous, or if a baby is breech after thirty-four weeks (see "Breech Presentation" on page 430). If that's the case, we talk about ways she can make a scheduled C-section a better, more family-centered birth experience. (See "Preparing for a Scheduled C-section" on page 476.)

But sometimes for no medical reason at all a woman is convinced she'll have a C-section. Maybe her mom had a C-section and she always assumed she would need one, too. Maybe she thinks her pelvis is too small and the baby will get stuck. (A surprising number of my patients believe they will need a Cesarean because an incidental comment about their "small" pelvis size made during a pelvic exam when they were in high school or college has stuck in their minds.) Or maybe she's heard one too many stories about Cesarean deliveries and she can't imagine not "ending up" with one.

Whatever the reasons, if you feel like a C-section is inevitable, it's important to start talking with your care provider about your belief and your wish to avoid surgery. Also consider talking with an experienced childbirth educator or doula, who may be able to give you a different perspective on your upcoming birth (see "What Is a Doula?" on page 402).

If your discussions bring up powerful emotions, consider talking to a therapist or someone you trust who won't feed your fears. No matter what, take time to sort through your assumptions about the inevitability of a surgical birth. (For more on C-sections, when they're necessary and what happens during one, turn to page 475.)

- *Who's in the room?* Often, there are two different groups of people in each drawing. A sister, mother, doula, or friend might be in the picture of the birth a woman wants to have, but not in the drawing of the birth she thinks she'll have. If this is the case for you, ask yourself: What would this person bring to my birth experience? What need does she fill that's not getting met? Can she be at the birth? If not, what are the barriers? If they're logistical, is there a way to arrange for her to be there? Or is there someone else who might be able to fill the role you feel this person would fill? Are the barriers emotional? For example, maybe your partner doesn't want anyone else at the birth, but you do. Can you talk it over and come to some kind of compromise or better understanding? (For more on who you'd like to be at the birth, see "Creating a Birthing Team" on page 397 and "Using Guided Imagery and Creating a Birthing Team" on page 399.)
- *Where's your partner?* A striking difference that can show up is where a laboring mother and her partner are in relation to each other. I'll look at a picture of how a woman wants her birth to be, and her partner (most often a husband) is beside her, but in the picture of how she believes it will be, her husband is farther away. Sometimes, the woman doesn't even notice the difference, and I'll simply ask, "Why is your husband standing over there?"

Thinking about childbirth can trigger powerful emotions about a relationship—feelings of intimacy or longings that highlight difficulties in a relationship. If this exercise exposes issues in a relationship, try to use what you learn to address them well before labor begins. (See "Creating a Birthing Team" on page 397.) Couples typically enter a labor/birth room with all their best intentions along with their emotional "baggage." I've seen couples at odds in labor too many times, and the experience isn't good for anyone involved. But talking about these concerns before birth (either on your own or with the help of a marriage counselor) can help bring you closer together and lay the groundwork for a positive, life- and love-affirming labor and childbirth.

Common Fears About Labor and Birth

✦ Some women feel only excitement and confidence when they think about labor and birth. Others have specific fears mixed in with——or dominating——their excitement or anticipation. Sometimes a fear is reinforced by the "horror stories" people love to share about labor and birth; other times a fear is simply present or deeply ingrained. Here are some common fears that crop up as women prepare for childbirth:

• *Fear of death:* In my own experience, this very basic fear is expressed more often in the childbirth classes we offer than in either prenatal visits or the drawing exercise. One of the best ways we've found to work with it is to reinforce the facts. First, a woman's body is designed to give birth. Second, while complications do happen and must be guarded against, a skilled care provider can use the tools of modern medicine to prevent a tragedy. The incidence of maternal death in childbirth in the U.S. is extremely low (12 per every 100,000 live births), and many of these heartbreaking events happen when women don't have access to consistent prenatal care. Third, in real life, unlike on TV or even "reality shows," it's extremely unlikely that a life-threatening complication will develop without any warning. With consistent prenatal care, a care provider either knows about preexisting risk factors or, once you're in labor, can identify trouble spots and intervene before things reach a critical stage. If you find you can't trust your body's ability to give birth, the statistics, or the experience of your caregiver, you might consider exploring your fears with a therapist or clergy member. Discussing this kind of fear could be an opportunity for you to examine how you feel about the profound questions of faith and the human condition.

• *Fear of pain:* By nature's design, pain is a part of the birth experience.

Everyone feels and responds to pain differently, and it's impossible to predict what kind of pain you will experience in labor and childbirth. So much depends on how quickly your labor progresses, whether or not it's induced, your own attitude toward pain, and your pain threshold. If you're very concerned that you won't be able to manage the pain, talk about your options with your caregiver. A "pain-free" labor may not be possible, but medication certainly can help make the pain manageable.

It may help to remember that while the pain of contractions and birth can be intense, it's part of a natural process. If you can, try to cultivate trust in your body's natural abilities and your own inner strength. By doing so, you may find it easier to cope with whatever pain or sensations you experience.

• *Fear of exposure:* When you're laboring and birthing, you're going to do things, and be in positions, that aren't typical in everyday life—but they *are* typical in the life of a maternity floor or birthing center. What might be considered "gross" somewhere else is simply part of the sacred process of giving birth. That goes for everything from moving your bowels to vomiting to moaning, yelling, or doing whatever it is you need to do. No professional or support person will (or should) judge you for anything you do—especially when it comes to your bodily functions. For example, if you vomit, the nurses, doctors, and midwives won't be offended or upset. They'll only be worried about how you're feeling and will want to help clean you up—it's part of what they do every day.

REAL VOICES

It turns out that when I was pushing, there were ten people in the room because I had very low platelets and a lot of people were interested in . . . I don't know *what* they were interested in, and I didn't care. Before I went into labor, I was really worried about that self-conscious thing: "Am I going to poop? What's going to happen?" But when you're there, you're so exposed, and you couldn't care less. I *so* didn't care. In fact, I was delighted by everyone else enjoying it. It was really cool. I look back on feeling that way and think, "What was I, nuts?" But everyone was so celebratory when Milo came out. I mean, there were so many people in the room, none of whom I knew except my husband, and it just felt great. Everyone was like. "Oh my god! He's beautiful! He's got so much hair!" It was really neat.

Asha, mom of one, pregnant

Creating a Birthing Team

Over the years, I've given a lot of thought to the interpersonal dynamics of child-birth and how they affect a woman's labor and her overall birth experience. I've seen couples that were completely in sync throughout the whole labor and birth, and how positive that can be for everyone involved. I've also seen couples go through birth with a constellation of support—maybe a doula is there, a dear friend (or friends), a sister, or a mother—and that's also amazing for everyone. In both scenar-ios, a birthing mother feels love from and trusts in those around her.

On the opposite end of the spectrum, I've seen couples in which the partner and the birthing woman had very different expectations, needs, or wishes, and they sim-ply could not work together. Maybe a woman felt responsible for how her partner felt during labor; maybe a partner felt overwhelmed by the reality of labor and couldn't commit to being there. In situations like these, the babies were usually fine and healthy, but the birth experiences were either not happy or not as happy as they could've been for the parents. And I've observed where unresolved conflict in a cou-ple that emerges during birth can even hinder labor's progress.

Looking back, I've come to realize that a crucial element of laboring and birth is for a woman to feel support from and confidence in the people who are with her in labor in addition to her care provider and the hospital staff—in other words, her "birthing team," whether it's made up of just her partner/labor coach or a bigger group of people. Let me be clear: A care provider and nurses play extremely impor-tant roles, but so, too, can a birthing team.

As you think about what's important to you during birth, consider the question of whom you want there. Try to assemble a birthing team of people who can give you emotional and physical support throughout labor and birth. With your team in place, you'll have the people *you* want there with you.

• *A primary support person:* At the cornerstone of the birthing team is the *one* per-son who can be the primary support person. Others can fill in at different points, but it's tremendously helpful when you're in labor to have constant companionship, and the more continuity the better. With one person to rely on, you can develop a rhythm and a routine as you move through the stages of labor. Any one of a number of people can fulfill this role—your partner, a doula (see page 402), a dear friend, or a family member.

• *A communicating couple:* The process of laboring and giving birth is emotionally and physically demanding. For some couples, there's no doubt that a woman's partner will be her primary support person throughout the entire labor. For other couples, however, a woman's partner isn't necessarily the best choice.

I've mostly worked with married couples, and for some, it's easier for both if they can plan on the husband slipping in and out of the room throughout labor as opposed to him being there all the time. Much more often than I would expect, a patient has told me that her husband said explicitly he didn't want to be there for the labor. I don't think this means he doesn't want to be there at all. But it may mean he isn't comfortable with the responsibility of being the *primary* support person. Some women are comfortable with this; others are deeply disappointed. Either way, it's important to be honest with each other about what choices will work for both of you. Even when you and your partner agree on who will do what during labor, it's useful to talk about what you imagine it will be like to experience labor and birth together.

There's no doubt that talking about childbirth can be difficult. First of all, there's the fact that, especially if this is a first baby, neither of you knows what your labor will be like. And no matter how many times you've given birth, nobody ever knows what will happen once a labor begins.

Beyond the unknowable facts, sometimes it seems to me that people think about labor and birth as a kind of play or performance, with a woman and her partner each filling prewritten roles. This can leave precious little room for two people to honestly explore their individual needs and expectations, because the weight of external expectations can be so heavy. (Many patients have told me that if they could give birth away from home, and the perceived judgment of friends and family, they wouldn't expect their husbands to be with them throughout labor.) Unfortunately, if a couple *doesn't* share their *true* feelings about what they need and want from each other before labor begins, divisive situations can unfold: husbands on cell phones, wives furious—and the last thing any woman needs is to be furious at a "support person" during labor. Childbirth then becomes a breeding ground for resentment instead of an extraordinary life passage.

If you can find a way to talk about each of your needs and approach the great unknown of labor and birth from a place of mutual understanding, then there's a much greater potential for you both to experience the wonder of birth in a way that will bring you closer together.

From My Office: Using Guided Imagery and Creating a Birthing Team

✦ If a pregnant woman I'm working with describes a very strong sense of anxiety or fear, it sends a signal to me that she could be struggling with a deeper conflict that she's possibly unaware of. When this happens, I'll often recommend she set up an imagery session with Monique Class, our nurse practitioner and childbirth educator who is certified in using imagery and visualization as a healing technique. From my perspective as a doctor, I believe guided imagery offers a woman access to feelings and fears that she might not otherwise recognize or acknowledge.

Jennifer was one such patient. Around thirty weeks, she came in for a prenatal appointment, and it was obvious that she was on edge. When I asked if there was something bothering her, she said she was really concerned about a number of things, but she didn't get specific. Because I could see and feel her anxiety, and because I felt it would help her to address what was bothering her before childbirth, I recommended she see Monique for a guided imagery session.

Monique Class: Joel referred Jennifer to me for imagery work in her third trimester. Before we got started, I asked her why she thought she was there, and she said she was very anxious about having a hospital birth, which she'd never imagined for herself. She was worried about what the nurses and doctor would do, and that it would be too medicalized. She also mentioned, in passing, that she felt she hadn't really connected with her baby.

Because she was so anxious, I began the imagery session by bringing her into a gentle, but deep, relaxed state where she could really let go. I asked her to put her hands on her belly and breathe deeply. Then I did a progressive relaxation exercise where she would tense and release one part of her body at a time, starting with her toes and ending with her head. When she'd relaxed her body, I asked her to imagine going to a safe place. This turned out to be quite hard for Jennifer, so I slowly brought her out of the relaxed state, and we started over. The second time we went through the relaxation process, she was able to find a safe place more easily.

When her breathing was calm and steady, which signaled that she was in a place where she could visualize freely (a hypnotized state), I asked her if she was in her safe place. She said yes. I asked if there was anything she wanted to add to make it safer or if she wanted to bring someone in with her. Her first response was that she wanted to bring in her husband, but then, suddenly, she started to cry. Jennifer quickly emerged from her relaxed state and cried hard for a long time. Eventually, she caught her breath and said she didn't feel safe with or supported by her husband. She said he *never* asked how she was feeling or offered to give her a back rub. He didn't seem connected to her or the baby, and she was really nervous about going into labor and childbirth with him. In fact, she had wanted to hire a doula, but her husband didn't want someone he didn't know there. She realized that they needed to talk about this, and that she was also partly responsible for the breakdown in communication, because when he withdrew, she wouldn't try to talk to him. She only distanced herself further from him.

At this point, we agreed it would be a good idea to go back into a hypnotized state to see what she'd learn. This time, I asked Jennifer to imagine herself in a labor and delivery room. When I asked her who was with her, she said her husband and her sister. After spending some time with the image, she came out of the hypnotized state, and she was ecstatic. Jennifer had never thought of having her sister at the birth before, but she had always felt a deep connection to her, and her husband was really fond of her. Jennifer thought that with her sister there, she would feel much safer even with the doctors, nurses, and residents all around her. She then said that she thought she'd been projecting her concerns outward onto the medical staff in order to keep herself from moving inward, so she wouldn't have to confront the gap she felt with her husband or connect with her baby. She left with a plan to: (1) try to talk with her husband about how she'd been feeling, (2) spend time each day focusing on and connecting with her baby, and (3) ask her sister to be with her at the birth.

I next saw Jennifer a few weeks after she gave birth, when she came in for a breastfeeding consultation. She was thrilled. She said the birth was better than she'd imagined, that she and her husband had done a lot of work together beforehand and were able to work as a team in the labor room. And, she said, having her sister there really helped her feel safe. Her birth experience, which had filled her with so much anxiety, turned out to be phenomenal for her on many levels.

• *A third person:* Just as Jennifer and her husband were helped, probably in very different ways, by having her sister at their birth, many couples feel having another person with them in the labor room makes a big difference in the quality of the experience. For Jennifer, it was her sister. At my own first son's birth fourteen years ago, it was my wife's mother. At the time, even though I'd been a practicing obstetrician for two years, I had never spent an entire labor with one woman, and honestly, I wasn't quite sure what to do or say in all that time. (I was also a very different kind of doctor then.) My mother-in-law naturally slipped into the role of primary support person for my wife, and I was able to come and go as I needed—which was better for both my wife and me. It worked beautifully for all of us.

A third person can help a laboring woman and her partner in a number of ways. She or he can step in for the primary support person when that person needs a break. If a woman is laboring without pain medication, particularly if the labor is long, a third person can stay awake with the woman while her partner sleeps, or she can help defuse any tension that may develop when two sleep-deprived people (the laboring woman and her partner) have to make medical decisions.

A labor nurse can sometimes fulfill this role, though whether or not one will be available depends on how many patients she has to attend to. If you're working with a midwife, particularly a solo practitioner, she might provide the extra consistent support. (Talk with your midwife directly about how she supports laboring women and what she does when she has more than one woman in labor at a time.)

Having a third person with you and your partner/labor coach isn't for everyone. Many women and couples feel that labor and birth is too private to share, and some women are concerned that they'd feel responsible for anyone besides their partner in the room. But if you think having a third person would be helpful for you and your partner, you can arrange in advance for someone to be there. This can be a friend, family member, or a doula (see box, page 402).

What Is a Doula? An Interview with Penny Simkin

✦ Penny Simkin has been a doula and childbirth educator for over thirty-five years. One of the founders of DONA (Doulas of North America, *www.dona.org*), she's the author of many books, including *The Birth Partner* and, most recently, *When Survivors Give Birth*.

Q: What does a doula do?

Penny Simkin: A doula is usually a woman, not always, but usually, who is trained and experienced in childbirth. Her role is to accompany a woman or couple through the birth experience by providing *continuous* emotional support, physical comfort, and assistance in getting the information they need to make good decisions by facilitating communication between the client and the care provider.

Q: You emphasized emotional support. Why is that so important?

PS: Continuous emotional support is an ingredient that's missing in most conventional maternity care. The stress and vulnerability experienced by laboring women, combined with the fact that they hardly know anyone else who's at the birth, means that it can be enormously helpful to have a person who doesn't leave (a doula leaves just to go to the bathroom, essentially, not otherwise), who can reassure and support the partner, and who can say, "This is normal." And then there's the encouragement and empathy—helping a woman if she's having a difficult labor or if a problem arises that requires action. A doula can often guide a couple through and keep them calm.

Q: Would you say that in general being surrounded by people you trust, even if they're relatively new to you, is another key ingredient in labor that's overlooked?

PS: Would I? Yes, I would. Absolutely. Can I tell you a story? I was at a birth on Monday. This is a woman having her second baby. She had planned a home birth with the first and was unable to have that. She had had a very long, nonproductive labor, which ended in Cesarean. Well, this time she was going for a VBAC (vaginal birth after Cesarean), and this woman, who had had an orientation towards natural birth, actually wound up with every intervention you could imagine shy of vacuum, forceps, and a Cesarean (see chapter 22). During pushing, which she did for three and a half hours, she looked up and said, "This is like a home birth in the hospital." Now, she had an epidural, she had continuous monitoring, she had IV fluids, she had a bladder catheter . . . You name it, she had it. But, you see, the essential ingredient was that she was surrounded by people who loved her and that she totally trusted, including the wonderful nurse who was there, and her husband and her best friend and her doula. Those were the things that made this *such* a special, special experience for her.

Q: What do you think makes a good match between a doula and a woman?

PS: If a doula is comfortable hearing the woman's choices and taking on the woman's values as her own values for the extent of their relationship—that's what makes a good match. It depends more on what the doula brings than what the woman brings.

Q: Is there a red flag to watch for when interviewing a doula? Sometimes you don't know what somebody's like in the trenches . . .

PS: That's right—I think it's probably a bit of a gamble with anybody. But a woman's gut feeling towards the doula—it's like when she's choosing a pediatrician for her baby—she really wants to listen to how her questions are answered and how the answers make her feel inside. She should ask herself, "Does this doula seem like someone I want to trust with my emotional well-being?" Sometimes she can't point to anything; the doula has given all the right answers, but there's a discomfort. I think she ought to pay attention to that. If she can, interviewing more than one doula would give a woman a sense of who might be a better choice.

Q: How do you respond to charges that obstetricians feel like doulas interfere or are too directive in the labor process?

PS: I find it very troubling. The charge relates to the advocacy role doulas play, which is important, but very tricky.

Doulas who think it's their responsibility to make sure the staff behaves a certain way are mistaken. But, in our defense, one of the most frustrating things for a doula—and I'll speak for myself as well as everyone else—is sometimes we have that sense of standing by and seeing things done against a woman's will. This is *not* the norm, but there are care providers who really want a woman to be induced or they want to give her Pitocin, and there isn't a clear medical reason for it, or at least they can't explain it to the woman in a way that makes her realize that it's a good idea. It can be very hard for a doula to stand by and watch in this situation.

I do think sometimes the doula is a contributor to a poor relationship with a care provider, but I don't think it's only the doula. Everyone—provider, nursing staff, doula—has to look into their hearts and examine if they have an agenda. The providers and staff might ask, "Am I doing this for the well-being of this mother and baby, or do I really want to get to bed?" or "Am I worrying about my clientele piling up in my office?" or "Am I upset with this woman because she's being difficult and I want to make her behave differently?" And doulas have to look into their hearts and ask, "Am I pushing the way I want this woman to give birth onto her and the staff?" The advocacy role of a doula is really one of trying to facilitate communication; the mother and father or partner are the ones who *must,* in the end, ask the questions and give the consent and be sure it's informed.

Q: Does a doula ever give medical advice?

PS: No. That's something in the letters of agreement that DONA doulas draw up. We make it clear that we can give nonclinical advice, but we can't give clinical advice. Even if a woman calls me up and says, "Should I go to the hospital now?" I don't say yes or no except if her bag of waters is broken and she's pushing. Mostly I say, "If you go now, this could happen; if you stay home, this could happen." So I toss it back to her, having given her a little more information to make her decision with.

Our philosophy is emotional support, physical comfort, helping the woman communicate—those are the things that have been proven to help obstetric outcome. There are fewer Cesareans when women have doulas. There are fewer requests for pain medications, not that the doula's keeping her from it, but that she doesn't feel the need. So there are improvements in outcomes, and it isn't from taking over clinically, and it isn't from fighting over the woman in the labor room—having the doctor, nurse, and doula at odds. That isn't what improves outcome. It's having a woman feel that everybody is on her side.

REAL VOICES
We chose our doula, who was our childbirth instructor, when we were doing hands-on labor practice. She was rubbing my back and I thought, "Wow, she's really good!" Even though she had a very big personality as a teacher, in the hospital environment she was very subdued and wonderful. At first we were a little resistant to the idea of a doula because my husband wanted to be very hands-on. But we talked about it and proposed to the doula that he would

take care of me, and she would take care of us and help at the hospital. That's how it went, and it was great.

Trina, mom of one, pregnant

I didn't want to have a doula. I'm personally someone who when I'm in pain I just want to be left alone. I just go into a very internal space and I really just want privacy when I'm in pain. I know this about myself, and it was very true my first time in labor. I know it's really different for different women. There are some women for whom a doula is really a very comforting presence, and I'm sure that maybe if I'd been more open about it some of the biofeedback approaches to managing pain would've been helpful, but I just relied on my usual, habitual approach.

Kathleen, mom of two

Connecting with Your Baby Before Birth

I believe there's a natural energetic connection between mother and baby that extends beyond the physical. Another step you can take toward preparing for childbirth is to tap into that energetic connection, creating a sense for yourself and your child that you'll be going through this labor and birth together.

• *A longer exercise:* This is a relatively simple exercise that you can start in the six weeks or so before your due date. To begin, make yourself comfortable either sitting or lying down. Turn off the ringers on your phones. Sit in a relaxing space where you won't be disturbed for ten or fifteen minutes. Start by doing belly breathing: Breathe in deeply through the nose, out through the mouth. You can say "soft" on the inhale and "belly" on the exhale. (For a full description of belly breathing, see page 63.)

When you feel calm, open yourself up to your baby (or babies). Do this in whatever way comes naturally—you can imagine opening a door to the baby's room, or traveling into an imaginary womblike space that's filled with warm light, or maybe just a feeling. Go with whatever happens. Once you've established a bridge, you can start to talk with your baby. If you've picked a name, you can use it. Tell him whatever you like—that you love him, a funny story, something about your day. Use language that comes naturally to you. See if you "hear" anything back—if you get some kind of sensation. If it doesn't feel weird, go ahead and ask him something, for example, "How are you doing today?" or "What do you need?" or "What would you like to tell me?" You might not get a response, and then again, you might. (When patients do work like this in guided imagery sessions with Monique Class—see page 399—they often ask a relatively specific question—and get answers like "I need more time," or "I'm ready." When a baby lets a mom know he needs more time or attention, we recommend adding an affirmation like "I'm here for you, I love you" to the end of this exercise and repeating it a few times every night before going to sleep.) But it's not important to focus on getting a specific answer to any questions you ask your baby. What's important is just taking some time out of your day to be with him.

When you feel complete with the experience, slowly start to deepen your breath again. Focus on your breathing for a few minutes, then return to your day.

• *With multiples:* If you're having twins or more, do this same exercise, but spend some time focusing on each baby. If you have some sense of where each baby is, breathe with your hands where one baby is, move your hands to the next baby, and breathe there. Try to spend the same amount of time with each baby.

• *A shorter exercise:* If you don't have the time or opportunity to do the longer exercise on a regular basis, you can try a shorter version of it. Wherever you are—in the office, at home, or even in the waiting room for a prenatal visit—take a few minutes and start to breathe calming, deep, nourishing breaths. Place your hands on your belly, and let your baby know you love her and that you're there for her—either by talking out loud or silently directing your words and love toward her. Let her know little things about the day, like where you are right now, what you're doing, or reassure her about birth, telling her with spoken or silent words that you're looking forward to meeting her, that it'll be safe, and that you'll be in it together. When you feel done, linger with a few quiet, gentle breaths before returning to your day.

• *Recognize the challenges:* As straightforward as these exercises are, they can be challenging to do. First, there's always the problem of time. We lead time-pressured lives, and whatever it is that keeps you busy—working, preparing your home, caring for other children—can make it easy to forget to slow down even for five or ten minutes and just *be* with yourself and your baby.

Then there's how you feel physically and how much energy you have. In the last weeks before you give birth, you may be more tired and physically uncomfortable. When you slow down at the end of the day, lying on the couch may seem like plenty of activity! Directing any extra energy toward anything, even your baby, may feel like too much.

Finally, in these last weeks, the romance of pregnancy may become more complicated. You may feel like you'll miss being pregnant and the special connection you have with your baby. Or you may feel like you're absolutely ready to give birth and have this pregnancy come to an end—regardless of how the baby feels.

Take all of these challenges into account. These exercises shouldn't feel like one more thing on your "to do" list, but instead like something you could do that would feel good.

• *Listen to your gut:* It's crucial to acknowledge the time constraints, exhaustion, and conflicting emotions that fill the weeks before birth. Taking every feeling you have into account, ask yourself whether sitting and talking to your baby (or babies) to connect energetically makes intuitive good sense to you *today*. It won't make sense for everyone, or it might not feel right to do this every day. Don't force yourself to do anything that doesn't ring true. If your gut tells you not to focus too much on your baby or birth right now, then don't. But if you feel that either the short or long exercise is a good idea, then set aside a few minutes to sit quietly and tap into the energy you and your baby share.

Childbirth Classes

In my opinion, there's a basic difference between classes in childbirth education and those in childbirth methods. *Childbirth education* involves learning about the nuts and bolts of labor, vaginal birth, and Cesarean delivery. *Childbirth method* classes teach techniques and philosophies for managing labor and birth—e.g., breathing and relaxation exercises, various positions that might make labor more comfortable, etc.—in addition to covering the basics of childbirth education. Classes in a particular childbirth method may also present a distinct philosophy of labor and birth (how it should or shouldn't be managed, what is an ideal experience). How rigidly that philosophy is adhered to depends to a large degree on the childbirth educator.

There are no rules for how much or how little childbirth education you should have. I would encourage everyone to get to know the basics of labor and birth so at least the vocabulary isn't entirely new to you when labor begins (see chapters 21 and 22).

• *Timing:* Plan to complete childbirth education classes by thirty-four weeks, or six weeks before your due date (eight weeks for multiples). Some classes take ten or twelve weeks and others take a day, so when to start really depends on what kind of class you're planning on taking.

• *Hospital tours:* Many hospitals hold regularly scheduled tours of their facilities separate from childbirth education classes. No matter what kind of class you plan to take, I strongly recommend touring the facility where you plan to give birth or the backup facility for a home birth. (For more on home births, see "Birthing Locations," page 416.) It's useful to know what the environment looks like and to have a general idea of where to go when you arrive in labor.

• *Hospital childbirth classes:* Hospitals usually offer some kind of childbirth education. Most often, these classes take place over the course of one day or several evenings. They tend to review the basics of labor, vaginal birth, and Cesarean sections as well as hospital procedures. They should also include a tour of the hospital facility.

• *Birthworks:* Birthworks focuses on the individual's process of laboring and giving birth, and encourages couples to begin preparing for birth very early in pregnancy. (For more information, go to *www.birthworks.org.*)

• *The Bradley Method (also known as The American Academy of Husband-Coached Childbirth):* An intensive childbirth class, the Bradley Method emphasizes how women and their partners can prepare for and work together through a natural, medication-free labor and birth by changing positions, relaxing, and preparing for contingencies. A standard Bradley class is taught by a Bradley-certified instructor, has ten to twelve class meetings, and six to eight people per class.

Bradley instruction is quite thorough, but a frequent comment about it is that instructors tend to have a bias against conventional obstetrics and its techniques. If you're concerned about this, feel free to explore the issue with the instructor you're thinking of working with. How "rigid" any class might be will depend to a large degree on her approach and mind-set. (For more information, go to *www.bradleybirth.com.*)

• *Lamaze:* Founded in 1960, Lamaze is popularly associated with specific breathing techniques. While breathing is part of Lamaze education, the twelve hours of classes now cover a range of relaxation techniques, comfort methods, general education, and partner preparation. The goal is to help women have a low-intervention labor and birth, and to make informed decisions throughout. Lamaze publications emphasize their openness to whatever pain-relief techniques will work best for a woman—breathing, relaxation, medication, whatever she wants. Classes will be small and taught by Lamaze-certified childbirth educators. (For more information, go to *www.lamaze.org.*)

• *Combined methods:* In many communities, birth centers, doctors' offices, independent childbirth educators, and childbirth associations offer a variety of childbirth education classes that don't adhere to a specific method or philosophy. Instead, they blend primarily Lamaze and Bradley techniques with other approaches to labor and childbirth. These classes can be extremely informative and useful, but as with any class, the quality of the material depends to a large degree on the skill and knowledge of the instructor. Look for someone who has medical credentials, such as a labor and delivery nurse, and/or someone who's accredited by the International Childbirth Education Association, a voluntary accrediting organization that certifies lay childbirth instructors who incorporate labor and birth techniques from a range of sources. (For more information, go to *www.icea.org*.) Ask around about instructors. Your doctor or midwife may know about a particularly good teacher, or friends may be able to suggest a class.

• *Picking the right childbirth class for you:* Picking a childbirth education class means first thinking about what kind of birth you want to have and, second, how much time, money, and energy you want to commit to the process. If you want to have a natural, medication-free labor, more preparation than a one-day class can provide is probably better. Similarly, if you want to be very involved with every aspect of your labor, a more in-depth class would be a good choice. But whether you decide to take a long or short class, when you complete it, you should feel both well-informed about labor and childbirth and physically able to have a baby. In other words, when you finish class, you should ideally feel like "I can *do* this!"

If you leave a pre-class discussion with an instructor or the class itself and feel fearful or overwhelmed, look for another class or talk to your care provider about your concerns.

REAL VOICES ON CHILDBIRTH CLASS
I took a Lamaze class, not so much for the technique but because I really wanted to meet other parents. I met some really nice families, and I ended up forming a mom's group with them that stuck together for over two years. I also read a ton about birth. I just loved reading about women's experiences; I loved hearing people's birthing stories; and I loved watching a TV show called *The Baby Story*. I was totally obsessed with it! It actually really helped me. I learned that birth wasn't so scary, that usually when you're birthing, it's just a few people in the room, unless you're having a problem. It helped to see women going through a regular, vaginal childbirth. It's not so frightening, there's not a lot of fanfare—in a good way. Just being exposed to these stories actually helped me give myself over to the experience completely.

Mary, mom of two

We didn't take a class, mostly because I missed the deadline to sign up for it. But we got a doula who came to our house a couple of times. We watched some videos with her, and she had a doll to show us what happens, and we talked about different possibilities in labor, which gave me a sense of what to expect. I didn't feel prepared, exactly, but I also didn't feel like I was turning a corner with no idea what was behind it. I had a friend who did hypnotherapy, and she spent an enormous amount of time in these classes and it really helped her and that's what she needed—but it's not something that I would've benefited from. What did help, though, was prenatal yoga, because I really learned a lot about my body, especially as it got bigger and bigger. When it came time to actually deliver, I used a lot of my yoga breathing, and the sense of knowing my body was really helpful. I know it sounds sort of cheesy, but it's true.

Jane, mom of one, pregnant

I took a birthing class that I loved even though it scared the shit out of me. I had been pretty laid back about everything and when I learned what could go wrong, I realized the true meaning of "ignorance is bliss"!! Still, I would advise people *not* to get overly nervous about childbirth. My sister gave me amazing advice before my first child was born, and it really stuck with me. She said that so many people worry so much about labor/childbirth and really, the hardest part comes in those first two weeks when it's all so exhausting and new, and you're healing. The other thing to remember is that the labor/childbirth is so finite! It ends and the pain is forgotten.

Kate, mom of one, pregnant

I would definitely recommend taking a class, and definitely take it with your partner. The thing that I learned from it was that my body could do this. The wonderful thing about Birthing from Within (the class I took) is that they really do give you a connection to all the women throughout history who've given birth, so you don't feel like you're doing something that isn't possible. You really do think that this is something that women do, and we've always done it, and so we'll all be fine. I really did believe it. And also I learned to let my body take over. They say trust your instincts and that your body knows what to do. The nurses at the hospital were great about letting me be in any position I wanted during labor. You don't have to think about what to do, you just kind of do it.

Maia, mom of one

A Birth Plan

• *What it is:* A birth plan is primarily a statement about your preferences and feelings around birth and labor. It's useful in several different ways. First, the process of writing a birth plan can help you clarify and articulate your ideas about labor and birth. Also, you can use either the process of writing a birth plan or the written plan itself to initiate a conversation with your care provider about your preferences, concerns, and general outlook as labor nears. Finally, if you're planning to give birth at a hospital or birthing center, a birth plan can give the staff some important information about you, your background, and what's important to you.

• *What it isn't:* A birth plan can't bind your care provider or the hospital/birthing center staff to a particular course of treatment. The document goes into your chart, and most, if not all, of your preferences will be respected as long as they don't create a medical concern (which is unlikely if you've discussed the plan with your care provider). But the hard fact remains that if complications develop, the legal and ethical obligations for your well-being and that of your baby rest in the hands of the medical professionals you'll be working with. By the time you're in labor, ideally you'll have a high level of confidence in your medical birthing team, and you'll be able to trust that your care provider and her partners/covering physicians (who may be attending your labor) understand your approach to and overall expectations for labor and birth. In this situation, if you have to have a procedure or intervention that's not in your plan, or that you've said beforehand you didn't want, you'll be able to participate in the decision to change course, and trust that it's being done out of necessity.

• *Communicating with your care provider:* Just as the process of creating a birth plan gives you the chance to identify what's most important to you, the process of discussing your birth plan with your care provider can be an equally important step in creating a positive birth experience. Before you bring in a birth plan, let your care provider know that you're planning to write one or that you'd like her input into the plan itself.

When you sit down to talk about your plan, try to stay open to your care provider's perspective. If you can both really listen to what the other has to say, you can establish a mutual understanding for your labor and birth—even if your care provider doesn't typically work with birth plans.

If you're in a group practice and you're not sure who will be on call when you go into labor, ask the care provider with whom you discuss your birth plan to share the most important points of your conversation; you can decide together what those are. (It's standard in group practices to discuss issues concerning patients who might go into labor with the physicians or midwives who will be "on call" at a specific time.)

• *Communicating with the nursing staff:* This is an important function of a birth plan because once you're in labor you may not be in any mood to present your feelings and wishes about labor and birth to the hospital staff. If you clearly, concisely, and respectfully present your mind-set and preferences concerning labor and birth, the nursing staff will have a better idea of how best to care for you.

What Makes a Birth Plan Work

✦ We asked Penny Simkin, author, doula, and birth plan advocate, about what makes a successful birth plan.

Q: Ideally what should—and shouldn't—be included in a birth plan?

Penny Simkin: I really urge an introduction in which a woman tells the hospital or birthing center staff about herself. Nurses don't know the clients at all; they're total strangers. They may not know that this woman is terrified that her baby is going to have Down syndrome because she had a triple screen showing a possibility of Down. They may not know that she's been infertile for nine years and this pregnancy means everything and she wants every heartbeat monitored, every intervention that could possibly make a difference. Or they may not know that a woman's only experience in the hospital was to visit her dying grandmother, and she has all these negative associations with the hospital. These are things that are important, and learning about them enables the staff to take the woman as a human being and an individual.

It's also important for her to be up front about any fears that she has. For example, a lot of women have a phobia of needles, of blood draws. Well, if a woman knows she panics when she has a blood draw, she can tell the staff that in a birth plan and then the nurse isn't completely caught off guard when it happens.

Q: Do you feel that presenting your emotional context for the birth is just as important to the birth plan as details like "I want to move around" or "I don't want an IV"?

PS: More important. I think explaining a general approach is probably more appropriate than those details of "I'll have this kind of monitoring but not that." Those checklists that are on Web sites are terrible; I don't think they're clarifying to anybody.

The most significant points in birth plans are: an introduction, an explanation of any fears or concerns, and a general statement about how you want your care to be handled. In other words, many people say, "I'm no expert on this, I want the doctor to run the show, and I'd appreciate being informed of what you're doing and why." Others will say, "This is a life-altering experience for me. I'd like to be an active participant in my care. I'd like to minimize the interventions, have maximum communication, and do as much self-coping as possible." When a woman gives a general approach like that, then the care provider, who, let's face it, really has the power, can put things together when the time comes.

There's *so much* potential in talking over a birth plan with a care provider, and when doing so, care providers can often simplify a very detailed birth plan with the woman's trust and appreciation.

• *Specifics to consider when writing a birth plan:* Once you've figured out your general approach to labor and birth (see "What Makes a Birth Plan Work," page 412), it's worth considering a few specific aspects of labor and birth so you can discuss your preferences with your care provider. These include:

— *Standard protocols:* What are the standard protocols where you'll be giving birth? What are your caregiver's protocols? If they include steps that you have questions about, such as putting in an IV right away or setting up continuous electronic fetal monitoring (see page 468), talk to your doctor or midwife about your options with those or any protocols you wonder about.

— *Birth team:* Find out if your birthing location limits the number of people you can have in the labor room/birthing suite. If they do, and if your birth team exceeds the allowed number, discuss whether or not an exception can be made and what options you might have.

— *Pain medication:* If you'd prefer not to be offered medication or an epidural for labor pain, talk with your caregiver about the best way to handle that, particularly if you'll be giving birth in a hospital. Also, talk with your care provider and your birth partner, doula, and/or team members about situations in which you might want pain medication. For example, some people like to come up with a code word for when they're *really* sure they want drugs. Others just want to be able to say, "I want an epidural."

— *Episiotomy:* If you have strong feelings about this procedure (see page 474), bring it up with your caregiver. If you'd like to avoid an episiotomy, when you discuss your birth plan, ask your care provider what steps she might be able to take to help minimize the chances you'll either need or have one if another doctor/midwife attends your birth.

— *Cesarean section:* Find out what the standard procedures are during and after a C-section. Can your labor support person be there? Can your doula join you and your partner in the operating room? How quickly will you be able to hold and/or nurse the baby after surgery?

— *Post-birth:* If you want someone other than your care provider to cut the umbilical cord, tell your caregiver and include that in your birth plan. Also, review the standard post-birth procedures where you'll be delivering, discuss your preferences with your care provider, and include them in the plan. (See page 452 for a description of what happens right after a baby is born.)

— *Breastfeeding:* Include whether or not you plan to breastfeed. (See page 496 for more on breastfeeding immediately after birth and in the hospital.)

• *An effective birth plan:* When you pack your bag for the hospital or birth center, include several copies of your birth plan to give to the staff. If you don't live in an area where birth plans are standard and you want the staff to take the document seriously, I recommend three things:

1. Adapt the general approach we've described here, using the document to present who you are, what's important to you, and your preferences.

2. Try to avoid being too directive or negative. For example, if you write "Don't offer me an epidural" or "No IV," you set an oppositional tone. Instead, try to state your preferences clearly and positively—e.g., "I hope to have a natural childbirth, and I'll ask for an epidural if I need it" or "I'd prefer to only have an IV if it becomes medically necessary."

3. Keep the document relatively brief (about one page) so the staff can incorporate it into your care easily.

Preparing the Pelvis: Kegels and Perineal Massage

• *Kegels:* Developed by Dr. Arnold Kegel to help women with problems controlling urination, "Kegels" build the muscles of the pelvic floor. Specifically, Kegels strengthen the pubococcygeus (PC) muscle, part of a set of muscles that extend from your pubic bone to your tailbone. To do the exercise, simply contract the muscles around your vagina as if you were stopping the flow of urine, count to ten, and release. Do ten repetitions two or three times daily. (You may have to work up to this; these muscles tire easily.)

Some natural childbirth instructors advocate doing Kegels throughout pregnancy to strengthen your perineum (the area between the vagina and the anus), learn to relax the muscles there, and avoid an episiotomy (see page 474). A recent study of 301 first-time mothers in Norway showed that when women do a regular routine of pelvic-floor exercises from week 24 through week 36, it can help shorten the "pushing" stage of labor. (For the "pushing," or second, stage of labor, see page 451.)

In my experience, however, some women build up their perineal muscles to such a degree that they have difficulty relaxing them enough in birth. And when you start to push, you won't be using those perineal muscles as much as the large muscles of your diaphragm and abdomen. Therefore, when you do Kegel exercises—I recommend three to five sets of ten each day—bring as much attention to the release phase as the tensing phase of the exercise. Let the muscle relax completely, pause, notice what it feels like to relax these muscles, and then contract again.

• *Always do Kegels:* If you have any urinary incontinence during your pregnancy, do three to five sets of ten Kegels daily.

After you give birth, whether vaginally or by C-section, do three to five sets of ten Kegels each day. Kegels are useful after a Cesarean because even if the perineum wasn't strained in labor, the pelvic floor was strained by being pregnant.

• *Perineal massage:* Perineal massage is another way to prepare the perineum for childbirth and help avoid an episiotomy. The goal of doing this is to gently stretch the perineum while learning to relax it.

Starting at around thirty weeks, do the massage described below three times a week. At thirty-four or thirty-five weeks, you can either increase to nightly massage or maintain the routine that you have.

You can do the massage yourself or have your partner do it. Whoever does it should have trimmed nails and clean hands, and should use a lubricant (either a pure vegetable or fruit oil, like olive oil, or a water-based lubricant like K-Y jelly).

There are two methods for perineal massage:

1. Imagine the opening of the vagina as a clock face. Using lubricant, gently insert one or two fingers around four o'clock. Slide the fingers down and up to around eight o'clock. Around six o'clock, apply a little extra pressure until you feel some resistance. That's where the perineal body is strongest, and that's what you want to relax in order to open the vagina. Slide your fingers up to eight o'clock and then back to four o'clock, pressing down gently again at around six o'clock. Keep doing this for up to five minutes.

2. Again, think of the vagina as a clock face. Using a lubricant, slide both thumbs in at six o'clock. Gently press down until you feel some resistance and then simultaneously slide your thumbs outward, with one thumb going up to four o'clock and the other up to eight o'clock. Bring both thumbs back to six o'clock. Keep going for up to five minutes.

With either method, breathe deeply and try to *relax* as the fingers press into your perineum. It might feel weird, and you might experience some tingling, but you shouldn't feel any real discomfort or burning. The next day you might feel some muscle soreness, but that's fine and normal.

When you do this massage regularly, you or your partner will find that you have to press down a little harder to get some resistance. For example, at first you might only be able to press down about one millimeter. As the weeks go on, you may be able to press down as much as one centimeter (but don't worry about specific measurements—these numbers are just meant to give you a sense of the change in muscle resistance). If perineal massage turns into sexual foreplay, it's absolutely fine and safe.

Birthing Locations

In the United States today, you can choose to give birth in a hospital, birthing center, or at home. Each one has its pros and cons. When deciding where to give birth, you need to figure out what kind of care will best meet your needs and make you the most comfortable. The vast majority of births (between 85 and 90 percent) happen without complications, and there's no reason to assume your birth will be anything but normal. Still, it does make sense to have a contingency plan in place for the small but real possibility that complications will develop. Therefore, when you consider where you want to give birth, think about where you'll feel most confident and cared for. In other words, ask yourself what the right balance is for you between assuming all will be well and creating a "just in case" plan.

Here's an overview of the basic choices for birth locations:

• *Hospitals:* In the U.S., hospitals offer the most comprehensive maternity care, and most can handle any emergency situation that might develop during labor and birth. But hospitals are not exactly inviting places. They're big institutions; they're impersonal; the food isn't great; and they may have bureaucratic procedures that are baffling at best and frustrating at worst. Also, it can be strange to go to the hospital when you're not sick.

Often people choose hospitals for birth because they feel good going to a place that's equipped to handle any emergency that might arise. Plus, these days, many hospitals have created birthing rooms that look a little homier, so you can have a less hospital-like hospital experience. For example, the medical equipment is behind cabinet doors, and the furniture can be quite comfortable. But you may not have access to amenities like a tub to labor in or a wider bed to share postpartum (see "Birth Centers," page 419).

As I've mentioned, touring the birthing/maternity unit of a hospital to see what it looks like will help on several fronts. If you're unsure whether or not you want to give birth in a hospital, it will give you a little more information with which you can make that decision. (If this is the case for you, I'd recommend going on a hospital tour early in your second trimester so you'll have time to change care providers if that becomes necessary.) If you know you'll give birth in a hospital, a tour will make the experience of going in a little less intimidating and overwhelming.

What to look for in a hospital:

— *Anesthesia:* An anesthesiologist on site twenty-four hours a day is ideal but not always necessary or possible. Smaller hospitals may only have an anesthesiologist on call, not on site. Find out what the staffing is where you plan to deliver, and how quickly an anesthesiologist can be there in case of an emergency C-section, when immediate access to an anesthesiologist is crucial. Also, ask if the hospital will call in additional anesthesiologists to the labor floor to place an epidural if the on-call anesthesiologist is busy in the operating room. Sometimes hospitals will only call in additional anesthesiologists for emergency C-sections, not routine labor epidurals.

— *A neonatal intensive care unit (NICU):* Since you may be choosing to be in a hospital to reduce your risk on every front, find out what kind of newborn care a hospital offers. NICUs and nurseries have three classifications:

1. *Level III NICU care unit:* These provide the latest in pediatric care for newborns, and will have a neonatologist (a doctor specializing in the care of newborns with health problems) on staff 24/7. They are usually found only in large university hospitals.

2. *Level II NICU:* These can handle *almost* all of the situations that a level III NICU can, and they will have a neonatologist either on call or on site 24/7. (If you're giving birth at a level II hospital, ask your care provider which it is.) These units are typically in more advanced community hospitals.

3. *Level I nursery:* This is a nursery that provides basic, routine newborn care and may or may not have a neonatologist on call. (Ask your care provider if they do and what happens in case of an emergency.) No intensive care can be provided in a level I nursery.

— *The labor/birth environment:* Can you dim the lights? Bring your own music? Are there birthing bars or stools available? (A woman can use a birthing, or squatting, bar during the pushing phase of labor (see page 451) to help her stay in a squatting position, or she can brace herself against it instead of having someone hold her legs or using stirrups. Birthing stools allow a woman to actually sit upright in a squatting position while she's pushing.) Are there showers or tubs to labor in? Do you give birth in the same room you labor in?

— *Relatively flexible protocols:* Can the hospital adapt to the protocols you and your care provider agree to? For example, if it's hospital policy to set you up with an IV and you don't want one, can you choose to have a heparin lock instead? (A "hep lock" is when a needle with a closed tube is inserted into your arm and taped there without being attached to an IV pole.) Or not have one at all?

— *Relatively flexible postpartum protocols:* Again, if you want more time with your baby than hospital protocols typically allow, can they adapt to your wishes? (For example, if you want to spend time with your newborn right after birth and before he's cleaned up or has eyedrops, can you? See chapter 23 for a rundown of postpartum procedures.)

— *Lactation support:* Find out what kind of breastfeeding support is offered in the hospital. Many hospitals have lactation consultants on staff and offer breastfeeding classes to new moms.

— *Is it a teaching hospital?* If so, it means they have the latest technology and are always fully staffed. It also means there might be residents and/or medical students around for some part of your labor and birth. If you're giving birth in a teaching hospital, you'll be asked to sign a release allowing students and residents to attend. You can opt not to sign; discuss this with your care provider.

REAL VOICES

We were in bed around eleven at night around three weeks before my due date when I heard a pop, and I knew it wasn't gas but it kind of sounded like it. Then I felt this gush—not a huge one—and I said to my husband, "Oh my gosh, my water broke." And he said, "No. No way." We looked on the sheets, and I knew I hadn't peed. I thought maybe it could be discharge, but it was a lot of fluid. After that I had about a half an hour of shaking, sitting on the toilet letting the amniotic fluid just drip out of me, and diarrhea. I called my doctor and he said go to the hospital because they'd want to deliver within twenty-four hours. It wasn't a huge rush, but we definitely wanted to get to the hospital. We lived five minutes away, and we felt more comfortable there—especially with my water breaking and it being my first baby, there wasn't any reason to stay home.

Mary, mom of two

Actually, the first time with my twins, I labored a little too long at home . . . Let's just say I got to the hospital just in time. I did most of my laboring in the bathroom, and I kept kicking my husband out of the room, so he missed my transition. I kept waiting for the pain to get absolutely unbearable. It hurt, but I kept waiting for it to get worse. You know, you hear these terrible stories . . . So I was waiting for it to get even worse, and then I needed to push! We got to the hospital in a big hurry.

Rochelle, mom of three

• *Birth centers:* Birth centers are typically staffed and run by midwives with OB consultants for emergencies and certain complications. If you opt for a birth center, you'll probably have your prenatal care there from the staff midwives. Some birth centers are owned independently by midwifery practices.

A birth center may be freestanding, near a hospital (across the street, for example), or physically within a hospital building. The labor and birthing rooms are likely to be homier and more family-oriented than on a hospital maternity

HIGHER-RISK BIRTHS

Most often, vaginal deliveries in these categories are absolutely safe. But they do have some risks associated with them that make a hospital a better choice for a birth location. A birth center located in the same building as a hospital would also be a safe choice for these situations.

- *Vaginal birth after Cesarean "VBAC" or other uterine surgery:* Scars on the uterus may rupture during childbirth. (See page 482.)
- *Breech:* You may have to sign consent forms before a vaginal breech delivery. (See page 430.)
- *Twins:* Vaginal delivery of twins is standard when the first twin is head down. (See page 457.)
- *If a mother has gestational diabetes:* There's a greater chance the baby could be large and need medical attention immediately after birth.
- *Preeclampsia or hypertension*
- *Large fibroids:* How large depends on where they are in the uterus.
- *Too much or too little amniotic fluid:* Polyhydramnios and oligohydramnios, respectively. (See page 334.)
- *Preterm labor or birth:* In which case, you'd want access to an NICU. (See page 417.)
- *Intrauterine growth restriction (IUGR):* In which case, you'd want access to an NICU. (See page 345.)

floor. You will probably have access to a large tub in which to labor, bigger rooms, and a bigger bed. Birthing centers embrace a philosophy of birth with minimal medical interventions. (For standard medical procedures used during labor, see page 468.) A birth center will not typically have an anesthesiologist on call to provide an epidural, but a certified nurse midwife can administer narcotic—or "systemic"—pain medication (see page 461). Birth centers are appropriate for low-risk pregnancies and childbirths.

If you're considering giving birth in a birthing center, research the center's history, accreditation, and reputation. How many births do they handle in a year? Who serves as OB backup? At what point would they transfer you to a hospital setting? How long does an average transfer take? What happens if you decide you would like to give birth in the hospital instead of the birthing center? What's the center's C-section rate? What kind of neonatal/pediatric care is available? First-time mothers should consider how close the birthing center is to a hospital and how easy it is to transfer to a hospital facility, particularly in case of an emergency.

REAL VOICES
I went to the birth center at around ten-thirty at night—it's just kind of a wing on the eleventh floor (of a hospital), and labor and delivery is on the twelfth floor, so if they need to transfer you it's just one floor. I preferred to be in the hospital and have a safety net around me. Why not? When I got there, the midwife on call opened the door to the floor. She had a big smile on her face and said, "Welcome!" It was so nice.

Miranda, mom of one, pregnant

• *Home births:* In the U.S., home births are controversial. Some people consider home the ideal environment in which to labor and give birth; others think it's too risky.

HIGHER-RISK BIRTHS *(continued)*

• *A known anatomic or genetic abnormality:* In which case, you'd want access to an NICU.
• *Large size baby (larger than nine pounds):* A care provider may suspect a baby is big, or her size can be estimated by ultrasound in the weeks before birth. Large babies are more likely to have metabolic problems (low blood sugar), which would warrant medical attention, and their shoulders are more likely to get stuck on the way out of the birth canal (shoulder dystocia). The latter can lead to serious complications, including the need for immediate resuscitation, permanent nerve damage in the baby's neck and arm, or more severe damage.

Still others think that while there are risks, it's a relatively safe choice if you've already had one vaginal birth without complications. Most often, home births are attended by midwives who specialize in them and provide all prenatal care during the pregnancy. Deciding on a home birth means figuring out how much risk you're comfortable with and what's most important to you in a birth experience.

You can minimize the risks associated with a home birth by doing some advance planning:

1. *Look for a highly experienced, certified midwife and have a consulting OB in place:* (See pages 86–90.) All certified midwives have an OB backup on call. I strongly recommend meeting with the OB in advance so that if an emergency situation unfolds, you're not meeting for the first time in that context.

2. *Have a backup plan in place:* You should not be more than twenty minutes from a hospital. (In some rural areas, this means that you may labor and

give birth in someone else's home or a hotel.) The twenty-minute access window is important if an unforeseen problem develops. Plan a route to the hospital and ask your midwife if you need to make any advance arrangements with the hospital.

3. *Do your homework:* Research the ins and outs of home births thoroughly and learn as much as you can about labor and childbirth. Talk with your midwife about the contingencies and what situations would mean you would go to the hospital.

REAL VOICES

Part of the reason we decided to have a home birth the second time was our crazy cab ride to the birth center the first time I gave birth. It was rush hour, and there were contractions every two minutes. I was on my hands and knees in the backseat moaning and yelling. Very uncomfortable. The other reason was that, for me, the fact that I could only stay in the birth center for twenty-four hours really sucked. My daughter was born at 10:50, and we left the next day at 6 P.M. I was like, "Now I have to pack again!" There was all this packing and unpacking and all this traveling. It just was so rushed! I didn't really feel like I wanted to have some special, meaningful thing with my family in my home; it was just the hassle of traveling when I didn't have a good alternative nearby. As it turned out, after my second daughter was born on the third floor of our house, I just went down into my own bed and that was *heaven*.

Erin, mom of two

I'd done a lot of reading, as many older mothers tend to do, and I really wanted to have a natural childbirth. I thought that would be less likely in a hospital because I thought the minute things started not conforming to hospital protocols—like "dilate one centimeter per hour" or "give birth within twenty-four hours of water breaking"—I would feel pressure to take steps that would take me further and further away from the birth I'd envisioned. And while having a hospital birth is important for some women, hospitals make me nervous. So I was faced with just two possible models: a hospital birth with a doula or a home birth. The two seemed at such extremes, but there weren't any in-between options because the closest birthing center to where I live is at least an hour away. It was a difficult decision, particularly since my husband wasn't crazy about the idea of a home birth. But we met with a friend who was studying to be a midwife, and she allayed my husband's fears about home birth. I also got parallel prenatal care with an OB and my home-birth midwife, since my insurance covered the OB, and I paid for my midwife's care out-of-pocket. That meant that if I had to go to the hospital, or if things changed during my pregnancy, I had a doctor of record who knew me and my pregnancy, and this seemed like a viable backup plan. It also enabled me to have access to a variety of medical tests—for example, amniocentesis—that I couldn't get through my home-birth midwife.

Sue, mom of two

20

The Last Weeks of Pregnancy

As childbirth nears, your body starts to change subtly, and your inner world begins to shift, too. You may find that you're more introspective and your emotions are even more intense. Your dreams may be more vivid, and your moods may swing more easily.

In this chapter, I talk about some of the typical physical and emotional changes of the last few weeks of pregnancy. I describe signs that labor is approaching, what early labor is like, how you can encourage it, and how and why labor is induced. I also review some of the basic questions that come up when a baby is in the breech (buttocks first) position.

✦ ✦ ✦

In this chapter you'll find:

- The Last Month . . . or So: The Countdown Begins
- The Body Prepares for Labor and Birth
- Breech Presentation
- Signs of Labor
- Encouraging Labor
- Inducing Labor

The Last Month . . . or So: The Countdown Begins

As you head into the last few weeks of the third trimester, you may feel bigger, and more cautious, than ever. The pregnant women I work with often ask if they can keep up with their hectic daily routines, and for the most part, my advice is to keep doing what you're comfortable doing, with the caveat that you should try to carve out a little bit of time both to connect with your baby (see page 405) and to rest. Fatigue can be a problem late in pregnancy. Your body is working at full capacity during the day, and you may be having trouble sleeping at night for a few reasons: It can be hard to find a comfortable position; the baby may keep you awake with kicking; and you may have to go to the bathroom frequently. (For dealing with third-trimester insomnia, see page 185.) So if you have a chance to lie down and relax during the day, even for a fifteen-minute catnap, take it.

• *Work:* You can continue to work as long as you like and as long as your commute is feasible. Work might help keep you centered and engaged at a time when it's natural to start feeling impatient for the birth. If you're planning to return to work after your baby is born, you probably have a limited number of weeks for maternity leave. Most of the women I work with say that while it's nice to have the time off before they give birth, they *really* want that time at home with their babies afterward.

Keep in mind that it is *not* safe to drive while you're having contractions, so if working means driving, it may make sense to stop at thirty-eight weeks unless you can work out a plan with a coworker who'll drive you home if contractions begin (even if it turns out to be "false" labor) or you can take a taxi. (For more on when to stop work, see page 329.)

• *Exercise:* Some women exercise up until the very end of their pregnancies; others find that they're too uncomfortable or tired to keep working out. This is another situation where you really need to listen to your body. If you want to keep working out in these last weeks, you don't have to hold back, but this isn't a time to push yourself. As long as you've exercised consistently throughout your pregnancy, you can continue to do low-impact activities like walking, swimming, riding a stationary bike, yoga, Pilates, etc., up to the very last days of your pregnancy *as long as you feel comfortable.* In fact, it can be a good idea to keep exercising for as long as you can. Even a gentle workout can help clear your mind and relieve any anxiety that you might be feeling about childbirth or parenting. Plus, exercising will help you both sleep better and feel more energetic during the day.

Waiting Out the Wait: Finding Inner Peace

✦ Waiting for labor to begin can be tough. You're big, uncomfortable, and overtired. Plus, you could be living with many different layers of intense emotions. You may be excited to meet your baby, and at the same time you may feel some nostalgia about your pregnancy coming to an end and trepidation either about the birth and actually having a baby. No matter what your emotional landscape looks like, by this time it's not at all unusual to be a little overwhelmed by the potent mix of physical discomfort, excitement, anticipation, and even fear that accompanies the transition to parenthood.

To help keep things in perspective, I recommend repeating a simple "mantra" (traditionally a verbal phrase repeated in meditation or prayer). Take a few deep breaths and say to yourself, "All is well. All is as it should be. All will be well." Repeat this phrase to yourself as you go to sleep, when you wake up, and at any point in the day when you find yourself thinking you can't take another minute of being pregnant, you start to get nervous about labor, you find yourself having a face-off with your "to do" list (and the list is winning), or all of the above.

Often when I talk to patients about trying this, they'll ask, "Do you really believe that all will be well?" The truth is, I really do. After all, you won't be pregnant forever. The really important things will get done. Even with labor, while there's no way to know what will happen, the odds are that it will go relatively smoothly and you'll come through it healthy with a healthy baby.

• *Cleaning the house:* Here's one area where, if it's possible, you definitely can start to scale back (unless you're nesting and can't!). The bending and lifting involved with heavy cleaning stresses your joints and can injure your back. The time you would spend cleaning is better used for rests, walks, even work. Ask your partner or a friend to help you keep your house in order, or if you can afford it, hire someone to come in and clean for you. Asking for help and letting go of housework now is good practice for what you'll need to do after the baby comes.

REAL VOICES
I went to my midwife for an appointment today and she said, "Okay, so we'll have just three or four more of these." And all of a sudden it hit me: I'm going to have a *baby*. So much of this has been about the pregnancy—getting pregnant, staying pregnant, being pregnant. But the pregnancy isn't the point. Soon I'm going to have a baby!

Margaret, pregnant

The Body Prepares for Labor and Birth

Throughout the last few weeks of pregnancy, your body starts to prepare in subtle and not-so-subtle ways for labor and birth:

• *Braxton Hicks contractions:* You may notice that you're having many more Braxton Hicks contractions, which by definition don't lead to labor. (For more on Braxton Hicks contractions, see page 193.) As labor draws closer, you may have days when you have Braxton Hicks contractions for several hours. When this happens, contractions come at regular intervals, but they don't get longer, stronger, or more painful. And then they stop. These are considered "pre-labor" contractions, and even though it can be discouraging if they don't progress into labor, they help the uterus prepare for labor and birthing.

If you start having Braxton Hicks contractions during the day and you feel emotionally and physically ready to deliver, then take a walk to try to encourage them to continue and "flip" into early-labor contractions. If they start in the middle of the night, try to keep sleeping (you need all the rest you can get before labor). Or if they start and you're not quite ready for labor (if, for example, your baby shower is later that day), try lying down on your left side and drinking one liter of fluid over thirty to sixty minutes. This will help them stop if you're actually not in very early labor.

• *The baby drops:* As childbirth nears, the baby moves lower into the pelvis. Usually you can feel the drop because you feel more weight, pressure, and even discomfort in your pelvis, and you have to urinate more frequently. Ironically, this phenomenon is sometimes called "lightening" because after the baby drops, your stomach and lungs have more room to do their work.

Your care provider will know this has happened because when the baby drops, your fundal height (the distance from the top of the pelvic bone to the top of the uterus), which he has been tracking since twenty weeks, shrinks; for example, you can go from thirty-eight centimeters to thirty-seven centimeters. When this happens, your care provider will probably perform a pelvic exam to evaluate the length of your cervix (see "Effacement" and "Dilation" below) and to see if he can feel the baby's head.

• *Effacement:* As the baby presses downward in the pelvis, the cervix, which is a tube made primarily of a thick, fibrous substance called collagen, gets shorter and thinner; this is known as "effacement." On average, a cervix is normally two centimeters long when measured by hand during a pelvic exam. When your doctor or midwife tells you that you're, for example, "50 percent effaced," it means that your cervix is 50 percent shorter, or one centimeter long, and thinner than usual. In labor, your cervix will be paper-thin when it's "100 percent effaced."

• *Dilation:* As your cervix shortens (effaces), it can also start to open up, or "dilate." As with effacement, the dilation process often begins before you're technically in labor. It can be exciting to learn that your cervix is a few centimeters dilated or somewhat effaced, but you can't predict when labor will begin based on the state of your cervix. In fact, you can walk around for a couple of weeks with a cervix that's two or three centimeters dilated. (In my practice, the record is held by a woman who was five centimeters dilated for two weeks.)

• A *burst of energy:* In the week or two before labor begins, many—not all, but many—women experience a burst of energy, famously known as "the nesting instinct." If this doesn't happen to you, it doesn't mean you're not about to go into labor. But the phenomenon is real—it's not just an old wives' tale—and if you experience this rush of energy, you may find yourself cleaning nooks and crannies in your house, updating all the addresses of everyone you've known since high school, or scrubbing every floor. You certainly don't have to resist these urges. But try not to overdo it and exhaust yourself.

REAL VOICES

I stockpiled an entire freezer full of food before my second daughter was born in January. The fact that she was two weeks late didn't help. Suffice to say, my husband once caught me making four meals at once, including one that had me carving up a pork butt bigger than the baby I eventually delivered.

Mary Elizabeth, mom of two

I'm not a nester, and I didn't get a huge burst of energy in either pregnancy. I did, however, feel a growing sense of panic as my due dates approached that I had not even begun to finish any of the tasks on my list of things to do. In fact, those tasks are still not done, but the list has been destroyed, probably by one of my daughters.

Suzanne, mom of two

The so-called nesting instinct did kick in, but, in my opinion, it was only because I couldn't rest—I was anxious, uncomfortable, and impatient. (These are qualities I tend to have anyway.) So, to pass the time (often in the middle of the night), I'd clean, seriously: mopping, painting, washing the baby's clothes in Dreft for the twentieth time, rearranging furniture, organizing the baby equipment . . .

Jane, mom of one, pregnant

• *More physical signs that labor's on the way:* In the week before labor begins, additional signs start to appear. These include more frequent and more painful Braxton Hicks contractions, the baby dropping even farther into the pelvis, worsening hip pain, more frequent urination (yes, it's possible!), vaginal pain, and more low back pain. Right as labor begins, the body releases prostaglandins, which causes the uterus to contract. Sometimes prostaglandins make the

WHAT TO PACK

If you're planning to give birth in a hospital or birthing center, you'll probably pack a few things for your childbirth and time away from home. Here are some suggestions.

- *For you for birth:*
  - Music and CD/MP3/tape player
  - Candle (if you want and it's allowed by hospital)
  - Lip balm
  - Lotion/massage oil
  - Massage device (tennis balls, rollers), if you're planning on using one
  - Toothbrush and toothpaste
  - Hairbrush/ponytail holders (if you've got long hair)
  - Socks/slippers
  - Gown/robe (if you prefer your own)
  - Juice, sports drink, lollipops, bottled water, and/or popsicles, if possible
- *For you postpartum:*
  - Nursing bra
  - Nightgown/shirt/robe that opens in front (if you prefer your own)
  - Basic toiletries
  - Something to wear home
- *For baby*
  - Diapers (usually these are given by the hospital, but ask your caregiver what's standard)
  - Two layers of clothing (e.g., kimono shirt/onesie and outer layer) (Bring

WHAT TO PACK *(continued)*

warm clothing if it's cool/cold. Here's a good rule of thumb: No matter what time of year, the baby will need one more layer than you do. So if you'll be wearing a shirt, sweater, and jacket, the baby will need four layers and a hat.)
  – Receiving blanket
  – Crib blanket
  – Car seat (install in advance)
• *For your partner/labor coach:*
  – Toothbrush/toothpaste/toiletries
  – Change of underwear/clothes
  – List of phone numbers of people to call
  – Cell phone/phone card (A hospital may or may not let you use a cell phone near equipment; ask about the policy when you tour the facility.)
  – Snacks

bowels contract, too, and the result is diarrhea.

Breech Presentation

Care providers use the term "presentation" to describe how a baby is positioned in the uterus. The part of the baby's body that's directly above the cervix is the body part that will emerge first during birth; it's called the "presenting" part. Most babies are head-down in what's called "vertex" or "cephalic presentation." This is the preferred position for birth because the biggest part of the baby, his head, leaves your body first—so everyone knows that it *can* get out. When a baby's bottom is the presenting body part, he's considered breech, a riskier position for a vaginal birth.

(See "The Risks of a Vaginal Breech Birth" on page 434.) A care provider can usually figure out if a baby is breech by feeling your abdomen, and an ultrasound exam can confirm the diagnosis.

Before thirty weeks, a breech isn't really a concern, because the baby is likely to turn on his own. (Twenty-five percent of babies are found to be breech before twenty-eight weeks. By thirty-two weeks, 7 percent of pregnancies are breech, and 3 to 4 percent of women in labor at term have babies in a breech position.) Basically, between thirty-two and thirty-four weeks, there's a good chance that a baby will turn on his own. In my experience, after thirty-six weeks, it becomes less likely that a baby will turn, simply because he has less room to maneuver.

• *Turning a breech:* There are several ways to encourage a baby to turn from breech into a vertex position. The following are techniques I use regularly and have had the most success with:

— *Exercise:* Starting in week 30 and continuing for four to six weeks more (or until the baby turns), do the following exercise twice daily on an empty stomach.

Make a nine- to twelve-inch pile of pillows or folded blankets on the floor. Lie down with your back on the pile. Shift so your buttocks are near one end of the pile, with the middle of your back at the opposite end and your head and shoulders on the ground. Stay here, with your pelvis nine to twelve inches above your shoulders and head, for ten to fifteen minutes.

This exercise has been shown to encourage a breech baby to turn into a vertex position, or if the baby has "dropped" in a breech, it can dislodge her from the pelvis just enough to make it easier for another turning method to succeed.

— *Acupuncture/traditional Chinese medicine (TCM):* There are many different protocols in TCM for turning a breech. One that's relatively widely used and well studied for both safety and effectiveness involves applying heat from a burning moxibustion stick to the acupuncture point on the outside corner of the fifth toes ("Bladder 67") for five to ten minutes. (Moxibustion uses the herb *Artemisia vulgaris,* also known as mugwort.)

A practitioner may warm one toe for five to ten minutes and then the other, or he may warm one toe for one minute, switch to the other side, and then go back and forth for five to ten minutes. You may have several treatments each week, or you may be given a stick of moxibustion to use at home daily. The details of when to start the treatment—and how often it should be repeated—will vary from practitioner to practitioner, but in clinical studies, treatment usually begins at thirty-three weeks.

In my practice, we typically start moxibustion treatments at thirty-four weeks and continue them once a week until thirty-six weeks. When we do a moxibustion treatment, a woman is on continuous fetal monitoring so we can be sure there's no fetal distress. But monitoring is not essential for the procedure to be safely and effectively performed. (In one study, pregnant women had a non-stress test at the same time as a moxibustion treatment. The study showed babies were active during a treatment and were not distressed at all by it.)

From my perspective as a doctor of Western medicine, using moxibustion to turn a breech baby is a wonderful option. It poses minimal risk to a mother and baby, and it's been shown to be effective in many clinical studies. (There's no standard statistical rate of success because of the variety of methods used. Estimates of success rate range from 50 to 84 percent.)

From My Office: An Acupuncturist's Perspective on Turning a Breech

✦ "Theoretically, moxibustion encourages a baby in breech position to move because it literally sends energy, or qi, directly into the mother's meridian, which boosts the mother's and baby's energy. But it's useful to remember that a version with moxa also works because the baby wants it to. That's a basic idea in Chinese medicine—it doesn't force anything on people; for a treatment to work, it has to work on both sides."—Jacques Depardieu, MSOM, L/Ac

If you're interested in trying TCM to turn a breech, look for a practitioner who has a lot of experience with this technique, even if it means going to someone other than your regular acupuncturist.

— *External version:* This medical procedure involves physically turning the baby from breech to vertex by pressing on a woman's abdomen. Most often external versions are done by doctors.

Before starting the procedure, a woman has an ultrasound exam to make sure that the baby hasn't already turned and there's adequate amniotic fluid. Next, she may be given a regional anesthetic (an epidural) and/or a drug to relax the uterus (such as Terbutaline). Alternatively, she may undergo this procedure with no drugs at all. A doctor will then start to press on her abdomen with both hands in order to encourage the baby to somersault into a head-first position. An external version can be painful because the care provider must press fairly hard for the baby to shift. The version should take around a half hour, and you'll likely be monitored for about a half hour after it's done, to ensure that all is well.

Statistically the chances of the external version succeeding are 50 to 60 percent, though with a skilled care provider the success rate can be higher. The procedure tends to be more successful if it isn't a first baby. Since this is an acquired skill, it's worth looking for someone who has had a lot of experience—and success—doing it. Ask your doctor or midwife if she's experienced with it or if she would recommend someone who could do it.

It's my strong belief that an external version should be done in a hospital setting in case the baby becomes distressed and you need an emergency

C-section. (This is rare, but not unheard-of.) However, some care providers might perform external versions in their offices.

— *Ask yourself why:* At the end of a prenatal visit with a woman whose baby is breech after thirty-two weeks, I'll throw out the question: "Why do you think your baby is breech?" Most often the first response is a bewildered "Huh?" Then we agree to talk about it during the next visit. Those conversations are often extremely interesting because this simple question can tap into strong feelings about the upcoming birth, anxiety about the world, or a sense that the baby is somehow not quite ready to be born.

David Cheek, MD, an obstetrician, first pioneered this technique in the 1950s. He wrote the first academic paper ever to address the phenomenon of fetal perception in utero, and he felt that exploring the issue of why a baby is breech was an effective way to encourage him to turn into a vertex position. Whether exploring the issue of why a baby's breech results in a statistically significant turn rate or not, I think it's worth asking yourself the question just to see what comes up for you.

— *Other techniques:* Studies of both chiropractic and hypnotherapy have shown that each method has some success in turning breeches. Again, seek out practitioners who are very experienced in using these techniques to turn breeches.

• *Vaginal breech birth:* A breech baby can be delivered vaginally when these criteria are met:

1. *Your care provider is experienced in vaginal breech deliveries, and the birth will take place in a hospital:* Unfortunately, because fewer and fewer breech babies are being born vaginally, fewer residents (doctors in training) are taught how to safely manage vaginal breech births. Therefore, depending on where in the country you live, it can be hard to find a care provider who's both experienced with breech deliveries and affiliated with a hospital that will allow him to perform them. This can affect midwives, too, since a midwife attending a vaginal breech should, ideally, be working with a consulting obstetrician who's also skilled in vaginal breech deliveries.

2. *The baby is in a frank or complete breech position:* There are three basic breech positions.
   • A *frank* breech means a baby's hips are bent and his legs extended—he's basically folded in half; this is the most common breech position and in it a vaginal delivery is safe.
   • A *complete* breech means a baby's buttocks are nestled in the mother's

pelvis, and his knees are bent into his chest. It, too, is safe for a vaginal delivery.

- An *incomplete,* or *footling,* breech means the baby's hips and knees are bent as in a complete breech, but a foot, or two, and not his buttocks, is the presenting body part in the mother's pelvis. Incomplete breeches are always delivered by C-section.

3. *A baby's neck is flexed so his chin is against his chest:* If his neck is extended, a vaginal delivery is more dangerous. An ultrasound done during labor can determine the position of the baby's head.

4. *A mother's pelvis is considered "adequate":* This is a judgment call a care provider must make about whether or not a woman's pelvis is wide enough for her baby to fit through. There are no absolutes to this, but an experienced care provider will have an opinion about whether there's an anatomical issue with the mother's pelvis. This is less likely to be a concern if a woman has given birth vaginally before.

5. *The baby isn't too big.* It's difficult to get an accurate assessment of a baby's weight at the end of pregnancy. That said, every care provider will have her own criteria for how big a baby can be to attempt a vaginal breech delivery. Whether or not a woman has given birth vaginally already will also come into play in deciding how big a baby can be before attempting a vaginal delivery.

6. *Labor itself progresses well:* The labor should unfold without any stalls or interventions. I want to emphasize that this last point is *my* own belief and practice. There are obstetricians who would use Pitocin (see "Inducing Labor" on page 440) in a labor with a breech baby.

Note: If you know your baby is breech and your water breaks before labor begins, go to the hospital *immediately.* Call your caregiver once you're in the car on your way there. With a breech and broken membranes, you're at risk for a prolapsed umbilical cord (see below).

- *The risks of a vaginal breech birth:* There are two reasons why vaginal breech births are considered risky, and they're not insignificant:

1. *A prolapsed umbilical cord:* When the membranes of a breech baby rupture, there's a risk that the umbilical cord will drop down through the cervix. This is known as a prolapsed cord. If it happens, the cord could become kinked or compressed, which in turn would limit the flow of blood and oxygen to the baby. This scenario is highly unlikely when the baby is head-down because his head fits snugly into the opening of the cervix, and there's

very little room for the cord to slip through before the baby. But with a breech, a baby's buttocks don't always block the opening of the cervix entirely. While this is extremely rare even with breeches, if it happens, it can be catastrophic for the baby. (If your water breaks and the cord comes out, get on your hands and knees, put your chest on the ground, and stick your buttocks into the air, to keep pressure off the cord. Stay in this position until you get to the hospital.)

2. *The baby's head will get stuck:* Because his head comes last, and it's the biggest part of the baby, there's no guarantee that it will fit through the birth canal. By making sure the baby's head is flexed (with his chin against his chest) and assessing the size of the mother's pelvis in advance of labor, a care provider can reduce the risk that the head will get stuck or that the baby's neck or nerves will be injured during delivery.

Note: In the current legal environment, obstetricians, midwives (CNMs and CMs), and hospitals often require a woman and the baby's father to sign an informed consent document that lists all the risks of a vaginal breech delivery.

Signs of Labor

Most often, labor doesn't start at one particular moment. Rather, there's a slow buildup of signs and symptoms until you reach the point where you just know, "This is it." Here's a list of the common signs that labor is getting under way:

• *Very early labor:* Well before you realize that labor is getting under way, you may feel kind of "off"—for example, your back may be more sore than usual, you may feel menstrual-like cramping, and you may have some diarrhea.

• *Bag of water breaks:* Membranes surround the baby and contain the amniotic fluid in which she's floating. They can break very early in labor with a pop or gush. The membranes that hold the "waters," or the amniotic fluid, serves as a barrier, protecting the baby (and mother) from bacteria that can cause infection. Therefore, most, but not all, care providers and hospitals follow a protocol in which labor begins or the baby is born within twenty-four hours of the membranes breaking. (If your water breaks before your contractions are in full swing, call your caregiver right away.) Membranes rupture before labor begins only about 10 percent of the time; the other 90 percent of the time, they break (or are broken, see "Artificial Rupture of the Membranes" on page 449) while labor is in full swing.

THE TRUTH ABOUT THE MUCUS PLUG

The cervical canal is a tube that connects the uterus to the vagina. The mucus plug is a blood-tinged gob of mucus that functions like a cork inside the outer end of the cervical canal. As your cervix softens to prepare for labor, you can pass the mucus plug. There's a widely held belief that if and when you pass it, you're either in the early stages of labor or will go into labor almost immediately. Unfortunately, this simply isn't the case. The only thing that passing a mucus plug demonstrates with any certainty is that the cervix is preparing for labor by opening slightly, which allows gravity to pull the plug through. Therefore, if you pass a mucus plug (not everyone does) after a pelvic exam, or after intercourse, for example, it doesn't mean you'll go into labor in the next twenty-four hours, but it is a sign that labor is getting closer.

- *Bag of water starts to leak:* You may notice that amniotic fluid starts to leak from your vagina in something like a trickle well before labor truly begins. If you have a very thin, watery discharge that doesn't smell at all like urine, and if you suspect that it's your amniotic fluid leaking, call your caregiver right away. If your membranes are leaking, it means that they've ruptured and your risk of infection goes up, just as it does when the membranes break with more of a gush.

- *Contractions (the clearest sign):* When labor contractions begin in what's known as "early labor," they may be uncomfortable but relatively mild. They will become more intense and come closer together over time. Then you'll *know* that labor has begun. Every caregiver will have her own guidelines for when to call after contractions have begun in earnest, but with a first baby, if you don't have any bleeding and/or your water hasn't broken, I recommend calling when you've had painful contractions that you can't speak or stand through every five minutes for at least an hour. With a first baby, it's likely to take at least several hours for contractions to progress to this point. (For "Early Labor," see page 445.)

Q: How do I know if my amniotic fluid is leaking or if my water has broken?

Dr. Evans: Amniotic fluid is thin and either clear or straw-colored. (Occasionally it's tinged green if there's meconium in it; see page 146.) If you have an intermittent or continuous trickle of fluid (enough to make you want to wear a panty liner) that's *not* white or mucuslike, you may be leaking amniotic fluid from a broken bag of waters. A "popping" sound or sensation and a gush (sometimes big) of fluid are also signs that your bag of waters may have broken. Either way, if you suspect your membranes have ruptured, give your care provider a call.

A doctor or midwife will check to see if the membranes have broken by performing a vaginal exam with a sterile speculum. The speculum allows her to see if there's any fluid pooling in the vagina. If there's fluid, she'll test to see if it's alkaline. (This is called a nitrazine test; the vagina is usually acidic, and amniotic fluid is alkaline.) She also might take a sample of the fluid and look at it on a slide under a microscope. If it's amniotic fluid, she'll see crystalline structures that look like fern leaves. (This is known as "ferning.") If those tests are inconclusive, she might inject some blue dye into the mother's abdomen to see if blue fluid ends up in her vagina. This is safe, but it's not that common.

REAL VOICES

You can feel like you know what to expect in labor, but how can you? I had no idea. I was convinced my water broke one day, and really, I'd just peed. Once I was in a false labor, and I called my OB and said, "I'm in labor." She said, "No, you're not." "Yes, I am! I'm having these contractions," I said. And she said, "If you were in labor, you would not be able to talk to me." I was like, "How do *you* know that?" "Just trust me on this," she said. She was right, but there was no way that I could've known that. It's not a feeling that you've ever had before. And that's the thing. You're this person who feels like you have everything under control, and then this thing is completely out of your control, which is both miraculous and devastating at the exact same time.

Asha, mom of one, pregnant

Encouraging Labor

For all we know about the process of labor and childbirth—and we know quite a lot—we still haven't figured out why labor begins when it does. But we do know the substances the body releases once labor starts and those that keep labor going. Most of the strategies for encouraging labor to begin try to increase those substances, either through natural or medical means.

• *Intercourse:* Prostaglandins are chemical messengers that stimulate contractions. A woman creates them, and they're also found in semen. In fact, semen has the highest concentration of prostaglandins, which come in a variety of types, of any bodily fluid. When you have intercourse, prostaglandins in the semen are "delivered" right to the cervix and to the lower segment of the uterus if the cervix is even slightly dilated. In addition, the uterus contracts when you have an orgasm. Between the prostaglandins in semen and the natural contraction of the uterus from orgasm, intercourse can encourage labor to begin.

Intercourse and orgasms are absolutely safe at the end of pregnancy, unless your caregiver has recommended you avoid sex for a specific reason (for reasons to avoid intercourse during pregnancy, see page 309) or you think your water has broken—in which case you would not want to introduce any bacteria into your cervix because it could cause an infection. I've been asked many times if a penis can hurt a baby's head when the cervix is dilated, and the answer is no.

• *Nipple stimulation:* When you stimulate the nipples, the body releases the hormone oxytocin, another chemical that triggers contractions. (Pitocin, the agent used in hospitals to induce labor, is a synthetic form of oxytocin; see "Inducing Labor," page 440.) To stimulate the nipples, squeeze them for thirty seconds to a minute. The squeezing should be intermittent and quite forceful. You can expect some mild-to-moderate discomfort, but squeezing the nipples shouldn't be excruciatingly painful.

Some care providers express concern over using nipple stimulation to induce labor because there's no way to know how much oxytocin it releases. As a result, you could end up with very strong contractions that distress the baby. To be on the safe side, only try this under the guidance of a midwife or with the advance knowledge of your doctor.

• *Acupuncture/acupressure:* There are several acupressure points that are traditionally used to induce labor. An acupuncture practitioner will assess how you're doing—for example, if you're fatigued or anxious—and select points based on your individual situation. Two acupressure points you can stimulate on your own are:

1. *Large Intestine 4:* The point between your thumb and forefinger. (This is a powerful point that also relieves headaches; pregnant women should avoid it before they want to go into labor.)
2. *Spleen 6:* Located about the width of three fingers above the ankle bone on the inside of the shin, just behind the bone, this is a fairly tender spot for most people, and you might be able to feel a slight indentation at the site of it.

For acupressure to work, you must press *very* hard, so hard that it's actually uncomfortable. Press for five minutes per side every half hour to forty-five minutes, up to ten to fifteen times. You may want to ask your birth partner or a friend to do this.

• *Herbs:* Certain herbs are known to induce labor either by softening the cervix or bringing on contractions; midwives use them more often than OBs. In my own practice, we offer an herbal tonic blend to women who are thirty-nine weeks or more and interested in a natural way to induce labor. The tonic includes ginger, partridge berry (*Mitchella repens*, also known as squaw vine), cotton root (*Gossypium herbaceum*), spikenard (*Aralia racemosa*), and red raspberry leaf (*Rubus idaeus*). (See "Resources," page 523.) If you decide to try an herbal approach to inducing labor, do so under the care of an experienced, reputable, and preferably American Herbalist Guild–certified herbalist or midwife with extensive experience using herbs.

Other herbs commonly given to induce labor:

— *Evening primrose oil* (Oenothera biennis): This may be taken orally or vaginally; the latter prepares the cervix for labor. It's thought to contain a substance that acts as a precursor to prostaglandins.

— *Blue cohosh* (Caulophyllum thalictroides): This herb is thought to bring on both menstruation and uterine contractions. Its use in pregnancy is controversial in the United States because its safety and efficacy have not been well studied and there are some conflicting reports about its potential to cause harm. Because the data are confusing, I can't recommend using it. If you decide to take it, do so only under the strict supervision of a knowledgeable, experienced herbalist and a care provider who knows your plans.

— *Castor oil* (Ricinus communis): A laxative, castor oil is sometimes used to bring on labor. Some studies have shown it to be effective, but reviews of its use by midwives note that it can bring on a very fast labor. It's also associated with meconium staining, diarrhea, and irritation of hemorrhoids. I wouldn't recommend using it. If you choose to, do so with caution and only under the care of a practitioner who is very experienced with it.

• *Stripping the membranes:* When a woman is at least thirty-nine weeks, her cervix is at least one centimeter dilated, and she's anxious for labor to begin, I'll offer to perform a manual procedure known as "stripping the membranes." To do it, I put my finger into the cervix, through the internal os (the part of the cervix that opens to the uterus), until I reach the membranes, which lie between the baby and the wall of the uterus. I then try to put my finger between the membranes and the lower portion of the uterus; this will release prostaglandins. The procedure can be very uncomfortable, and I only do it if a woman requests it or agrees with my recommendation that we try it. Over the twenty-four hours following a vigorous pelvic exam during which the membranes are stripped, you may experience a small amount of spotting and/or contractions, which may or may not mark the beginning of labor. (If the procedure works, labor will begin within twenty-four hours.)

Note: No one but a doctor or midwife trained to do this procedure should attempt it.

Inducing Labor

- *Why labor is induced:* From a medical perspective, there are several reasons labor might be induced:

  - *Medical condition in the mother:* High blood pressure, preeclampsia (see page 357), and gestational diabetes (when a woman has difficulty controlling her blood sugar levels) are conditions in which it might be safer for mother and baby to induce labor. Also, if a mother has herpes and has had outbreaks during her pregnancy but, as her due date nears, is lesion-free and wants to have a vaginal delivery, labor may be induced. (A vaginal delivery with an active herpes outbreak is extremely dangerous for a baby.)

  - *Concerns about the baby:* If a caregiver is concerned that a baby is no longer thriving in the womb, she might recommend inducing labor. Reasons for this include low, or no, amniotic fluid (or oligohydramnios, see page 336), IUGR (or intrauterine growth restriction, see page 345), or if late pregnancy fetal testing (non-stress test, contraction stress test, biophysical profile, see pages 299, 294, and 288) is not reassuring.

    If a mother notices that the baby is moving less, even when a non-stress test and biophysical profile are normal, sometimes she or her caregiver might feel the decreased movement is enough of a reason to induce. (See "How to Track Fetal Movement" on page 347.)

  - *Membranes have ruptured:* About 10 percent of the time, the "waters break" before labor begins—in some cases *days* before contractions get going. When that happens, mother and baby are at risk of developing an infection. There's no agreement about how long it's safe to wait before inducing labor after the membranes have ruptured. Every care provider and hospital will have its own protocol. But, as mentioned above, it's not uncommon for caregivers and hospitals to expect labor or birth to occur within twenty-four hours of when the membranes rupture.

  - *Postdates:* After you reach forty-one full weeks (or seven days past your due date), the risk of the baby developing a serious complication starts to go up, and therefore many, but not all, care providers will recommend inducing labor. After forty-two full weeks (or fourteen days after your due date), the risk to the baby—and here we're talking about a risk of dying—goes up significantly because the placenta no longer functions as efficiently as it has up until this point. (The placenta itself seems to have a specific time span in which it works at its peak efficiency, and that seems to end at forty-two weeks.) The question becomes, At what point between forty and forty-two weeks does it make sense to induce labor? There's little agreement on the answer, and the decision depends on your situation, your history, and your care provider's clinical judgment.

If your pregnancy extends beyond your due date, you may be asked to have several non-stress tests and biophysical profiles (see pages 299 and 288) to make sure the baby isn't in distress. If the baby is doing well, you can probably wait to go into labor spontaneously. With this reassurance, some care providers will wait for you to go into labor spontaneously if you go past forty-two weeks. If there are signs of a problem developing, however—if, for example, the baby starts moving less, or if the amniotic fluid is low (or gone)—you will probably be induced.

Note: The state of your cervix—that is, if it's effaced and dilated—can be an important factor in making the decision to induce or not.

If you and your caregiver are considering induction because you're physically uncomfortable or for some other nonmedical reason, the state of your cervix is an important consideration. If it's "favorable," in other words if it's more than 50 percent effaced and three or four centimeters dilated, then induction makes more sense, because your body is clearly getting ready for labor and you're statistically more likely to give birth vaginally.

If, however, your cervix is minimally effaced or dilated, your body isn't preparing for labor, and induction is not as good an option, because your chance of having a C-section would go up significantly.

If there's a clear medical reason that labor should be induced, for example, if the baby is showing signs of distress or you've got no amniotic fluid, then you will be induced regardless of how thin or dilated your cervix is.

In general, without a medical reason to induce, it's best to wait for labor to begin spontaneously. Since we don't fully understand what triggers labor—what role the position of the baby plays, for example, or what subtle signals mother and baby exchange—when we induce labor, we're just choosing a moment to artificially start a process that most often has no trouble starting itself naturally. As a result, the baby may not be in the best position and the mother's body may not be ready to labor, both of which contribute to a higher C-section rate for induced labors.

• *How labor is induced medically:* There are several different ways labor can be induced medically, and which protocol a care provider will follow depends on what he's seen work, what, if any, protocols a hospital uses, and the woman's particular pregnancy and medical history.

Often the first step is to put a ripening agent, such as a prostaglandin gel, directly onto the cervix in the form of a vaginal suppository, in order to help the cervix efface and dilate in preparation for labor. It can be applied once, or every four to six hours, depending on the situation and the protocol being followed. (Generally speaking, a ripening agent shouldn't be used in the case of a vaginal birth after Cesarean, or VBAC, see page 482.) Then, around twelve hours later, Pitocin, a synthetic version of the hormone oxytocin, which triggers labor, is given intravenously. (Exactly when Pitocin is given depends on both the ripening agent used and the particular protocol at your hospital.) Pitocin is administered very carefully in relatively low doses to minimize the risk of overly strong contractions that could distress the baby. Once Pitocin is started, it's most likely that it'll be administered throughout your labor, and you'll be continuously monitored (see "Electronic Fetal Monitoring" on page 468). At some point either early in an induction or to get labor going, your membranes may be ruptured. (See "Artificial Rupture of Membranes" on page 449.) Again, exactly when depends on your situation, your care provider's experience, and the protocol being followed.

Q: I've heard that induced labor is "worse" than spontaneous labor. Is that true?

Dr. Evans: Because we're all unique, and because there's no way to know what one person's experience of pain is compared to another's, it's impossible to predict how any woman will respond physically or emotionally to labor, whether it's induced or spontaneous.

A major difference between induced and spontaneous labors, though, is your time in the hospital. With induced labor, instead of going through early labor in the comfort of your own home and coming to the hospital once you're in active labor, you must come to the hospital before labor even begins. As a result, you end up spending more time in a hospital bed (which is always less comfortable than your own bed) and more time hooked up to an IV and fetal monitor. And if you're being induced for a medical reason, you might (reasonably) be more anxious about how the baby is doing. In this situation it can be more difficult to trust in your body, which is such an important part of laboring and birth.

Also, when labor is induced, doctors try hard to manage the medication so your contractions mimic those of a natural labor in strength, frequency, and duration. Sometimes, however, the contractions brought on by Pitocin are very intense and regular from the start, unlike those of spontaneous labor, which tend to build more gradually. All of these factors contribute to an overall experience that can be more challenging than spontaneous labors, and many women find they benefit from an epidural when labor is induced.

REAL VOICES

I was induced for a few reasons. The baby was measuring over eight pounds, and I was past my due date. I had this great relationship with one doctor in my practice who I knew would be on call that day. She'd been there for my son's birth, and we had a great experience with her. And, with three other kids at home, it felt like it was time to get the show on the road. So I got up, took a shower, put on lipstick, and walked in the front door of the hospital, which was totally weird. And still, when I got in the room, I started to cry because it just didn't feel right. My husband said that if I wanted to go we could go, but let's talk to the doctor first. Then she came in and held my hand, we talked, and I felt like I was right where I needed to be . . . Emotionally the buildup for an induction is totally different. But being induced didn't take anything away from the birth experience. It just gave me a whole different kind of experience that was just as powerful and amazing. My first choice is always for the baby to come on its own time, but considering everything, being induced was a really positive experience.

Ami, mom of two, stepmom of two

21

The Stages of Labor

Your labor, like every labor, will have predictable stages. But the details of it—how long each stage will last, when your water will break, when you'll be ready to push, whether or not you'll want pain medication—nobody can know any of that in advance. If you learn about what labor and birth typically involve, at least you'll have some familiarity with the processes and choices you may encounter along the way. Here, I describe the stages of labor, ways to cope with pain, and typical medical procedures.

◆　◆　◆

In this chapter you'll find:

- The Stages of Labor
  - The first stage of labor
  - The second stage of labor
  - When your baby is born
  - The third stage of labor
- Pain Management
  - Coping methods
  - Self-coping
  - Medication
- Some Common Medical Procedures Used in Labor

— Electronic fetal monitoring
— Intravenous fluids
— Vaginal exams

The Stages of Labor

Labor breaks down into three stages:

- *The first stage:* Also known as the *dilation* stage, during which the cervix fully effaces (thins) and dilates (opens) to ten centimeters.
- *The second stage:* Also known as the *pushing* or *birthing* stage. Your baby moves completely through the birth canal and is born during this phase.
- *The third stage:* The placenta and fetal membranes are delivered.

The first stage of labor

This stage of labor is usually the longest. In a typical labor, it can last anywhere from a couple of hours to twenty-four hours or more. The first stage of labor is subdivided into three phases: *early labor* (or the latent phase); *active labor*; and the *transition phase*.

- *Early labor (latent phase):* This is the initial phase of labor. You may not be sure that you're in labor when early labor begins; or you might not have any doubts. Some women find their early labor contractions are relatively mild and build up slowly. Initially, they may be as short as five to ten seconds and come at twenty- to thirty-minute intervals. For others, contractions start off relatively strong and come more frequently.

If you're planning a hospital birth, it's often a good idea to spend much of early labor at home *if you're comfortable there.* While at home, you

---

HOW THE UTERUS WORKS

When you're in labor, the uterus, which by this point in your pregnancy is big and strong, contracts purposefully. The top of the uterus presses down, while the bottom, or the cervix, pulls *back*. The baby doesn't push through an open cervix as much as the cervix moves backward over the baby's head. Effacement and dilation mark the start of this process.

Eating and Drinking in Early Labor

✦ If you're hungry and feel like eating early in labor, it's fine to eat small, easily digestible snacks like crackers, toast, or scrambled eggs. Your caregiver will let you know if and when you should stop eating solids entirely.

From a caring perspective, the caution regarding eating in labor stems from the fact that normal, active labor can trigger nausea and vomiting, and vomiting can be prolonged if there's a lot of food in your stomach. Not everyone experiences vomiting in labor, and your comfort, needs, and appetite should guide your eating in early labor.

From a medical perspective, you'd be asked to stop eating in early labor as a precaution if it turns out that you need an emergency C-section. During the procedure, you could have a tube put down your throat (intubation), which can be dangerous if your stomach is full because you can, theoretically, vomit into the tube and be unable to breathe.

There's no problem whatsoever with drinking fluids in early labor. In fact, because labor is so physically taxing and you can easily become dehydrated, it's a good idea to drink as much liquid as you *comfortably* can.

Drink whatever appeals to you. If you drink juices or sports drinks, you'll take in calories that you'll need for energy later on. Drinking water or herbal iced tea can help keep dehydration at bay. If you don't feel like drinking, you could suck on a lollipop or Popsicle.

If you're only drinking water and your labor becomes long, you may need IV fluids to give you the calories you'll need to have the energy to keep labor going and to push.

can do whatever gives you the greatest sense of ease—walk, rest, try out different positions during contractions, or sit and breathe quietly without distraction. (Very early in labor, when contractions can be mild, you may be able to stay relatively active and go about your day.) Review this plan with your care provider at a prenatal appointment; some conditions, like borderline high blood pressure, make getting to the hospital earlier in labor a safer choice. (If your water breaks before you have regular contractions, call your care provider, who'll give you guidelines for what to watch for and when to go to the hospital/birthing center if you're planning to birth outside your home.)

Early labor ends and active labor begins when you're contracting regularly and the cervix has dilated to three to five centimeters. Once you're in active labor (see below), your cervix will start to dilate steadily. As I've noted, you can be a few centimeters dilated for weeks before labor even begins. But even in that situation, during early labor contractions will build up until they become strong and coordinated enough to get the cervix dilating at a somewhat regular pace.

At what point in early labor should you call your care provider? You'll get instructions for when to call, but typically, a care provider will ask you to call when you've had contractions that last at least a minute and come at five-minute intervals for an hour.

REAL VOICES

There's a huge mind-body connection in birth. You have to be in a place where it feels safe to labor and birth; there might be something going on that slows you down. For example, when I went into labor with my second child, my water broke three and a half weeks before my due date, but I had no contractions. My husband was out of town, and there was no way he could get back to me for at least twelve hours. We were planning a home birth, and I couldn't imagine having this baby without him—but my midwife had warned me that my second labor could be much quicker, even half the time, than my first (twenty-four hour) labor. I really think I stalled my labor knowing that. But once my labor got going, it went really fast.

Sue, mom of two

• *Active labor:* In active labor, the cervix starts to dilate more rapidly and regularly. (The standard labor curve states that women in active labor dilate at a rate of about one centimeter per hour, but don't expect to dilate at that exact pace—it's an average.) In active labor, which generally starts when you're three to five centimeters dilated and continues until you're ten centimeters (fully dilated), contractions typically last about a minute and come every three to five minutes. While the contractions of early labor aren't always described as painful, these almost always are. Most women aren't able to speak or stand up straight during an active labor contraction. (Keep in mind that pain is a very subjective experience. Some women don't find active labor to be that painful.) It's hard to predict how long active labor will last; during a first labor, it can take anywhere from two to twelve hours.

REAL VOICES

I remember standing in the parking lot underneath the hospital where the birthing center was. I was bending over and holding on to one of those columns and thinking, "Okay, in childbirth class they said I wouldn't be able to speak or stand in active labor. This is it!"

Erin, mom of two

I walked into the hospital thinking I had been having contractions at five minutes for a while, but that they would turn me away. They were really busy, and I was very apologetic. I kept saying, "I'm really sorry, I don't mean to take up your time." And they said, "Well, you're here, let's take a look." It turned out I was dilated to seven centimeters, and I didn't even know that I had been in labor for the last twelve hours. I was able to walk through my contractions and talk through my contractions—it wasn't overpoweringly painful.

Martha, mom of two

• *The transition phase:* In this stage, your cervix completes the process of dilating, and shifts into pushing. It typically begins when you're around eight centimeters dilated, and it ends when you're fully dilated at ten centimeters.

During the transition, the baby prepares to move from the uterus through the cervix. Once you're ten centimeters dilated, the baby begins his trip past the cervix through the vagina. By this point in labor, contractions can sometimes last more than a minute and come very closely together. Because contractions come at a fast and furious pace, the transition phase can be the most challenging part of labor, but it's also the shortest, lasting on average anywhere from fifteen minutes to over an hour.

Sometimes, women feel the "urge to push" before the cervix is fully dilated; when that happens, they're asked to grunt or pant to keep themselves from pushing, because pushing before full dilation can cause the cervix to tear.

REAL VOICES

The way my labor went, I was in labor for a couple of hours and the contractions were getting stronger and stronger, and then all of a sudden my water broke and I went right into transition. It was like I went from zero to sixty. I remember my head flew back and it hit the back wall and I was like, "AAAAHHHHH!"

Miranda, mom of one, pregnant

I was surprised to find that while I was in labor I didn't want to be touched at all . . . I had a home birth and I had this vision of myself, like, "I'm not going to lie on my back, that's what they make you do in hospitals." But I was also surprised to find that all I wanted to do was lie on my back.

Lisa, mom of one

When the Waters Break (or the "Rupture of Membranes")

• *What it is:* As you know, your baby has been floating in a protective sac of amniotic fluid. During active labor, the sac, which is a membrane, will break from the pressure of the contractions. When this happens, the amniotic fluid can come out in a stream or a gush.

• *When it happens:* It's impossible to predict when the membranes will rupture. They most often rupture spontaneously during active labor; about 10 percent of the time they rupture before labor begins. Very rarely, a baby is born with the "bag of waters" intact; this is considered a sign of a miracle in some cultures. (This almost happened to me only once in my entire career; the membranes burst just as I was catching the baby.)

• *Artificial rupture of the membranes (AROM):* In this painless procedure, a doctor or midwife uses a long, thin hook to break the amniotic sac. Whether or not a caregiver *should* rupture membranes is a controversial question, and every care provider will have her own protocol for if and when to do so. Here are several reasons caregivers perform AROM:

— *To check for meconium:* Meconium is a baby's first bowel movement. Sometimes the baby passes meconium into the amniotic fluid before birth. Because the baby breathes in amniotic fluid while he's in the womb, there's a chance he'll breathe in the meconium, which could irritate his lungs and airways. If there's meconium in the amniotic fluid, a care provider will prepare for the birth by having either a pediatrician or specialist on hand to suction out any meconium that the baby may have inhaled. (Meconium is found in amniotic fluid in 5 to 10 percent of births.)

There's no correlation between how long the membranes are intact and the likelihood of the baby passing meconium. In other words, just because a woman's membranes are intact through active labor, it's not more likely that the baby will pass meconium before birth. On the flip side, rupturing the membranes doesn't necessarily remove the risk that the baby will swallow meconium, because there could still be enough fluid in the womb for the baby to swallow some if she had a bowel movement before birth.

If a care provider wants to be fully prepared for the potential complications that meconium creates—and they can be serious—he may choose to rupture the membranes when a woman dilates to seven or eight centimeters just to see if there is any meconium in the fluid. That way, if meconium is present, he'll have time to reach a specialist to care for the baby.

— *To strengthen labor:* Rupturing the membranes releases prostaglandins, which stimulate contractions. If labor is stalled or going slowly, a care provider might rupture the membranes to try to get labor going.

— *To induce labor:* Because AROM releases prostaglandins, a care provider might rupture the membranes before labor begins as a way to induce either with or without using Pitocin, a synthetic prostaglandin gel. (See "Inducing Labor" on page 440.)

— *For internal fetal monitoring:* The membranes need to be ruptured for an internal electronic fetal monitoring device to be used. (See "Electronic fetal monitoring," page 468.)

• *Arguments against AROM:* There are several arguments against rupturing membranes, particularly early in labor:

— Breaking the membranes introduces the possibility of infection where it didn't exist before.

— It doesn't always speed up or bring on labor.

— Once the amniotic fluid is gone, there's an increased risk that contractions will compress the umbilical cord, possibly causing distress to the baby.

— Some care providers object to AROM on a philosophical basis, believing that rupturing the membranes is a step toward a more medicalized birth. (I don't object to AROM, and I don't believe that any one intervention *necessarily* leads to more interventions. See my answer to the question "Once I get an epidural, are more medical interventions inevitable?" on page 467.)

The second stage of labor

During the second stage, also known as the pushing or birthing phase, your baby completes her trip through the birth canal and is born. Pushing, which is instinctual, involves bearing down with the diaphragm and abdominal muscles to move the baby through the vagina and into the world.

The birthing stage can last anywhere from fifteen minutes to three hours. First-time moms, on average, push for two hours. In subsequent births, a mom might push for an hour or less.

Q: What does "crowning" mean?

Dr. Evans: During the pushing stage, a baby is said to "crown" when his head remains visible in the cervix between contractions.

> REAL VOICES
>
> I only pushed for an hour. "Only an hour." It's super, super intense, but it wasn't that long. Although one thing I didn't know about pushing—I guess I didn't know what I thought—I thought pushing would be more like having an orgasm. Really, it's like pooping. Didn't know that.
>
> Marjorie, mom of one, pregnant
>
> At around five in the morning, I had this tremendous urge to push, and it felt amazing. The last hour and a half of pushing went so fast—I swear it felt like ten minutes. It was such an incredible feeling—to feel yourself birthing your baby.
>
> Susan, mom of two

Note: One of the many theories about the G-spot that I first heard in my medical training is that its primary purpose is for childbirth, not sex. At the moment of greatest discomfort during labor, when the baby's head begins to crown and a woman feels a burning sensation known as the "ring of fire," the head presses against the G-spot and releases endorphins in the mother's brain to counteract the pain message. There's no literature on this, but undocumented doesn't necessarily mean untrue!

Water Births

✦ I've been fascinated with water births ever since medical school, when I first saw a remarkable video of one, but I've never attended one. Water births became popular in Europe (especially Russia and France) in the 1970s as a way to ease a baby's transition from the womb. Laboring in water can help ease a woman's pain. And the idea that a baby who has been floating in liquid for over nine months can enter the world more gently in water makes very good sense intuitively. After being birthed underwater, the baby continues to get oxygen through the umbilical cord and gently emerges into the air in her mother's—or father's—arms.

But I am aware of some risks associated with water births. There are reports of babies drowning during water births and complications arising from water in the lungs—and I've seen babies gasp for air immediately upon being born, which makes me wonder what would have happened in a water birth.

That said, if you're at all interested in a water birth, I'd recommend investigating it thoroughly and pursuing it if it makes good sense to you. With a doctor or midwife experienced with water births and a sound backup plan in place, a water birth can be a safe option.

When your baby is born

• *Suctioning:* After your baby's head emerges, your care provider will probably suction his nose and mouth quickly and gently to prevent him from inhaling the mucus that covers his face when he's born. (Not every care provider does this as a matter of course; some wait to see if the baby needs suctioning to start breathing.)

• *Guiding the baby's body:* After the head emerges, a care provider will gently guide the baby's shoulders and body the rest of the way out. (If things are going smoothly, once the shoulders are out from under the pubic bone, I'll occasionally ask a woman's partner to assist with the rest of the birth—i.e., "catch the baby.")

• *Skin-to-skin contact:* Once born, the baby may be placed on your belly, and you'll both be covered with a warm blanket. Immediate skin-to-skin contact is a great way to regulate a newborn's body temperature, which can fluctuate.

• *Cutting the umbilical cord:* The umbilical cord may or may not be cut right away, depending on your care provider, the length of the cord (it may be too short for a baby to reach Mom's belly with it attached), whether it's around the baby's neck, and the protocol where you're giving birth. In some hospitals, the umbilical cord is cut immediately and the baby is taken to be cleaned, tested, and swaddled before being returned to the mother. If this is the protocol where you'll be giving birth and you'd prefer the baby to be put on your belly for twenty minutes to an hour before being cleaned, ask your caregiver if this would be possible.

When exactly to cut the cord is subject to some controversy. Some make the argument that while the cord is pulsing, the baby is still getting blood, oxygen, and nutrients from it, so it's better to wait until it stops pulsing altogether to cut it. No scientific data show that the baby will be hurt in any way if the cord is cut immediately after birth, but if you'd prefer to wait for the cord to stop pulsing for it to be cut, let your caregiver know. Once the cord is cut, cord blood can be collected for either personal banking or donation. (For cord blood banking, see page 454.)

After the cord is cut, your caregiver may check the pH level of the cord blood, which will tell you the oxygen level of the blood in the umbilical cord (and your baby) at the time of birth. (I do this routinely as a way to reassure new parents that the baby had enough oxygen throughout labor and birth, but not all caregivers do. The test does require cutting the cord fairly soon after birth, because the sooner it's cut, the more accurate the oxygen reading will be.)

• *A baby's first cry:* While the baby's on your belly, she'll be gently wiped off, and after about fifteen seconds or so, she should let out a cry. If not, some gentle stimulation usually works.

• *Breastfeeding:* If you plan to breastfeed, the baby might be able to start nursing within twenty minutes to an hour. Breastfeeding, whenever it happens, will release oxytocin, a hormone that causes contractions, which will help your uterus contract back to its normal size.

New mothers often have high expectations that a newborn baby will try to nurse shortly after being born. In studies of newborns born after a medication-free labor, it sometimes took up to an hour for them to "crawl" over to the breast and start to nurse. In my own experience, the baby often prefers to "hang out" on Mom's belly, which is wonderful, and he's simply not ready to nurse right after birth. Please don't panic if this is the case with your baby; he'll nurse when he's ready. (For a description of the tests and treatments a baby typically receives within an hour or so of birth and a description of what happens to you the first twenty-four hours after giving birth, see page 490.)

Cord Blood Banking

✦ Right after the umbilical cord is cut, blood from it can be collected and saved for future medical use. Cord blood is special because it's made up of unspecialized blood cells, which, if needed, can produce any kind of blood cell—such as blood-clotting platelets and red and white blood cells—at any time in the future. Umbilical cord blood can be used to treat various genetic disorders and immune disorders, as well as certain cancers (like leukemia). Currently, about forty-five disorders can be treated with stem cells from umbilical cord blood.

• *Should you bank your baby's cord blood?* Only you can make that decision. On the plus side, cord blood banking is something of an insurance policy. You may never need it. (The odds are about 1 in 2,700 that a child will need her own stem cells by age twenty-one for currently available treatments; the odds that a family member will need them are about 1 in 1,400.) But if your child develops one of those life-threatening diseases that can be treated most effectively by cord blood, it's worth having. On the downside, it can be very expensive (between $500 and $2,000 for initial banking and then yearly maintenance fees; however, insurance companies are beginning to cover some of these costs).

Talk with your caregiver about your options, which include banking or donating cord blood, and consider setting up a consultation with a genetic counselor, which will help you evaluate your family history and level of risk.

REAL VOICES
She was up to her waist—her shoulders were out and her head was out. The midwife was suctioning her and said, "Miranda, do you want to deliver your baby?" I started weeping and nodding, so she took my hands and put them underneath her arms and I pulled her legs out and I held her up and saw that she was a girl. I screamed, "It's a girl!" And then I was crying, Michael was crying—that part was amazing, pulling her out myself. It was unbelievable.

Miranda, mom of one, pregnant

The third stage of labor

During this final stage of labor, the placenta and fetal membranes are birthed. After the baby is born, rhythmic contractions basically stop, with maybe just one or two ushering out the placenta and membranes. Usually, new mothers are occupied with their babies at this point and barely notice what's happening. The third stage can last anywhere from ten to thirty minutes.

In the unlikely scenario that the placenta hasn't emerged about twenty minutes or so after birth, I (like many care providers) switch into medical mode because I want to be sure the placenta isn't "retained," or stuck, which can cause serious bleeding. If a woman's had an epidural, I can reach in and gently remove the placenta. If she hasn't had one and there's time, I strongly recommend calling for an anesthesiologist to provide her with pain relief before removing the placenta by hand, because it can be quite painful.

Q: Is labor different after a first baby?
Dr. Evans: Every labor is different. The pattern that we most often see is that a first labor is long, a second labor is shorter, and a third or subsequent labor is unpredictable, though usually it's relatively short and certainly not as long as a first labor.

Q: What happens in a vaginal twin birth?
Dr. Evans: Even though scheduled C-sections for twins are increasingly common, vaginal births are a safe and viable option when certain criteria are met.

• *Presentation:* The first thing to consider when deciding whether or not to pursue a vaginal twin birth is the presentation of Baby A (the first baby out). If Baby A is vertex, or head down, then a vaginal birth is possible. If Baby A is breech or transverse (lying across the uterus), then a Cesarean is the standard of care.

The importance of Baby B's presentation depends on the care provider. For some, it doesn't matter—they feel that if Baby B doesn't flip into vertex on his own after Baby A is born, they can flip him or deliver him breech. (Some actually prefer Baby B to be breech.) Others insist that Baby B be vertex to attempt a vaginal delivery. Talk with your care provider about his guidelines for presentation, experience with breeches, and his thoughts on the likelihood that if Baby B is breech or transverse, he'd be delivered by Cesarean.

• *Who's there:* Twins are most often delivered in a hospital by either a doctor or a certified nurse midwife with a consulting OB present. In addition to the care

Labor and Birth with a Midwife

✦ Libby Cohen, CNM, has been a midwife in solo practice for eighteen years.

Q: Can you give an overview of midwifery's approach to labor and birth?

Libby Cohen: There's a nursing foundation to almost all—not all—but almost all midwives that means we're always going to look at the person first and then at the process. In other words, midwives see the locus of control during labor as with the woman.

Also, for me, and I think for midwives in general, labor and birth are a continuum; one flows into the next. I'm there supporting the labor, and I'm there for the birth. That's the work for me, and that's different from labor and birth with an OB, because an OB will show up intermittently throughout the labor and then be there for the birth.

Q: What do you do when labor stalls?

LC: First, trust that it'll work out; second, try to fix things like hydration (dehydration can stall contractions), going to the bathroom, etc. As a last resort, Pitocin almost always works, eventually. The classic labor curve says you should dilate a centimeter every hour, but no one is on that curve. I think the smartest thing you can do in a labor is have faith in the process, which means letting it unfold.

Q: Can you have an epidural with a midwife?

LC: People think you're not going to get an epidural with a midwife, and that's not true. Some midwives may discourage you from getting an epidural, but my own feeling is that I'm there to support a woman in what she wants and to bring my expertise to help her figure out what would be right for her. I'm not there to make the decision *for* her. I don't offer an epidural, but I don't withhold it, either.

Q: Are there times when you've felt an epidural was helpful?

LC: Yes. Some women need to be able to concentrate, to labor in their heads, and for that they need an epidural. There are times when we've done everything we can to move labor along and nothing's happening. Then, an epidural makes a lot of sense because you're starting to talk about a C-section; which means you're talking about an epidural, anyway. So if the baby is fine and the mom is fine, let's get the epidural, take a nap for four hours, and see what happens. I've heard people say epidurals make it harder to push, but the pain can make it hard to push, too.

Q: Are there labors/births you won't or can't attend?

LC: Other than the ones I'm not qualified to attend? I can't perform a C-section. Otherwise, if I'm not qualified to provide prenatal care, I won't manage the labor. Protocols and guidelines for prenatal care are determined by the state. So I don't provide prenatal care to women with any unstable and/or serious medical condition such as insulin-dependent diabetes, chronic kidney disease, or lupus. Also, multiples greater than twins are always delivered by C-section.

For twin births, there's always an obstetrician in the room. For VBACS (vaginal births after Cesarean), labor management is the same as for a regular labor, but I keep in very close contact with the backup doctor on call.

Q: What advice would you give someone considering using a midwife?

LC: Think about what you want from your prenatal care and your birth. The midwifery model means you'll spend more time with your midwife during prenatal visits and during labor. But if you view pregnancy and birth as a medical event, and you don't want to do anything touchy-feely, then an obstetrician could be fine. If you're more comfortable thinking that the person who'll deliver the baby can do it either way (vaginally or surgically) then it makes sense to go with an OB, as long as you keep in mind that a doctor who can do a C-section is more likely to do a C-section.

provider, there will be two pediatric care providers and an anesthesiologist. In some hospitals, vaginal twin deliveries take place in the operating room just in case a woman needs an emergency C-section, either for both babies or the second.

• *What happens:* The stages of labor are the same for a twin birth, except that since twins usually weigh less than singletons, the pushing stage is shorter. A mother will usually have more monitoring than with a singleton. (See "Electronic Fetal Monitoring" on page 468.) Assuming Baby A is vertex, he'll be born just like any other baby. Then, the uterus will stop contracting and, ideally, Baby B will drop down, headfirst, into the pelvis (you'll have a quick sonogram to figure out her position). Then her heart rate will be assessed to make sure she's not in any distress. Things can get complicated in this period between the birth of Baby A and Baby B. Ideally, labor would start up again on its own within twenty to thirty minutes (although I personally have waited as long as six hours) and Baby B will be born without any problems. (Management of Baby B's labor varies among care providers.)

Usually, both placentas, or *the* placenta if they shared one, will be delivered after both babies are born, but sometimes Baby A's placenta is delivered before Baby B emerges.

• *Combined twin deliveries:* A combined twin delivery means Baby A is born vaginally and Baby B is born by C-section. This happens in approximately 6 to 10 percent of attempted twin vaginal births. The likelihood of a combined delivery goes up when Baby B is breech and there's a long interval between the birth of Baby A and Baby B.

Pain Management

Labor and birth involve physical pain. (The pain is caused first by the cervix dilating and second by the contractions themselves.) Because pain is subjective, everyone will experience, and describe, the pain of labor and childbirth differently. That said, labor pains do have some distinct characteristics: They are rhythmic; they get more intense as birth nears; and, gloriously, once you give birth, the pain ends.

There's no "best" way to manage the pain of labor and childbirth. Some women don't want to imagine labor and childbirth without medication; others are very committed to a medication-free, natural childbirth; and still others want to "see how it goes" without labor medication but would be willing to use it if necessary.

However you feel about medication in labor, the decision to use it or not is an intensely personal one based on your own needs, your philosophy of birth, and your actual experience in labor.

Coping methods

Just as labor pains have a few consistent characteristics, in my experience positive labor experiences share some distinct elements that are applicable whether or not you decide to use medication at any point in childbirth:

• *A positive attitude:* This may sound simplistic or redundant, but I truly believe that if you approach labor with more excitement and anticipation than fear and dread, your experience will be better and the labor itself might even progress more smoothly. This isn't to say that a good attitude guarantees that complications won't develop—nothing can do that. But cultivating a positive attitude toward labor certainly can't hurt and, in my experience, can help.

• *A supportive team and environment:* The beauty of emotional support is that you can take it with you wherever you birth. A birthing team that's brought together to support you—whether it's made up of just your partner/coach; or your partner/coach and a doula, dear friend, or family member; or an even larger group—can make an enormous difference while you're laboring. (For more on birthing teams, see page 397.)

• *Let your body lead the way:* Labor and childbirth are intensely physical and emotional experiences. Try to trust your body and your instincts over and above any preconceived notions or specific plan you made in advance. Let yourself really *be* in the moment and let your gut be your guide.

Please don't misunderstand me. For many women it's important to write a detailed birth plan, but if you do so, keep in mind that labor isn't something that can be controlled. Over the years, I've worked with many women who've had very explicit ideas about what should and shouldn't happen during labor, and I've found that what's most useful for everyone, but especially for a birthing woman, is to let go of the specifics of a birth plan, let your body take over, and embrace the unique rhythm of your own labor.

REAL VOICES

It was great to walk into the hospital with my partner the morning I was induced and just give myself over to the experience. Part of what made it so positive was I was with a physician who really knew what she was doing and I had a really great nurse. When you can entrust yourself to a really experienced team, it makes a huge difference.

Ami, mom of two, stepmom to two

In *Birthing from Within* they say to let yourself go into "Labor Land." You don't have to think about what to do, you just kind of do it. I kind of felt like I was almost like a spectator at this thing that was happening because I didn't have to control it. It never felt scary, which I think is so amazing, and it never felt like I couldn't handle it.

Maia, mom of one

I didn't have a lot of close friends that had gone through pregnancy, but the recommendations I did get were "Prepare for an epidural! You'll want it early like a cocktail and enjoy!" So the idea of unmedicated natural childbirth was sort of foreign to me. But after my childbirth class I really bought into that idea. I didn't know what would happen, and if there were complications, of course I would take a C-section and drugs if I needed them, but I just really liked the idea of being as in-tuned to the natural process as possible.

Trina, mom of one, pregnant

Self-coping

There are many techniques and approaches to coping with pain in labor without drugs. If you were to ask me if I've seen one that works more often and consistently than others, I'd have to say no. In my own experience, what's more important than a particular technique is a woman's attitude toward labor, her preparation for it, and her willingness to let her body lead the way. Here are a few approaches and techniques that are well known and relatively widely available:

• *Hypnotherapy:* Hypnotherapy during birth involves entering into a deeply relaxed, hypnotic state during labor. You won't be "zoned out"—that's a myth about hypnosis—but the hypnotic state calms you and allows your subconscious mind to redirect its focus away from the pain. Preparation for hypnotherapy involves classes that teach visualization exercises and meditation.

• *Position and breathing:* The positions you labor in and your breathing can ease the discomfort of labor as it intensifies. Many labor positions involve using gravity. For example, you can stand and sway with your partner/labor coach (slow dance) through contractions; sit on or drape over a birth ball while leaning into your partner/labor coach; lunge through contractions; or simply sit on the toilet. The Bradley Method and Lamaze are best known for combining breathing techniques, relaxation exercises, and shifting positions to help women and their partners cope with a medication-free labor. Classes and books will teach you a range of postures to try and exercises to help you prepare. (For more on both Bradley and Lamaze, see page 408; for recommended books about childbirth, see "Resources," page 522.)

• *Water:* A birthing tub with jets or even just a long shower can help ease the pain of active labor. Not all hospitals will have tubs/baths available, but most will have showers. Birthing tubs can be rented for home births, whether or not you're planning a water birth.

• *Massage:* When isn't massage soothing? Therapeutic massage done by hand or with old tennis balls can help relieve pain during active labor. Also, handheld massage rollers can be extremely helpful when a particular part of the body needs extra attention, for example if you feel contractions in your back (known as "back labor").

• *Find your rhythm:* One of the defining characteristics of contractions is that they're rhythmic. They come and go at a predictable and steady pace. When a contraction is over, you're no longer in pain, which gives you a chance to recover and prepare for the next one. You can use the natural rhythm of labor to create a pattern of actions with your partner/labor coach that help you ride the waves during contractions and regroup in between.

REAL VOICES

The midwife had told my husband that every time a contraction hit to put this ice-cold washcloth right on my face because it will give me another sensation—and it helped so much. It was an icy sensation like the minute the contraction would hit, but the contractions were unbelievable.

Miranda, mom of one, pregnant

Medication

As with most medical procedures, there are several protocols and procedures that are used for pain relief during labor. Here's an overview of the basic types of pain relief medication currently available and at what point in labor they can be given:

• *Narcotics:* In early labor (before you reach three centimeters), your OB or midwife might suggest a narcotic like Demerol, Stadol, or Nubain to take the edge off the pain. These are also known as "systemic drugs" because they diffuse through your entire body and cross the placenta. Given by IV or injection, these drugs are generally administered in low doses early in labor because if they're given too close to the birth, they can affect the baby's breathing.

  — *Risks:* These are powerful drugs, and some women find they become "loopy" and/or queasy after taking them. Plus, as noted, they cross the placenta, so they can affect the baby's responsiveness and ability to breathe if they're given too close to birth.

• *Epidural:* The dura is the membrane that surrounds the spinal cord. (*Epi* means "around" in Greek.) An epidural is an injection of local anesthetic medication into the space around the dura that provides pain relief through the lower half of your body. An epidural is also known as a "regional anesthetic" or "regional block" because it numbs only a specific region of the body.

Ideally, an epidural provides enough relief that you're not in pain, but not so much that you lose all sensation or the ability to move your legs. That's not to say you'll be able to walk around after receiving an epidural (see "Walking Epidural" on page 464), but, depending on the dose and when in labor it's given, you could be able to move your legs and feel when to push once the second stage of labor begins.

— *When it's given:* During active labor. Some caregivers don't recommend an epidural before you're at least three centimeters dilated, because they're concerned that the anesthetic will relax your pelvic muscles too much and slow down labor. (There's a long-running debate about the effect of an epidural on labor's progress overall, not just in early labor. Some argue that whenever it's given, an epidural could slow contractions and lead to a stalled labor.) Newer, sophisticated combination spinal-epidurals may be given in early labor, and the most recent data show that they don't slow labor's progress. (See "Combination Spinal-Epidural" on page 464.)

— *How it's given:* An epidural is administered between two vertebrae, usually in the lumbar spine. First you'll receive IV fluids to help prevent a drop in blood pressure, which is one of the risks of an epidural. Then you'll either lie on your side or sit with your knees curled into your chest to create more space between the vertebrae. The site of the injection is then cleaned (the antiseptic may be cold), and you'll be given a local anesthetic to numb the skin where the epidural needle will be inserted. Once the site is numb, the anesthesiologist will first put a needle into the epidural space, then insert a thin plastic tube (a catheter) and tape it in place. After the catheter is in place, the doctor will remove the first needle. Medication may be given through the catheter in one dose via a syringe or in a low, continuous dose that's maintained by a pump (this is known as a "continuous epidural"). An epidural typically takes about twenty minutes to work, and one syringe full of anesthetic (a "bolus") will last a few hours.

Note: Occasionally, the medication from the epidural flows to one side of the epidural space, meaning that only one side of your body will get pain relief. If you've had back surgery, the scar tissue around the spine could make the effects of the epidural patchy. Finally, sometimes, for an unknown reason, one area of the spine doesn't get bathed in the medication. This creates a "window," or a small area that hurts while the rest of your body is free of pain.

— *How it works:* In the simplest terms, an epidural stops pain by blocking the pain messages sent to the spinal cord and brain by the nerves that come from your uterus and the lower half of your body.

— *Maintaining the medication:* If you have a continuous epidural, a consistent low dose of anesthetic medication is delivered through an electronic pump. After the first hour on the medication, an anesthesiologist will adjust the amount you receive to your needs. If your legs feel too heavy, he can lower the dose; if the medication isn't strong enough, he can increase it. You can use the pump to self-administer small doses of medication if you have some "breakthrough" pain. It takes about four minutes for a self-administered dose of medication to take effect.

If you're given a bolus of medication instead of a continuous dose, it will last about four hours, after which you may or may not be given a second dose, depending on where you are in labor and what you want to do.

— *Disadvantages:* After receiving an epidural, you'll no longer be able to get up and walk around. You'll need IV fluids and consistent blood pressure monitoring. And if it becomes difficult for you to urinate because of the anesthesia, you may need to have a urine catheter put in. Some argue that your chances of a C-section may go up after an epidural because it can slow labor. Studies have never shown definitively that epidurals have that effect, and in my own experience, epidurals don't increase the chances of a Cesarean.

— *Risks:* No procedure is free of risks, and an epidural has its own. There's the risk of bleeding or infection at the site where the epidural is given. Your blood pressure can drop, which is why you're given IV fluids. (The extra fluids help you maintain your blood pressure; if necessary you could be given medication to boost your blood pressure.) There's a risk that the fetal heartbeat will slow down (known as fetal bradycardia—this is usually temporary). For some reason, an epidural increases the chance that you'll develop a fever (which may mean extra testing for the baby to rule out infection). Some women get shaky or shiver after getting an epidural, but this can happen in a labor without medication.

A bad headache, known as a "spinal headache," is a relatively rare side effect. If the needle nicks the spinal cord and spinal fluid leaks out, a headache can develop after the epidural catheter is removed and up to a few days following the birth. Spinal headaches happen somewhere between 1 and 3 percent of the time; the risk depends on the skill of the doctor administering the epidural. Even more unusual, breathing problems or damage to the spinal cord can occur.

• *Combination spinal-epidural (a "spinal"):* A "spinal" means a narcotic is injected directly into the dural space. When the spinal technique is combined with an epidural, you'll be prepped as if you were getting a regular epidural. After the wider needle is inserted to open the epidural space, a doctor uses a very, very thin needle to inject a low dose of narcotic (such as Fentanyl or, less commonly, Sufentanil) into the dura itself, which contains spinal fluid. This brings almost immediate pain relief that lasts up to ninety minutes, at which point, assuming your labor's progressed well, you'll receive local anesthetic in the epidural space through the epidural catheter as you would with a "regular" epidural.

A combination spinal-epidural has certain advantages. Since it uses a narcotic, it can be given earlier in active labor, because the narcotic won't relax the pelvic floor muscles, which could potentially slow labor. While the narcotic given in a spinal *could* have similar side effects to the systemic drugs described above, it typically doesn't, and the risks to the baby (problems breathing if given too close to birth) are minimized for two reasons: (1) the dose given in a spinal by an anesthesiologist is much smaller than that given via injection or IV by a doctor or midwife early in labor, and (2) when the medication is injected directly into the spinal column, it doesn't have to be metabolized by the liver and travel through your body to work. Combined with the smaller dose, this means much less of it crosses the placenta. As a result, you get the benefit of narcotics—quick pain relief—without the side effects of IV narcotics to you or the baby or the risk of relaxing the pelvic floor muscles and slowing labor from a too-early epidural. (See "How It Works" below.) After receiving the spinal portion of the combination spinal-epidural, you might need less of the local anesthetic, which means you'd have more sensation during the pushing phase.

An anesthesiologist will determine the appropriate balance of spinal (narcotic) and epidural (local anesthetic) medication based on her experience and your situation.

• *A "walking" epidural:* This is a version of a combination spinal-epidural. In it, more narcotic is given via spinal injection and very little local anesthetic is given through the epidural catheter. The combination allows for pain relief without slowing the labor, and you may be able to walk, with help, after getting it.

— *How it works:* The narcotics in a combination spinal-epidural work on a molecular level. At nerve endings, there are several "receptors" including "opioid receptors." (Receptors are proteins that can bind to a specific substance like a drug, hormone, or neurotransmitter.) When these receptors are stimulated, a chemical reaction occurs that causes the sensation of pain. But the molecules of a narcotic bind directly to the opioid receptors and stop the transmission of the pain message. When the narcotic is injected into the spinal column, all the nerves, with their opioid receptors, are right there, so a very low dose of narcotic can work quickly and effectively with minimal side effects.

— *Disadvantages:* With any combination spinal-epidural, even a "walking epidural," walking is difficult and IV fluids are necessary, as are constant blood pressure monitoring and fetal monitoring.

— *Risks:* The risks from a combination spinal-epidural are, for the most part, the same as those of an epidural. There's the risk of a "spinal headache," a severe headache from leaking spinal fluid where the needle was withdrawn. You could have some itchiness as well, which is treatable with an antihistamine. Finally, if the spinal needle brushes up against the nerves of the spinal column, you could experience a feeling of pins and needles in your hands and arms (paresthesia). This should go away in a few seconds. If it doesn't, the anesthesiologist will stop the procedure.

Note: If you have to have an unscheduled C-section, a higher concentration of local anesthetic would be given through the epidural catheter. The dose would be strong enough that you'd be unable to move your legs. After the surgery, you might receive an injection of narcotics through the epidural catheter, which would provide pain relief for twelve to twenty-four hours after the operation.

In addition to the epidural medication, women are sometimes given sedatives before an unscheduled C-section. If you're sure you won't want the extra drugs, tell your doctor or midwife at a prenatal visit and ask what would be the best way to prevent that from happening. (For more on C-sections, unscheduled and scheduled, see page 543.)

REAL VOICES
I had an epidural, but my idea before labor was "C'mon, I'm a runner, I can do this. I've lived through enormous amounts of pain." This pain was more than anything I've ever done, and it was three days long . . . After the epidural, labor became a really great experience. I took a nap. I rested. I prepared myself . . . It took six hours from when I got the epidural to when my son was born. By the time I was pushing, I could feel everything. I felt the

contractions—they just didn't hurt anymore. I was very aware of what was going on, and I was very aware of the movements the baby was making. I mean I really enjoyed birth after I had the epidural.

Asha, mom of one, pregnant

When I had my second baby, I kind of didn't trust my body. I knew this was going to be a bigger baby (than my first), and I didn't know what it was going to feel like . . . Plus it was a really busy night at the hospital; they were kind of pushing for me to have this baby. So I felt pressured into getting an epidural. Now, I definitely made that decision myself, but there's something that still doesn't feel right for me. I never really felt the pains of labor, and I ended up getting an epidural because I was at the stage where I could. They gave me a really light epidural so I did have feeling in my legs, but I was much more anxious with it. I didn't like it. It definitely took the edge off, but I didn't have that much of an edge to take off, and I shook a lot—you know, some women get the shakes—which made me feel out of control. Part of me wonders what kind of birth I would have had naturally, but my doctor said, "Mary, why do you have to be in pain to feel that this was a good birth experience?" So I have really mixed feelings about the epidural. Who knows how it would have been without it. Still, in the end, I had a great, controlled delivery, and I was totally with it.

Mary, mom of two

Q: Will an epidural affect my baby?

Dr. Evans: In this day and age, and in this legal environment, epidurals of any sort wouldn't be given if they weren't considered absolutely safe for both mother and baby. Still, this question sparks some debate and the answer to it depends on whom you ask. If you ask a doctor, you're likely to hear that epidurals do not affect newborns. In clinical studies of newborns whose mothers received the low doses of local anesthetic and/or narcotics that are currently the standard of care, the effects on the babies from the drugs were considered insignificant.

If you ask a lactation consultant or natural birth advocate, you could hear that they've noted that babies born to moms who had epidurals are less likely to breastfeed in the first hour after birth. For the first day or so they don't suck as strongly when they breastfeed, and they can be fussy. These side effects pass after a baby fully metabolizes any of the medication that passed through the placenta during labor.

Q: Once I get an epidural, are more medical interventions inevitable? Is it more likely I'll end up with a C-section?

Dr. Evans: In some cases, getting an epidural actually helps a woman avoid a Cesarean because it gives her a chance to rest and regain strength for pushing. Also, some women can't help but tighten their muscles in response to the pain of contractions; this tightening slows dilation. When they get an epidural, the pain relief allows their muscles to relax, and labor to progress more rapidly. I can't even count the number of times I've seen women who were either exhausted or in extreme pain dilate from five to ten centimeters in an hour or two after getting an epidural.

As for the "cascade" theory of an epidural leading to more medical interventions and complications, in my own experience it doesn't hold true. Sometimes labor and birth go smoothly. Other times, the road is bumpier. It's often impossible either to predict that a labor will become more challenging or to attribute the cause of the complications to one intervention or another. A labor that ends up with many interventions or a C-section may start with a single problem that needs attention, then something else happens, and so on. I think it would be intellectually dishonest to blame the series of events on that first intervention.

On the other hand, over the years I have seen rare cases where an epidural (or another intervention) created a complication—for example, it led to a drop in fetal heart rate. The baby's heart rate didn't rebound fast enough, and an emergency C-section became necessary. But I want to emphasize that, overall, epidurals rarely cause complications in and of themselves.

REAL VOICES

I was induced, and I had really hoped not to be. Once it began, I tried to power through the Pitocin for a couple of hours and that just was *not* happening—after two hours I'd dilated one centimeter. It was pretty bad. And then I had an epidural, and in another hour I had dilated like nine centimeters, and I thought, "Okay, I really like this epidural." I don't know, maybe it was wearing off, but when I got to the pushing phase, I definitely felt like I could push. Coming from a natural childbirth kind of place, I had gotten the message that epidurals always lead to eight million other interventions and you're not going to be able to feel and you're not going to be able to walk. No, they wouldn't let me walk, but at that point— where was I going?

Marjorie, mom of one, pregnant

Q: Is it ever too late to get an epidural?

Dr. Evans: Technically, it's never too late. However, if you're more than seven or eight centimeters dilated and you're almost ready to push, or if you're fully dilated (10 centimeters) and pushing, it probably isn't worth getting an epidural. By that point in labor, you wouldn't use it for that long. Plus, late in active labor it's difficult to stay as still as you need to for an epidural to be safely administered.

Some Common Medical Procedures Used in Labor

There are many variations in the medical protocols and procedures used during labor. Here's an overview of some of the more common elements of that care:

Electronic fetal monitoring (EFM)

• *What it is:* The baby's heart rate is monitored throughout labor with an external or internal electronic device to make sure she doesn't show any signs of distress from the labor. The monitoring may be intermittent (external monitoring only) or continuous (internal or external monitoring).

• *How it's done:* For continuous electronic external fetal heart rate monitoring, two belts hold two instruments on a mother's abdomen—one detects the fetal heart rate (by ultrasound) and the other measures the contractions (by a tocodynamometer). The belts produce "tracings" on paper and on computer screens that keep track of how the baby is doing.

Internal fetal heart rate monitoring is far less common. A little clip is attached to the baby's scalp, and it reads the fetal heart rate. The membranes must be broken for it to work.

• *When it's used:* Continuous electronic fetal monitoring is widely used as the standard of care in most hospitals. (If you have concerns about its use during your labor, see "Options," page 469.)

• *Why it's used:* Electronic fetal monitoring keeps tabs on the baby's heart rate. Medical reasons for it include:

  — When there are questions during labor about the baby's well-being
  — When labor has been medically induced
  — When a problem develops in labor or labor stalls
  — When consistent monitoring by a nurse or midwife isn't available

— High-risk pregnancies (This is a broad category; talk with your care provider about your particular situation and the role monitoring would play.)

• *The arguments for and against electronic monitoring:* The scientific data are clear that there's no benefit to continuous electronic fetal monitoring. Monitoring the baby's heart rate with a monitor or fetoscope every ten to fifteen minutes in the first (dilation) stage of labor and after each contraction in the second (pushing) stage has been shown to be just as effective as continuous electronic monitoring in keeping track of a baby's well-being.

That said, continuous electronic fetal monitoring can help doctors detect and avoid problems early in labor. But it can also lead to overly aggressive interventions and may be a contributing factor to higher C-section rates. (According to the American College of Obstetricians and Gynecologists [ACOG], fetal heart rate monitoring predicts fetal well-being 99 percent of the time, but it only positively predicts fetal compromise 50 percent of the time. In other words, when monitoring says that a baby's healthy, she's healthy 99 percent of the time. When monitoring says that a baby is stressed, she's born with signs of distress only half the time.)

From a practical perspective, a hospital may not have enough nurses to provide intermittent monitoring to every woman, and even a midwife attending to several women in labor may not be able to provide the appropriate level of monitoring. In this situation, electronic fetal monitoring is better than no, or not frequent enough, monitoring.

• *Options:* If you have questions or are concerned about electronic fetal monitoring, particularly if you plan a low-intervention labor without pain medication (in which case continuous monitoring would make it difficult to move around), talk with your caregiver about your options. You may be able to agree on a set amount of time per hour (for example ten to twenty minutes) during which you'll be monitored, and you'll be free to move otherwise.

Intravenous fluids (IV fluids)

• *What it is:* A needle attached to a bag of fluid is placed in your hand or arm. The bag hangs on a pole, and a long length of plastic tubing transfers the IV fluid to your arm.

• *When it happens:* When and if you'll be given an IV depends on your caregiver's protocol, the hospital's protocols, and the flexibility of the hospital's protocols. Some hospitals give everyone an IV right away in case an emergency unfolds later on and you need to be given fluids or medication immediately.

• *Why IV fluids are given:* There are a number of reasons to give IV fluids during labor:

— *If you become dehydrated:* If you labor for a long time or if you vomit frequently during labor, you can easily become dehydrated. Drinking clear fluids or sucking on ice chips or Popsicles helps stave off dehydration, but it can still happen. If you become dehydrated, your contractions can become less effective, slowing labor. Being dehydrated can also lower blood flow to the baby, and you can become dizzy or faint after the blood loss of birth (particularly of passing the placenta).

— *If you haven't had enough calories:* If you haven't eaten anything or drunk juice or a sports drink since your labor began, and you end up laboring for more than eight hours, you'll probably need calories to keep up your strength and have energy to push.

— *If you have an epidural:* Because blood pressure can drop when you're given an epidural, IV fluids are given proactively. The extra fluid will keep your blood vessels full, which will help maintain a stable blood pressure.

— *If you need medication:* Certain medications—Pitocin, antibiotics (see page 471), or medication to stabilize blood pressure—are given intravenously.

— *If you have a C-section:* With a Cesarean, you need IV fluids to keep your blood pressure up and maintain appropriate fluid levels to make up for blood lost during the surgery.

• *Options:* If you don't want to be attached to an IV when you get to the hospital, and you don't need IV fluids, you can ask your caregiver about a heparin lock ("hep lock"). A needle is placed in your arm above the wrist, and a plug is attached to it. A hep lock allows you to keep a vein open in case of an emergency or if you become dehydrated and need IV fluids, but your arm is free of tubing.

Note: If you're afraid of needles or simply don't want a hep lock, talk to your caregiver about whether you'd need it at all.

If you decide against an IV or heparin lock, ask your primary labor support person to keep tabs on how much liquid you're drinking and how often you go to the bathroom (it's easy to forget to do this while laboring). You should drink eight ounces per hour and try to go to the bathroom every hour or so. Pack your favorite drinks in your hospital bag, and ask your partner or someone on your birthing team to find the ice machine when you get to the hospital or birth center.

Q: Why would I need antibiotics during labor?

Dr. Evans: There are two main reasons. First, if you test positive for group B strep infection (see page 298), you'll be given antibiotics to keep the infection from passing to the baby during birth. (Since you will know this in advance of labor, I'd recommend bringing a probiotic like acidophilus to the hospital. Right after birth, dip your moist finger into the probiotic powder (you can moisten your finger with your own saliva and break open a capsule) and give it to your baby once a day for two days to help him maintain the good bacteria in his gut that the antibiotic could destroy. (The probiotic should be a reputable brand that guarantees 2.5 to 5 billion live organisms of *Lactobacillus acidophilus* through the expiration date.) Second, if, during labor, you develop an infection in the sac that surrounds the baby, the antibiotics will be given to control the infection in both you and the baby. Symptoms of an infection of the amniotic sac include a fever, feeling warm to the touch, elevation of the baby's heart rate, and a foul smell. If you develop such an infection, you should be able to continue laboring and have a vaginal birth after getting antibiotics.

Vaginal exams

Once you're either in the hospital or birth center or your midwife is at your home, you'll have vaginal exams intermittently throughout labor to determine how far your cervix has dilated; these are done by hand, without a speculum. (A speculum may be used to check on broken membranes.) You should not have too many exams, because they introduce the possibility of infection. But they're important because it's the state of the cervix (i.e., how dilated it is), not the duration and frequency of your contractions, that tells your caregiver how labor is progressing.

The problem with a vaginal exam is it can mean disrupting the rhythm of labor— particularly if someone is laboring without pain medication. There's no way around either fact: vaginal exams serve a purpose, *and* they can be disruptive for a laboring woman. If you're planning a natural labor in a hospital, talk with your care provider about the hospital protocols and how frequently you will be examined. Also talk with your partner/labor coach and/or doula about how best to manage the exams.

Note: Lauren Pueraro, MD, attending anesthesiologist at Stamford Hospital, Stamford, Connecticut, collaborated on the medical pain relief material.

22

Assisted Vaginal Births
and Cesareans

When labor doesn't go quite as smoothly as hoped and the baby doesn't progress down the birth canal, a doctor or midwife might recommend either an assisted delivery or a Cesarean. Here I review the basics of assisted deliveries, C-sections, vaginal births after Cesareans, and some of the controversies and complicated emotions that may accompany C-sections.

◆ ◆ ◆

In this chapter you'll find:

- **Assisted Delivery**
  - Forceps
  - Vacuum extraction
- **Episiotomy**
- **Cesarean Sections**
- **Vaginal Birth After Cesarean**

Assisted Delivery

Forceps

• *What it is:* A forceps is a tool used to assist in childbirth. It looks like two big spoons bound together.

• *Why it's used:* A forceps is used in the pushing stage of labor when it becomes clear that the baby can't finish the trip through the birth canal without some assistance. Reasons for this include: (1) when a mother is having trouble pushing because she is too tired, her contractions are no longer efficient, or possibly because anesthesia is interfering with her ability to push, and (2) when the baby shows signs of distress and is low in the birth canal.

• *How it's used:* A doctor places the forceps on either side of the baby's head and locks it into place so she can't squeeze too tightly. Once the forceps is locked, she can gently pull the baby down the rest of the birth canal while the mother pushes through a contraction. Forceps usually require an episiotomy (see page 474) and/or regional anesthesia (i.e., an epidural, see page 462). Midwives don't deliver with forceps.

Vacuum extraction

• *What it is:* A vacuum uses a little suction cup to gently pull a baby down the birth canal.

• *Why it's used:* As with forceps, a vacuum is used during the pushing stage when a mother can't push efficiently or effectively because she's tired, her contractions aren't productive, or possibly because of anesthesia. Or, a care provider might use a vacuum if the baby's head is at a funny angle or the baby shows signs of distress. An episiotomy may not be necessary with a vacuum extraction.

• *How it's used:* A little suction cup is placed on the baby's head; it will pop off if the care provider pulls too hard, protecting the baby from injury.

Note: The decision to use either vacuum or forceps should be made by the doctor and depends on her training, personal preference, and the position of the baby. Midwives (CNMs and CMs, see pages 86–90) may be trained in vacuum extraction, but its use isn't part of their core competency.

Episiotomy

- *What it is:* An episiotomy is a surgical cut made just before a baby is born to widen the birth canal. The cut starts in the vagina and most often proceeds toward the anus. (How far the cut goes depends on the care provider performing the procedure.) It's usually done with a local anesthesia, but may be performed without it in an emergency. Care providers almost always use a local anesthesia to stitch up an episiotomy. Midwives (CNMs and CMs) can perform episiotomies.
- *Why it's done:* An episiotomy is used to widen the vaginal opening if:
  1. It looks like it will be necessary—for example, if the baby's shoulders get stuck or if a care provider senses the shoulders could get stuck.
  2. The baby's in distress and a caregiver wants to speed delivery.
  3. It's necessary as part of a forceps or vacuum delivery (see page 473).
  4. It looks like the mother will have a significant tear either on her perineum (the area between the vagina and anus) or her labia (the folds on the sides of the vagina).
- *The debate:* There was a time when episiotomies were routinely performed. They're used much less frequently now. Many care providers (myself included) and several clinical studies have concluded that the use of episiotomies to prevent an imminent tear, the classic reason for the procedure, doesn't necessarily benefit a mother or baby. Plus, it's easier for a doctor to repair a natural tear than an episiotomy. That said, every care provider is different, and some will perform episiotomies more regularly than others. When you talk to your care provider about his approach to birth, ask what he thinks of episiotomies, why and how often he performs them, and what he does during a birth to avoid them.
- *Alternatives:* Perineal massage in the last two months of pregnancy and Kegel exercises (focusing on the relaxation phase) may reduce the likelihood of an episiotomy. (For perineal massage and Kegels, see page 415.) During labor, a care provider can stretch the perineum by applying pressure to it with the fingers. (This isn't the same thing as perineal massage and should only be done by an experienced doctor or midwife.) He or she might also apply a warm compress to the perineum to help protect it; midwives are more likely to use compresses than OBs.

Cesarean Sections (C-sections, Cesarean Delivery, Cesarean Birth)

• *What it is:* A Cesarean section is a surgical birth.

• *How it's done:* Most often a horizontal cut is made low on the abdomen (rarely, a vertical incision is made; it depends on the situation); the abdominal muscles are not cut. Next, an incision is made in the uterus, the amniotic fluid is suctioned, and the baby is carefully taken out, which is most often a two-person procedure, with the obstetrician assisted by a second doctor. Once the baby is out, the umbilical cord is clamped and cut, the placenta is removed, and the uterus is thoroughly examined. When a woman hasn't had any previous uterine surgery (such as another C-section or having fibroids removed), this takes about fifteen minutes, after which the doctor will take about a half hour to sew everything back up. If you've had uterine surgery before, the surgery could take a little longer, up to sixty minutes, depending on your situation and the doctor. When multiples are delivered by C-section, it takes about five minutes per baby once the uterus is opened.

• *Why it's done:* Cesareans may be scheduled for before labor is likely to begin, or they're performed either on an emergency basis or with some urgency during labor. Here are the basic reasons for each:

• *Scheduled C-sections:* C-sections are scheduled when a vaginal birth is considered too risky for mother and/or baby. Reasons include:

  — *Breech:* A baby is "breech" when his buttocks, or some combination of his buttocks and feet (instead of his head), will be the first part of his body to emerge. When that's the case and a vaginal breech delivery isn't possible or desirable, a C-section will be scheduled. (See "Breech Presentation" on page 430.)

  — *Multiple pregnancy:* In a twin pregnancy, if the first twin isn't head down, a C-section is considered the standard of care. (See "Vaginal Twin Births" on page 457.) For triplets and higher-order multiples, Cesareans are the standard of care.

  — *Placenta previa:* When the placenta covers part of or the entire cervix, a vaginal birth can lead to life-threatening bleeding in both baby and mother.

  — *A medical condition in the mother:* Preeclampsia, diabetes, a herpes outbreak, a chronic medical condition, or a large fibroid that could interfere with delivery are all potential reasons for scheduling a Cesarean birth. (*Note:* The risk created by a fibroid in labor depends on its size and position in the uterus.)

  — *A suspected problem with the baby:* If, after evaluations like non-stress tests and biophysical profiles, a doctor suspects labor would be too stressful for a baby, a C-section will be scheduled. An example of this would be when there's no amniotic fluid (oligohydramnios) and a baby has IUGR (see pages 336–345).

— *Repeat C-section:* Nearly half of all Cesareans are repeat C-sections. (For more information, see "Vaginal Births After Cesareans [VBAC]," page 482.)

• *The anesthesia:* With a scheduled C-section, many women receive a spinal, as opposed to an epidural (see page 464). This means you get one shot of pain medication as opposed to having an epidural catheter placed in your back. In addition to the spinal, you may receive pain medication (Duramorph) to relieve postoperative discomfort. If you're scheduling a Cesarean, talk over with both your doctor and the attending anesthesiologist at the hospital what kind of medication you can expect during and after the operation.

Preparing for a Scheduled C-Section

✦ It's not always easy to come to terms with having to schedule a Cesarean. Even though a C-section is most often planned to give a mother and baby (or babies) the best chance for a healthy outcome, some women feel a sense of loss at not having the opportunity to labor and birth vaginally. In this situation, it can be frustrating to hear "Just focus on a healthy baby and a healthy mom." It's important to be realistic about the full spectrum of emotions that a scheduled Cesarean can evoke, to both embrace the positive and accept the negative aspects of a scheduled C-section. The obvious positive is that the surgery significantly reduces potentially life-threatening risks that you and your baby (or babies) would face in a vaginal birth. The downside is not having the experience of a vaginal birth. No matter what people say about focusing on the positive, let yourself feel and express whatever sense of loss you may have. As with any feeling, by acknowledging it you can keep from getting stuck in a sense of loss and begin to embrace the excitement of meeting your child.

• *Steps you can take to improve the experience:* If you're scheduling a C-section, you may be able to make certain arrangements in advance that allow for a more family-centered experience. These include:

— *Have your partner there:* Many hospitals allow a partner to accompany you into the operating room. If you're unsure about whether or not your partner or a primary support person will be able to join you, talk it over with your doctor and make provisions to allow someone to be with you.

— *Ask for music:* If music will help you stay relaxed and at ease during the surgery, or if there's something you'd particularly like to listen to, ask your doctor if it can be played during the surgery. This can be beneficial for the baby as well; I believe that calm music soothes babies born by Cesarean.

— *Hold up the baby:* If you want to see your baby immediately after she's delivered and before she's cleaned, examined, and swaddled, ask your doctor to hold her up for you to see.

— *Ask if it's possible for your partner to be given the baby as soon as possible.*

— *Keep one arm free:* Typically, in an urgent or emergency C-section, one of your arms has an IV and the other arm is strapped down so your arms are spread in a "T" shape. If this doesn't appeal to you, ask your doctor if hospital policy will allow you to keep your second arm free during a scheduled surgery. Explain that you won't move it into the sterile field below your chest and you'd like to be able to touch your baby in the operating room.

— *Have skin-to-skin contact:* When you're given your baby in the recovery room, you can unwrap her, lay her directly on your bare chest, and place a blanket over both of you. If you can't do this, your partner can.

— *Breastfeed in recovery:* If you're planning to breastfeed, you should be able to do so in the recovery room. If you're having trouble maneuvering, a nurse will help you position the baby so she doesn't lie on your incision. (Later, you can place a pillow over your incision to protect it.) Breastfeeding will help your uterus contract to a smaller size, but you won't feel those contractions if you nurse in the recovery room, because the anesthetic will still be blocking any pain.

— *Placenta rituals:* If you'd planned on having a ritual around the placenta—for example, burying it in a special place—ask your doctor if hospital policy will allow you to have it.

Doulas and scheduled C-sections: If you'd planned to work with a doula in labor, she might still be able to help you in a scheduled C-section. A doula who has experience with Cesareans can help you stay calm and focused before surgery, and she can stay with you in recovery. This is more important if your baby has to go to the nursery after delivery and your partner goes with the baby. Once you and your baby are together, a doula can help you breastfeed if you plan to.

- *Urgent C-sections:* These C-sections take place after a woman has been in labor and a problem develops. Time is important for these surgeries, but they don't have to be performed immediately.

  - *Stalled labor:* A "stall" just means a woman stops dilating or a baby stops progressing through the birth canal; it can happen in the first (dilation) or second (pushing) stage.

    If labor stalls in the dilation stage of labor, a caregiver can give medication, such as Pitocin, to strengthen contractions, in the hopes that the mother's cervix will start to dilate again. There are other techniques to overcome a stall besides Pitocin—for example, giving IV fluids if a woman is dehydrated, or rupturing the membranes if they haven't broken already. If, after a few hours, nothing has worked, then a Cesarean delivery is warranted.

    If labor stalls in the pushing phase, a caregiver can decide whether a C-section or an assisted delivery (using a forceps or vacuum) is the safer and better route.

    Stalled labor is the most common reason for a first Cesarean. It can happen for several reasons—for example, if a woman's contractions become less effective, or if the baby is large and the mother's pelvis is small, or if the baby's head is in a funny position, or some combination thereof.

    Note: The position of the baby's head determines what part of the head will lead the way out of the birth canal: the narrowest, widest, or some part in between. Ideally, the narrowest part would come out first. For this to happen, a baby's chin would be tucked to his neck and he would face his mother's back. This is known as the occiput anterior (OA) position (the occiput being the crown of the baby's head). If a baby is in the occiput posterior (OP) position, the widest part leads. In the OP position, a baby is "sunny-side up," or facing his mother's front. It usually means back labor, and longer dilation and pushing phases.

  - *Fetal distress:* When a baby is distressed, her heart rate drops, and she gets less oxygen. During the pushing stage of labor, it's normal for the baby's heart rate to go down during a contraction, but it should bounce back to the normal range between contractions. If the baby's heart rate slows between contractions or if it's erratic (as measured by fetal monitoring), a C-section may become necessary.

- *The anesthesia:* If you already have an epidural catheter in place, you'll be given a boost of regional anesthetic before surgery. After getting the medication, you'll probably be unable to feel your legs at all. In addition, you might be given a sedative before the surgery. If you have a chance to discuss this with your doctor or the anesthesiologist, you can ask not to have the sedative. If you haven't had an epidural, you could get a spinal (one shot of narcotic pain medication) before an urgent C-section.

REAL VOICES

I really feel like the medical care I got supported me in trying to have the birth experience that I wanted, and then when it was the right time to change course, they helped me do it. You know, it's funny, a couple of months after I had my first kid (by C-section), I went to this baby store to pick something up . . . and they had a flyer up saying, "You have had a C-section. You are disappointed and distressed. You are sad and depressed," or something like that. And I thought, "I am grateful that my baby is alive. Thank you very much for telling me how I feel about this!" Actually, I *am* incredibly grateful. I mean I'm aware that there are problems with the C-section rate—but there are some times when it's really done for the right reasons.

Jill, mom of two

• *Emergency C-sections:* When one of the following situations emerges, a Cesarean must be performed immediately:

— *Prolapsed cord:* If the umbilical cord slips out of the cervix before the baby, it can become compressed or kinked, limiting the baby's blood and oxygen supply. This is a rare event. It's a greater risk when a baby is breech, but it can also happen when a baby is headfirst and the amniotic fluid gushes out with particular force.

— *Hemorrhage:* If a mother experiences severe bleeding because the placenta separates from the uterus (parental abruption, see page 349) or another reason, such as a uterine rupture (a tear in the uterine wall), immediate surgery is necessary.

— *Severe fetal distress:* If the fetal heart rate drops to less than 70 beats per minute (normal is 120 to 160 beats per minute) for more than a few minutes, an emergency C-section is necessary.

• *The anesthesia:* In general, anesthesiologists try to avoid giving general anesthesia, which knocks you out, during a C-section. Sometimes that's not possible in an emergency situation, and general anesthesia must be given. Otherwise, an anesthesiologist might be able to administer a spinal quickly.

Elective C-sections

✦ In the U.S., more and more women are choosing to schedule a Cesarean for a first birth instead of attempting a vaginal birth. Most women make this choice to avoid the risk of damage to the pelvic floor that could lead to incontinence or sexual dysfunction. But in the U.S., the great majority of women who give birth vaginally don't have pelvic floor damage. In other words, women are choosing an invasive surgical procedure over a natural process in order to guard against a future event (pelvic damage) that's unlikely to occur. At the same time, by choosing a C-section, they're introducing new risks from surgery. Even though Cesareans are safer than they've ever been, the risks involved with surgery of any kind shouldn't be minimized or dismissed.

According to the American College of Obstetricians and Gynecologists (ACOG), the decision of whether or not to perform an elective Cesarean section must be left up to the attending doctor who would be ethically and legally responsible for the health and well-being of a patient and her child during the procedure. A doctor's decision should be based on the concerns, needs, and actual risks facing the woman requesting the surgery.

There's no denying that in the United States (and indeed around the world) elective Cesareans represent a growing trend, and only time—and data—will tell if they are a good or bad thing.

Personally, as a doctor and surgeon, before I take a woman into an operating room, I need to believe that I have done everything possible to preserve her health and well-being. Therefore, all surgery should be performed only when medically indicated. An elective first-time Cesarean to prevent pelvic floor damage doesn't pass my own test, but that doesn't mean I think it's wrong for a woman to want it or for another doctor to perform it.

Note: Before you go into labor, if you're working with a midwife and/or doula, talk with them about what would happen in the case of a C-section. Your midwife or doula could either accompany you and your partner into the operating room (a doctor can facilitate this if it's important to you) or join you in the recovery room afterward. The latter is important so you won't be alone in recovery if your baby needs medical attention and your partner accompanies him to the nursery or NICU (newborn ICU). A midwife may have less time flexibility than a doula, especially if she's working with other women in labor. Include a Cesarean contingency plan in any agreement you draw up with a doula.

• *Adjusting to a Cesarean during labor:* Every woman responds to the need for a Cesarean differently. Some may not have any issues with having a C-section. Some have a relatively easy time coming to terms with any disappointment they feel. Others have much more difficulty emotionally with the surgery.

Adjusting to an urgent or emergency Cesarean tends to be most challenging for women who feel left out of the decision-making process in their labor and for those who began labor with very strong expectations about a vaginal birth. After a Cesarean, a woman may feel like she missed out on a very special life experience, or, worse, that the experience was taken away from her against her will or better judgment. While a care provider can't control a woman's expectations going into labor, she can offer clear, consistent, and honest information about what's happening throughout labor. That way, if surgery becomes necessary, a woman is more prepared emotionally.

If you feel you were left out of the decision-making process during your labor, I would encourage you to talk about it with your care provider. I know this may be difficult to do, but if you have strong feelings about how your labor was handled, it would help you and your care provider to talk through how decisions were made and why.

If you don't feel comfortable talking with your caregiver, try to talk about your feelings with someone to whom you can voice their full range—your partner, a trusted friend, or a therapist.

It can be confusing to feel excited and relieved that you and your baby are both healthy, yet disappointed about having had a Cesarean—but it's totally understandable. Just because people may be telling you that you "shouldn't" feel bad about a Cesarean doesn't mean that you don't. At the same time, if you feel bad about the surgery right now, it doesn't mean you always will.

• *When surgery is equated with failure:* As a physician, one thing that's particularly hard for me is when a woman tells me she feels like a failure because she had a Cesarean. As I see it, giving birth is the final part of the much longer process of pregnancy. Anyone who gives birth—whether vaginally or by Cesarean—has created a new life. Her body has done extraordinary work nurturing her baby throughout the nine months leading up to the birth. And if during labor and birth medical intervention was necessary, it doesn't mean that her body failed her, or that *she* was a failure.

After all, there are so many factors that influence how childbirth unfolds that to consider a surgical birth a personal failure seems unnecessarily harsh and self-critical. My hope is that after giving birth, a woman will treat herself with compassion and love as she heals from this great, but always demanding, experience—no matter what kind of birth it was.

REAL VOICES

We took hypnobirthing, the Bradley Method, and a hospital birthing class to prepare for a spiritual, natural delivery. It didn't work out that way. At one of my last prenatal visits, a senior doctor in the practice said she thought I'd need a C-section—and we thought she was just pro-Cesarean. A younger doctor encouraged us to try for a vaginal birth. I was induced, but our daughter just didn't descend. It was a difficult labor, and I ended up having a C-section—my daughter Davida was eleven pounds, six ounces. We later found out that the first doctor wasn't pro-Cesarean and that she thought a C-section would be necessary because of the position of Davida's head and the size of my pelvis. One great thing is that during the C-section, the doctor paused as she was lifting Davida out so we could say a prayer—a small hint of the more spiritual experience we had been looking for.

Katie, mom of one

Vaginal Birth After Cesarean (VBAC)

After a Cesarean, a vaginal birth is a viable option, but there are a few factors to keep in mind when making the decision to pursue a vaginal birth:

- *Your care provider:* Care providers don't agree when it comes to the question of how many previous Cesareans a woman can have had before a VBAC. Some will only support a VBAC if a woman's had one prior section, others will do so after two, still others will do so after more. Also, some care providers are simply more supportive of VBACs than others. Talk to your care provider about where he stands on the issue and his take on your situation. If a VBAC is important to you, but your care provider is hesitant about pursuing it, consider getting a second opinion from another doctor or midwife. (If you decide to work with a midwife for a VBAC, I'd recommend working with a certified nurse midwife (CNM) with hospital privileges, but that's a personal decision.)

Are Too Many Cesareans
Performed in the U.S.?

✦ C-sections represent a little over 26 percent of all births. While the Cesarean rate has leveled off in recent years (after climbing for years), many believe that there are still too many surgical births in the U.S. Why are so many Cesareans being performed?

Repeat C-sections, which represent nearly half of these surgeries, are the biggest reason the overall Cesarean rate is so high. This means we have to ask if too many C-sections are being performed in first births. The answer is yes, but for complicated reasons.

First, in the current medical-legal environment, more lawsuits are brought against doctors and hospitals for *failure* to perform a Cesarean than for doing the surgery. Doctors, therefore, may be more defensive in their decision-making than they might otherwise be. (In other words, they may decide a Cesarean is the right choice earlier in labor.)

Second, the current legal environment and the increasing legal and insurance costs incurred by teaching hospitals mean doctors are being trained differently. Young doctors in training (residents) are now less likely to get as much experience using forceps and vacuums because supervising doctors and hospital programs will opt for a C-section instead of an assisted delivery. As a result, more and more residents are trained to assist at either straightforward vaginal births or C-sections. When a forceps or vacuum delivery would help a woman have a vaginal birth, a young doctor might not have the training necessary to go that route, and the woman might end up in surgery. (*Note:* This is a general observation; trends in training vary by institution and state.)

Third, there's the issue of how labors are managed and whether or not continuous electronic fetal monitoring leads doctors to anticipate distress in the baby and decide on a Cesarean when there's not necessarily a problem. (Remember that 50 percent false-positive rate with monitoring, see page 468.)

Finally, the growing trend in elective C-sections will no doubt affect the overall C-section rate down the line as those women who choose a first Cesarean go on to have more children through surgical births.

- *The incision:* If you had a low-segment horizontal incision, which is the standard, a VBAC is a safe option. With a vertical incision, a scheduled C-section is the standard of care. (The type of incision used depends entirely on your medical situation and the doctor's decision. Vertical incisions, which are typically used in emergency situations, are relatively rare.)

- *Preparing for a VBAC:* It's always helpful to prepare emotionally, physically, and intellectually for childbirth, but with a VBAC, preparation plays a bigger role. Here are a few points to consider when deciding if a VBAC is right for you:
  - *Understand your priorities:* Consider what's most important to you as you approach your next childbirth. If your first Cesarean took place after a long labor, ask yourself if it's more important to you to have a vaginal birth or to avoid a prolonged labor. Every woman responds differently to this question. For example, when I work with a woman who had a very long labor before her Cesarean who says, "Look, I'd like to have a vaginal birth, but I *really* don't want to go through what I went through the last time," we'll work out a plan. I might suggest we see how labor progresses, and if things move along well, we'll keep going toward a vaginal birth. If labor stalls, then we agree to move into C-section mode sooner rather than try other interventions—*as long as when she's in labor that's still what she wants to do.* Alternatively, if a woman wants to have a vaginal birth and isn't concerned about having a long labor, then we'll go all-out to make that possible, accepting that there are no guarantees.
  - *Understand the risks:* VBACs have certain risks built into them. For example, when a scar from a previous uterine surgery tears, it's known as a *uterine rupture.* Labor contractions may make a uterine scar more vulnerable to tearing. Recent studies have shown that the risk of uterine rupture goes up in a VBAC when labor is induced using a substance such as a prostaglandin gel to ripen the cervix (see "Inducing Labor" on page 440). When labor begins spontaneously, the risk of a uterine rupture is about 1 percent. If a uterine rupture should occur, an emergency C-section would be necessary.

- *Repeat Cesarean:* Overall, between 50 and 60 percent of women who go into labor planning a VBAC have a vaginal birth. That number may be higher or lower depending on your personal history as well as your care provider and his approach to VBACs.

- *Choosing a provider:* Depending on the hospital, a doctor or certified nurse midwife (CNM) can attend the birth; whomever you choose should be experienced with VBACs and supportive of your wish to have one. You and your care provider should take the time to go over your history, the details of your last labor, and your priorities heading into this next labor.

If you decide to work with a CNM, look into setting up an appointment with the consulting physician who would perform a Cesarean should that become necessary. (Sometimes, insurance coverage and/or logistics, such as not knowing who will be on call when you go into labor, make it impossible to have such a meeting with a consulting physician.)

• *Choosing a location:* The warning signs of most complications in labor appear relatively early. An experienced doctor or midwife can read them and respond appropriately no matter where you're laboring (at home or in a birthing center or hospital). Some complications, however, appear out of the blue—and when they do, they're serious and need immediate medical attention. A uterine rupture is one of those complications that can happen without warning, and for that reason, I would not recommend attempting a VBAC at home. That said, there are midwives who will attend home VBACs. (They're sometimes called HBACs, or home births after a Cesarean.) Whether or not an HBAC is a reasonable option for you is an entirely personal decision that depends on how comfortable you are with the risks involved.

If you're considering a VBAC in a birthing center that's very close to a hospital—for example, across the street or actually housed in the same building—review the emergency procedures with the birthing center staff, including the average time it takes to transfer to the hospital (time could be of the essence), and talk over how they typically manage VBACs.

The American College of Obstetricians and Gynecologists (ACOG) recommends that all VBACs take place in a hospital equipped for an emergency Cesarean.

Q: Does a bigger baby mean a VBAC won't work?

Dr. Evans: All the medical literature says that a baby's size doesn't matter unless the baby is estimated to be over 4,500 grams (9.9 pounds).

Q: Is there anything that you've seen that gives a woman a better chance to have a vaginal birth when she plans a VBAC?

Dr. Evans: In my experience, the most important element of any birth is a woman's attitude toward it. When a woman goes into labor and she understands her priorities, accepts the possible risks, and is not too attached to a specific outcome, the chances are good that her overall experience will be positive—whether she delivers vaginally or not.

Whether preparing for a VBAC or a "regular" vaginal birth, I think it's important to accept that childbirth isn't the kind of life event that you can control. Nature and your body will take over any well-laid plan. So before a VBAC, it's important to try to cultivate trust in how your body works, in those who will be there to support you (your birthing team), and in your care providers.

REAL VOICES

We tried really hard for a VBAC with my second baby . . . I was trying to create the conditions for everything "right" to happen during labor. Eventually—I was in labor for twenty-four hours—one of the OBs on duty did this incredibly invasive exam and said, "This kid's head is stuck." And then he drew me a diagram: "Your bone is here, his head is there." At that point, even though intellectually I knew that having the second C-section was the right thing to do, I had some emotional stuff to work through, and I felt some time pressure to work through it quickly. It felt wrong to me to have really invasive surgery and be really upset about it at the same time . . . So I thought, "I need to be upset for a few minutes in this really intense way." I asked my doula to get one of the midwives I knew well. All I needed was to hear her say that in her opinion I was doing the right thing. She came in and said, "You're doing the right thing. It's time to get this baby out, and this is a fine way to do it. Let's go." And that went a huge amount of the way to get me feeling much better. I was able to go into surgery—I wouldn't say without anxiety—but I wasn't in this place of self-incrimination.

Jill, mom of two

I had had a very traumatic emergency C-section with my older daughter. The birth was hard on me, but it was *really* hard on her. I made the decision to have a VBAC after a lot of consideration and debate with my obstetrician. I looked at the literature and the complication rates, and I was very aware that there was a risk of a uterine rupture. As a physician, I knew what could go wrong, and I was really very clear that I wanted to be in a monitored, controlled setting . . . So with my second labor, I really was very interventional, where I hadn't been with the first . . . I really wanted the labor to progress because I'd gotten into a very arrested labor situation with my first, and my goal was to make sure that labor was moving along . . . Within seven hours of starting the Pitocin I was already almost fully dilated, and I pushed for an hour, hour and a half. For me, the contrast was just huge. For my daughter to emerge and immediately be able to be on my chest and my belly and I could nurse her within twenty minutes—it was an amazing experience, just wonderful.

Kathleen, mom of two

23

Postpartum

The initial hours, days, and weeks after you give birth are a time for you to get to know your baby, to take care of yourself, and to begin to adjust to this extraordinary new phase of life. The most important advice I can give is *slow down!* Try to resist the temptation to do, do, do (for the baby and others), and just be, be, be. By this I mean take time to catch your breath and reflect on the miracle of what you've just experienced. This is the time for you and your baby to get to know each other and for you to recover. All your baby really needs from you right now is love . . . The rest will follow.

◆ ◆ ◆

In this chapter you'll find:

- The First Hours and Days Postpartum: What Happens to Your Baby
- The First Hours and Days Postpartum: What Happens to You After a Vaginal Birth
- The First Hours and Days Postpartum: What Happens to You After a C-section
- Breastfeeding: The Basics
- The First Hours and Days Postpartum: Your Emotional World
- The First Six Weeks: Being Home
- The First Six Weeks: The Baby Blues and Postpartum Depression
- The First Six Weeks: Nutrition and Medication, Exercise and Sex
- The Six-week Postpartum Checkup

The First Hours and Days Postpartum: What Happens to Your Baby

Once your baby is born, your care provider will run through a series of tests and standard treatments. Whether this happens immediately after birth or twenty minutes to an hour or more later depends on the procedures of the hospital/birthing center where you are. If you're not sure of the protocol where you'll give birth, review it with your caregiver and ask if, assuming all goes well, you can make adjustments to suit your needs and wishes.

Here's a list of common procedures performed after birth:

• *Apgar test:* The Apgar test was developed in the 1950s by anesthesiologist Virginia Apgar to give a picture of a baby's well-being immediately after birth and help predict how much, if any, extra care your baby may need. Using a 1 to 10 scale, your caregiver will do the test at one and five minutes after birth by taking the baby's heart rate and evaluating her responsiveness, breathing, muscle tone, and color. A low score on either test doesn't predict anything about your baby's future health, intellectual development, or overall well-being. It's only used to assess how much care she might need right after birth. If you have questions about your baby's Apgar scores, ask the pediatrician when she comes to discuss your baby's newborn examination.

— *The one-minute score:*

7 to 10: The baby's condition is considered good to excellent. (Tens are rare—a baby's hands and feet are usually a little blue.)

4 to 6: The baby may need a little extra help; for some that means just a somewhat vigorous back rub.

Under 4: More intervention is needed.

— *The five-minute score:* This second evaluation helps your caregiver determine if the baby needs more care.

7 to 10: Normal.

Under 7: Your baby needs some attention and may be more closely monitored.

• *Eyedrops:* Antibiotic eye ointment is dropped in the baby's eyes within, or at the end of, the first hour after birth. The ointment prevents infection from gonorrhea and chlamydia, two sexually transmitted diseases that may be present in the vagina at birth (women are not always tested for the diseases) and can cause blindness. It's required by every state unless parents refuse it and the nurse or doctor agrees to withhold the medication. If you don't want the eyedrops, it might be worth getting tested for these sexually transmitted diseases shortly before delivery; talk to your caregiver about this. The eyedrops can cause temporary blurriness in the baby's vision, but it wears off quickly.

• *Vitamin K:* Vitamin K is given by injection or orally within an hour or so of birth. It's required by most states in the U.S. and Canada. Vitamin K helps blood clot, and newborns don't start producing it on their own until they are about a week old. The shot helps prevent any bleeding problems, which can be serious in a newborn.

• *Blood tests:* After twenty-four hours and usually within the first two days, a baby will be tested for metabolic disorders with blood drawn from his heel (see sidebar, page 490). It's important to identify these disorders as early as possible in order to minimize their severity. Every state requires that at least some of these tests be performed.

Other bloodwork a baby may have postpartum includes tests for jaundice (if the pediatrician suspects it because of the baby's color), blood sugar levels (if you had gestational diabetes or a large baby—

THE APGAR SCORE: WHERE IT COMES FROM

The numbers in each of these categories are added up to get a baby's score.

• *Heart rate:*
  0—No heart rate
  1—Fewer than 100 beats per minute (The baby is less than responsive.)
  2—More than 100 beats per minute (The baby is vigorous.)
• *Respiration:*
  0—Not breathing
  1—Weak cry; may sound like whimpering or grunting
  2—Good, strong cry
• *Muscle tone:*
  0—Limp
  1—Some flexing of arms and legs
  2—Active motion
• *Reflex response:*
  0—No response to airways being suctioned
  1—Grimace during suctioning
  2—Grimace and cough or sneeze during suctioning
• *Color:*
  0—Whole body completely blue or pale
  1—Good color in body, with blue hands or feet
  2—Completely pink or good color

---

how large depends on the hospital), blood tests and cultures, and possibly a spinal tap, to rule out an infection if you developed an infection or fever during labor.

POST-BIRTH TESTING: RARE METABOLIC PROBLEMS

The March of Dimes recommends that all newborns be given a hearing test and blood tests for nine disorders (see list below). Every state requires that at least some of these tests be performed, but not necessarily all of them. Only a few babies are affected by these extremely rare disorders, but if not identified and treated early, these metabolic conditions can have serious consequences, like mental retardation. If treated early, many of the problems these conditions cause can be avoided. For a state-by-state chart of tests required in each state and more information on each of the diseases, go to the March of Dimes Web site and the page on newborn screening tests (*www.marchofdimes.com*).

The disorders are:

- Phenylketonuria (PKU)
- Congenital hypothyroidism
- Congenital adrenal hyperplasia (CAH)
- Biotinidase deficiency
- Maple syrup urine disease
- Galactosemia
- Homocystinuria
- Sickle-cell anemia
- Medium-chain acyl-CoA dehydrogenase deficiency (MCADD)

• *Bowel movements:* Within a few hours of birth, your baby will have her first bowel movement, passing what's called meconium—assuming she didn't move her bowels during labor or delivery. Meconium is made up of waste that's built up throughout pregnancy, and it's greenish-black and sticky. (When a baby passes meconium before birth, it can be anywhere from light to dark green.) After she passes meconium, a baby's bowel movements will change color, going from dark greenish to yellowish. Nurses and/or the pediatrician at the hospital will give you instructions about how often your baby should have bowel movements and pass urine. Both are signs that the baby is healthy and getting enough nourishment.

The First Hours and Days Postpartum: What Happens to You After a Vaginal Birth

After your baby's born, your uterus stops contracting rhythmically, and usually within twenty minutes, you deliver the placenta (the third stage of labor, see page 455). Once the placenta is out, your caregiver will focus on helping your uterus contract to a smaller size and repairing an episiotomy or any tears you may have.

- *The uterus contracts:* After the baby and placenta are born, the uterus will start to contract in order to shrink and firm up, returning in about one to two minutes to about the size of a cantaloupe. Have your nurse or doctor show you how to feel your uterus shortly after birth. (It's very mobile.) Three things can help this process along:
  - *Nipple stimulation:* Either manual (with fingers) or stimulation from a nursing newborn will trigger the release of oxytocin, a hormone that generates contractions.
  - *Massage:* Kneading the uterus will help it contract. A care provider, nurse, or mother herself can do this—but it's not comfortable.
  - *Pitocin:* Your caregiver may give you a shot of Pitocin or put some in your IV (if you have one) in order to guarantee that the uterus contracts and shrinks appropriately. (Personally, I both massage the uterus and give Pitocin.)
- *Afterpains:* No matter the method your caregiver uses to stimulate uterine contractions, they can be uncomfortable—which is why they're called after*pains*. You have them whether you've given birth vaginally or by C-section. Generally speaking, afterpains are not that uncomfortable after a first birth; they are more painful with subsequent births.

Afterpains may continue for the first few days postpartum, particularly if you breastfeed (because nursing releases hormones that cause contractions).

If you're in pain, let your care provider or a nurse know, because she can give you some pain relief medication. If you find that you're very uncomfortable when you breastfeed, you can take ibuprofen or acetaminophen thirty minutes before you nurse, which will help take the edge off the pain.

- *Perineal exam/stitches:* Your care provider will examine the muscles around the vagina and rectum, first to make sure there aren't any tears and then to repair any tears he finds. If you haven't had any pain relief medication, this exam may be painful, but your caregiver will probably give you a local anesthetic (by injection) before putting in any stitches. If you've had pain medication, he may supplement the anesthetic in your epidural to relieve any pain from the stitches. The stitches themselves will be absorbed into your skin and/or fall out on their own within two to six weeks after you give birth.
- *Perineal care:* After giving birth vaginally, your perineum is likely to be sore. Here's how you can care for it:
  - *Ice packs* can soothe and numb the area, and they help bring down any swelling. Use them as much as you want and need during these first few days. Women who pushed for more than an hour often find it helpful to keep the ice pack on around the clock for the first day or so after delivery.

- *Warm soaks*, or sitz baths, also help soothe the perineum and keep it clean, which is your number-one priority in the days following birth. If you're very sore, try to soak at least two to three times a day.

- *Avoid* any topical ointments, even herbal ointments, which soothe the perineum, in favor of keeping it as clean as possible.

    Instead of ointments, take acetaminophen or ibuprofen to ease the pain, continue with ice packs and soaks, and if you find sitting very uncomfortable, a small inflatable donut pillow, which you can get at the hospital, should help.

- *The shakes:* Almost all women shake or shiver after labor. It's most likely your body recovering from the work it's just done. Ask for some extra blankets if you need them; the shaking should pass within a half hour or so.

- *Emptying your bladder:* You should urinate within four to six hours after a vaginal delivery. If you're in a hospital, you may be surprised by how often someone asks you about going to the bathroom. For many women urinating isn't a problem. After all, your body retains a lot of fluid during pregnancy, and the work of getting rid of it starts immediately. Plus, odds are you drank a lot of fluid during labor, or, if you had an IV or an epidural, you were given a lot of fluids.

    But urinating sometimes *is* a problem because the urethra and bladder are close to the uterus and birth canal, and the whole area may be sore or swollen. Running a faucet, walking around, sitting in a sitz bath, or standing in the shower may help to get things flowing. If you're still unable to urinate after trying the standard tricks, you may need to have a catheter put in; every hospital and birthing center will have its own procedures for how long to wait before doing so.

- *Cleaning after urinating:* Instead of wiping off with paper immediately after urinating, use a little spray bottle filled with warm water. After spraying the area, you can let it air-dry for a few moments (you'll be wearing a pad) or you can gently pat the surface with some toilet paper.

- *Emptying your bowels:* After all the pushing, the stitches, and the hemorrhoids, the idea of a bowel movement may make you cringe——but it's one of those things that just has to——and will——happen. To help make it easier to pass stool, try to eat foods and juices that ease bowel movements, like prunes, fruits, natural juices, and natural fiber supplements. I routinely recommend a stool softener, just to make sure that there are no hard stools, which can be quite painful to pass. If there has been a lot of trauma to the perineum (like a tear or episiotomy that approached the anus), you may need to be on stool softeners for a few weeks to ensure adequate healing can take place. You can take stool softeners as soon as you like after giving birth.

• *Sweating:* In the first hours and days after giving birth, you may sweat a lot. This is normal and not a problem as long as you don't feel achy or have a fever, in which case the sweating could be a sign of an infection. Once you're home, if you have a temperature higher than 100.3 or you feel "flulike" *and* you're sweating a lot, call your caregiver.

REAL VOICES
I was so waterlogged between having had (mild) preeclampsia and the IV from the C-section that the second day after I had the baby I lost eight pounds in a day and the third day I lost seven pounds. I just peed all the time and sweat a lot. It was funny, and it was totally satisfying. I wanted to get on the scale just to see what would happen; it was this crazy adolescent fantasy of weight loss. But my body was like: Done with this water, don't really need it. BAM! Gone.

Jill, mom of two

• *Vaginal Discharge:* Soon after giving birth, whether vaginally or by C-section, you'll begin to have vaginal discharge, or *lochia,* that resembles a period. In the first twenty-four to forty-eight hours, the discharge will be heavy, and you may fill a pad every hour or so. You'll continue to have periodlike discharge ranging from heavy to light for two to three weeks after delivery. Usually, the bleeding will ebb and flow, stopping for a day or two and then starting up again. It tends to slow down when you're sedentary and come on more heavily when you're active.

While there are all kinds of descriptions of what lochia looks like, the truth is there's a wide range of what's normal. It can be bright red or dark red at first; eventually it will become whitish, clear, or have a yellowish tinge. You may or may not have clots; if you do, they can be as big as pancakes or about the size of grapes. One thing that's consistent is that lochia has a very particular odor that's similar to the smell of menstrual flow (since both are made up of blood and the contents of the uterus), mixed with a little scent of perspiration—the smell is different for everyone.

If you're at all concerned about how much you're bleeding or the size and frequency of any clots you're passing, ask a nurse about them. She'll be able to tell you if what you're experiencing falls within the range of normal and get help if necessary.

Other signs to watch for, whether you're in the hospital or at home, include bleeding so heavily that it runs down your leg, a foul odor (like rotten eggs) from

Rest

✦ No matter where or how you give birth, in the first few days afterward, rest is the most important gift you can give your baby and yourself. While some women thrive on chatting with friends and family, I've seen over and over again how easy it is to fall into the trap of entertaining too many visitors for too long. When I make rounds at the hospital in the afternoons, I always clear a room of visitors, and often, new mothers thank me for getting everyone out. While a new baby is exciting for all your friends and family, everyone will have plenty of time to get to know the baby, and what's most important is for *you* to get to know your baby and recover from the physical and emotional strain of labor.

the lochia, or a fever above 100.3. If you have any of these symptoms, call your care provider.

REAL VOICES

I remember waking up the morning after giving birth and walking across the room to go to the bathroom and stopping to look in the mirror and starting to cry. I just thought to myself, "I'm a different person right now. I'm a totally different woman." Maybe that's because I was a mother. But I'd walked through this door, and I'd gone through this rite of passage, and I felt transformed.

Miranda, mom of one, pregnant

I'd say use those two to four days in the hospital to rest. You don't get them back, and there are so many people there to help you with the baby. My son was with us from the moment he was born. We'd go to the nursery if he needed a shot or to get checked out—and I wouldn't have changed that. But I probably would have scheduled visitors differently so I could've slept more while I was there.

Trina, mom of one, pregnant

The First Hours and Days Postpartum:
What Happens to You After a C-section

• *In general:* What happens after your C-section depends to some degree on what kind of surgery you had. If it was a scheduled Cesarean delivery, you may be able to see and hold the baby in the operating room, and certainly in the recovery room.

If you have an urgent or emergency C-section, a pediatric team may need to examine and take care of your baby immediately after the birth. After that, assuming everything is fine, your partner can hold the baby. Or, depending on the anesthesia you received, you might be able to hold her. After the surgery is finished, you'll be taken to the recovery room, where, depending on your condition (and how busy the labor and delivery floor is at the time), you could stay for anywhere from twenty minutes to a couple of hours.

If you plan on breastfeeding, you should be able to breastfeed in the recovery room. (You might still be numb from an epidural; if so, and if you're alert, it won't be painful.) If you aren't up to breastfeeding right away, ask your partner/labor support person to let the nursing staff know that you plan to breastfeed, and they'll help you until you're ready to nurse. (For more on C-sections, see page 475.)

• *Gas:* Usually after a Cesarean, gas builds up because your bowels have been slowed, first by being moved during surgery and second because you won't be moving around much during that first day.

Whether or not you can eat the day of surgery depends on your doctor. I feel it's a good idea to eat small amounts that first day *if you're hungry,* but some physicians won't allow you to eat for twenty-four hours afterward. When you do start eating, avoid gassy foods (cabbage, beans, etc.) and carbonated beverages. Drink a lot of water and juice. As soon as you can, start to walk around, which will help move the gas through your system and ease the pain and bloating.

• *Vaginal Discharge:* If you've had a C-section, you'll have the same vaginal discharge as someone who had a vaginal birth. (For details, see "Discharge" on page 493.)

• *The incision:* The incision from a C-section usually looks like a thin cut. In the days after surgery, it shouldn't appear inflamed, more than slightly red, or odd in any way. If it does, let your nurse or care provider know.

There's a risk that you'll develop a wound infection following a C-section; such an infection shouldn't create any major complications, but it needs to be diagnosed and treated relatively quickly. Usually, antibiotics alone will cure the infection, but occasionally pus or fluid collects beneath the incision. If that happens, the incision needs to be opened. Surprisingly, this procedure is often only minimally painful, because the fluid wants to be released. After it's opened, your incision will close on its own in a few days to a few weeks.

In general, treat your incision gingerly. In the shower, pay no more attention to it than you used to pay to that part of your belly—in other words, ignore it. Don't take a bath until the incision is healed (usually by the six-week postpartum visit). Try placing a pillow over it when you nurse, to keep it from getting irritated. Many women say that it feels good to press a pillow on the incision when they laugh or cough, because it eases the sensation of pulling. Your care provider and nurses will give you specific instructions for cleaning the incision.

• *Moving around:* Having a C-section is like having any other type of major abdominal surgery—only afterward you have to care for yourself *and* a new baby! As for your own recovery, the first day you won't be expected to move much. Starting the second day after surgery, you should try to get up and walk around for ten minutes or so at least four times a day. How easily and quickly you'll recover depends entirely on your situation—why you had a C-section, if it was scheduled, whether it was done as an emergency or after a prolonged labor, if you had an infection during labor, your own sense of pain, and your body's overall ability to recover. (If you felt fairly healthy going into labor or the C-section, the odds are good that you'll recover relatively easily.)

Breastfeeding: The Basics

Breast milk is the best food for your child. Whether or not to breastfeed is a personal decision only you can make, based on how you feel emotionally and physically, your philosophy, your work and family responsibilities, and the kind of support you have at home. The American Academy of Pediatrics recommends breastfeeding for at least a year, which is ideal, but however long you're able to do so, both you and your child will benefit from the experience of breastfeeding.

Breast milk is perfectly calibrated to the nutritional needs of a newborn, and as your baby grows, it adapts to his changing nutritional needs. Breast milk supports a baby's developing immune system, is anti-inflammatory, and helps fend off allergies, infections (colds, ear infections), and asthma.

For a mother, breastfeeding helps the uterus return to normal size. The same hormone that causes the uterus to contract, oxytocin, also releases a flood of good feeling toward the baby. And initially, it helps you take off the baby weight. From a practical perspective, breastfeeding cuts down on food preparation time and cleanup (including in the middle of the night and on family outings), and it saves money on formula.

Emotionally, it fosters a wonderful connection between mother and baby. (Once breastfeeding is established, many women find that pumping and giving breast milk in a bottle gives them more flexibility.) The bottom line is that no food source ever developed by humans has come close to the long-term nutritional value and complexity of breast milk, and no experience can substitute for nursing.

- *Maintain a basic, clean diet:* If you choose to breastfeed, I believe it's worthwhile to continue to eat a clean, basic diet just as before and during pregnancy. In fact, I think it's worthwhile to eat such a diet whether or not you decide to breastfeed, but especially if you do. As with maintaining any healthy diet, what's most important is figuring out the right balance for you. Eat as well as you reasonably can, and treat yourself (guilt-free!) when that feels right.
  - *Water:* Drink filtered spring water to satisfy your thirst.
  - *Dairy:* Don't have more than one or two servings per day of dairy; it might upset your newborn's stomach. If your baby is colicky, I'd suggest eliminating dairy altogether. If you're not getting 1,500 mg of calcium daily through food, take a calcium supplement. (For calcium-rich foods, see page 220.) When you buy dairy, look for organic products that are hormone and antibiotic free.
  - *Meat and chicken:* Buy organic meat and chicken if it's affordable and available.
  - *Fish:* Continue to avoid fish that's known to contain high levels of mercury—primarily swordfish, shark, tilefish, and king mackerel. (See page 231 for a complete list.)
  - *Produce:* If they're available and affordable, buy organic fruits and vegetables. If you buy conventional produce, wash it very well. (See page 29 for washing instructions.)
  - *Trans fats:* Avoid foods with trans fats (e.g., french fries and many commercial snacks), because trans fats pass easily into breast milk and can start to clog your newborn baby's arteries. (Check food labels to see if a product is free of trans fats.)
  - *Snacks:* Avoid snacks that you know contain preservatives; if a food has an

expiration date of a year from now, odds are it's full of chemicals (and trans fats) that you're better off not eating and that pass into your baby. Instead of choosing a packaged snack, try to have a whole food snack like fruit, or a slice of whole grain bread with avocado or organic peanut butter.

— *Vitamins and supplements:* Continue to take prenatal vitamins and eat foods rich in omega-3 essential fatty acids (like salmon and flaxseed, see page 29). Or take omega-3 EFA supplements to get up to 1,000 mg a day of combined EPA/DHA; try to get at least 400 mg of DHA to promote your baby's brain and eye development while nursing. Also take an iron supplement once a day until your iron levels are checked at your postpartum visit.

— *Alcohol:* You can have one or two alcoholic drinks a week. Alcohol cycles through the body quickly, and some women choose to pump after having a glass of wine or beer and then dump out the milk. (There's no research to suggest that this is necessary, but some women feel more comfortable doing so.)

After two hours, your milk should be alcohol-free. Other women *like* the fact that their baby is a little calmer if they nurse after having a glass of wine and wouldn't even consider dumping their milk after drinking. I don't believe nursing your baby after a glass of wine is harmful if it's done no more frequently than once or twice a week, but talk to your pediatrician about this.

• *Exercise and breastfeeding:* Take slow, easy walks in the first weeks postpartum. After that, try to exercise moderately and regularly because you'll have more energy and, of course, it will help you lose any excess weight.

• *Getting started:* It's nice to start breastfeeding as soon as possible, either in the delivery room or in the recovery room after a C-section. The skin-to-skin contact that regulates body temperature (see page 452) will also encourage breastfeeding.

If it turns out you can't breastfeed right away, it doesn't mean that you're off to a "bad" start or that you won't be able to breastfeed. You will. If you're at a hospital or birthing center, let the nurses know that you want to breastfeed; there's probably a lactation consultant on staff who can help you get started. Breastfeeding may be natural, but it's not intuitive, and it takes many women a couple of weeks to get comfortable with it. A lactation consultant can show you how your baby should "latch" onto your nipple (a proper latch helps prevent soreness and cracking), and she can teach you various ways to hold your baby while she's nursing.

If you find that you're having trouble nursing or the baby's latch doesn't seem quite right, call someone for help—a postpartum doula (see page 505), lactation consultant, or your local La Leche League. If you don't know anyone who can help, call your care provider. She should be able to recommend someone.

Nurse your baby when he shows signs that he's hungry. These include: turning his head toward something that brushes against his cheek, making sucking gestures and/or sounds in the air, putting his hand to his mouth, or crying and getting fussy. (Crying is a late sign of hunger.)

If you planned to breastfeed and it turns out that it's just not possible for you, try not to worry or feel bad about it. Breastfeeding isn't for everyone. Your baby will still thrive, whether he is fed from the breast or a bottle. (After all, generations of American kids—including me—were and are raised on formula and do beautifully.) As in every aspect of pregnancy and childbirth, every body works differently, and as much as you can, focus on the big picture: Enjoy being with your baby and feed him in whatever way works best for both of you.

- *Engorgement:* In the first few days after you give birth, your breasts will produce colostrum, a thick, nutritious substance that's the baby's first food. Then your milk will come in and your breasts will feel full, warm, and maybe tender—in other words, they'll be engorged. This can be mild or more severe; it can last for a few days or a couple of weeks. It will make your breasts less elastic and harder for the baby to latch onto, which is tough because a good latch will help relieve the engorgement! Ultimately, nursing will relieve engorgement and your milk flow will even out. In the meantime, here are some strategies to deal with engorgement (the nursing and lactation staff will help you, too):

   — *Apply warm, moist heat* for about five minutes or take a warm shower before breastfeeding.

   — *Apply a cold compress* for twenty minutes after breastfeeding. This will reduce swelling.

   — *Massage the breast* when the baby pauses and between feedings.

   — *Apply washed, cool green cabbage leaves* to your breasts for twenty minutes a few times a day.

   — *Ibuprofen* can help with the pain and reduce inflammation.

   — *Try both a supportive nursing bra and going without a bra*—one strategy may be more helpful than the other.

   — *Hand express* or briefly use a breast pump to relieve some pressure, which will soften your nipple and help the baby get a better latch.

- *What to watch for:* If your breasts are not just engorged, but also red, hot, and tender to the touch (this can be all over or in one spot), and especially if you have a fever and/or flulike symptoms, you may have an inflamed and/or infected milk duct. This condition is known as mastitis. Not every case of mastitis involves an infection, but if you have a fever over 100.4, it's likely you have an infection and will need antibiotics. If you suspect mastitis, call your caregiver, who can diagnose it and may prescribe an antibiotic for the infection that's safe to take while breastfeeding. Besides antibiotics, or instead of them, treat mastitis by:

— *Alternating hot and cold compresses* on the affected area. Use crushed ice or a bag of frozen vegetables for a cold compress, which will relieve pain, and a warm, wet cloth for a hot compress, which will increase circulation.

— *Resting:* As with any illness, rest will help you heal and fight the infection.

— *Drinking a lot of fluids:* Again, as with any illness, you need extra fluids.

— *Massaging the affected area:* When you're in the shower, massage the tender area very gently.

— *Trying to breastfeed or pump on the affected side:* This will relieve pressure that's built up in the breast.

— *Taking acetaminophen or ibuprofen* for the pain.

— *Going without a bra* when it's comfortable during the day or at night, so the breast isn't compressed.

— *If you take an antibiotic, take a probiotic, too:* A probiotic should contain two to five billion live organisms of *Lactobacillus acidophilus.*

— *Calling for help:* Call a postpartum doula, lactation consultant, or your local La Leche League for guidance.

• *Change in milk supply:* Most often, a woman's body adapts to the feeding needs of her babies, and she produces milk to meet demand. But some women have oversupply issues, and some sense that they're not producing enough milk. (Symptoms in your baby of oversupply mimic those of undersupply. They include fussiness, pulling at the breast, colicky crying, gassiness, and frequent nursing.) The first step in either instance is to once again ask for help from a postpartum doula, lactation consultant, or La Leche League volunteer. Also, talk to other breastfeeding moms about their experiences and what they've found to be most helpful in getting through challenging patches.

Lactation teas: Most natural food stores or trained herbalists will have botanical blends that help promote lactation, if you begin to feel that your milk supply is slowing down. There are also blends that may help if your baby seems to have an upset stomach or colic. Herbal blends work, but they do so very gently. If you try one out, don't expect results right away. (For a lactation tea source, see "Resources," page 523.)

Beer: One dark beer a day is an old-fashioned remedy known to help get your milk supply going again when it seems to be dwindling. In my own practice, I've found that it helps. If you like beer, it's worth trying.*

REAL VOICES

I breastfed for six months. It was *so* hard at first. I cried and got frustrated and wanted to shoot myself several times. I opted to have my son bottle fed for the two nights I was at the hospital so I could get that last little bit of sleep, and the lactation consultant made me feel awful for it, saying that I had blown my chances of him latching on and that my milk wouldn't come in and yadda yadda. So it blew all my confidence and optimism, and it took almost six days for my milk to come in. My son lost a pound, and I was so incredibly stressed about it. Once I finally did get my milk, I was like a nonstop milk machine, so I was constantly engorged and uncomfortable and leaking. It's a miracle that I stuck with it. Honestly, at first I found it lonely to be breastfeeding in the middle of the night, though I know plenty of women love that bonding time. It took until my son was about two months old for me to appreciate those middle-of-the-night feedings. But, when all is said and done, I am so glad I did it . . . . I feel like it's the best thing you can do for a baby. If I hadn't gone back to work full-time and hated pumping (for some reason it took me a good hour twice a day to get a significant amount of milk), I would've breastfed longer.

Kate, mom of one, pregnant

We had difficulty at first with latching on, and I went through a period where I thought I was not producing enough milk, but overall, it was a satisfying experience. I cherish the closeness I had with my son. When he was 5.5 months old, and I went back to work, he drank pumped breast milk when I was at work, and I nursed when I was home. He was able to stay on breast milk until nine months. Then on his eleven-month birthday two weeks ago, he self-weaned. Now he laughs when I show him my breasts.

Tina, mom of one

---

*For further reading on breastfeeding, see Resources, page 522.

The First Hours and Days Postpartum: Your Emotional World

There aren't any rules about how you should or shouldn't feel when you meet your baby after giving birth. Some women fall in love immediately; others don't—and then there's everything in between. There's no right or wrong way to feel. After all, you've just been through one of the most physically demanding experiences imaginable, and your expectations going into it—about how labor and birth would unfold and what it would be like to meet your baby—may have been very different from what's actually happening. Honor whatever emotions come up for you. Try not to pass judgment or think you're a bad mother if you don't feel like you've fallen in love with your baby right away. Give yourself time to recover physically and allow your emotions to unfold at their own pace.

Keep in mind that during those first days and weeks postpartum, your feelings about everything are likely to change fairly rapidly. Normally, we all have something of an emotional filter, but in the early postpartum period, that filter is gone and emotions can come to the surface very quickly. You may find yourself crying one minute and feeling great the next. Don't try to stop yourself from experiencing any particular emotion, and let the people around you know that what you need most is the time and space to let your feelings simply happen.

REAL VOICES

Three days after both my kids were born, I cried the entire day. I wasn't sure why then, and I'm still not sure. But I told my sister to expect the crying on the third day, and sure enough, it happened to her, too.

Wendy, mom of two

The First Six Weeks: Being Home

Over and over again you'll hear that nothing can prepare you for coming home with a newborn (or two, or more). The experiences of new parents run the gamut—some people have an easier time with the transition; some have a harder time. It's safe to say, though, that every first-time parent faces a steep learning curve. You must get to know your baby and her rhythms, needs, and signals, and you have to figure out how you will take care of this new being. On top of learning to care for your baby, you'll be recovering from the physical demands of pregnancy and childbirth. Taken together, this means the first six weeks with baby is a time to focus your attention on your immediate family and your needs. Here are some basics to keep in mind:

• *Prepare realistically:* If you can, cook and freeze meals in advance and stock up on the items you'll need for baby (see below). Most important, take some time to talk with your partner about household priorities and tasks. Even though you can't predict what you're going to want or need from each other once you're home with a new baby, you can still begin to sort out who will do what, when. That way, you'll have a basic plan to fall back on when you're home with your new baby and you have many new tasks suddenly at hand.

> REAL VOICES
> A group of moms I know generated this list, and I found it really useful.
> Amy, mom of one, pregnant

WHAT TO HAVE ON HAND FOR YOUR HOMECOMING WITH BABY

• *Drugstore stuff:*
  – Newborn diapers with space for umbilical cord stump
  – A&D Ointment: 1 tube for home/1 tube for diaper bag
  – Desitin for diaper rash: 1 for home/1 for diaper bag
  – Infant Tylenol
  – Digital thermometer
  – Baby nail clippers (Their nails grow so fast!)
  – Rubbing alcohol and alcohol wipes for umbilical cord stump
  – Bacitracin: good for belly button if it starts to smell a bit and if you circumcised.
  – Swisspers cotton pads (For some reason I found that these are the best for cleaning umbilical cord and all poops.)
  – Hand sterilizer
  – Panty liners if you don't have any
  – Dreft or Ivory Snow (Wash all baby clothes before.)
  – *No scented anything*
• *Clothing (not including layette):*
  – 5 kimono shirts
  – Receiving blankets
  – Outfits for baby that snap up front from the bottom

- PJs with easy bottom access
- Cotton diapers: great for spit-ups and cleanups
- Flannel diaper pads that go on top of your diaper table (These are easier to wash than the terry diaper cover, which you also end up washing, but not as frequently.)
- *Gear:*
  - Diaper bag with changing pad
  - Baby monitor
  - Front carrier or sling
  - Car seat(s)
  - Stroller
  - Infant tub (We bought ours a few weeks after our son was born.)
- *If you're nursing:*
  - A loose nursing bra (Don't buy anything fitted with cup size because you don't know how big you'll be when your milk comes in. A sports-type bra in s/m/l is a good bet until you have an idea the size you'll eventually be.)
  - Nursing pillow
  - Pump (purchased or rented)

REAL VOICES

I think the hardest part of it for me was probably communication with my husband. We had such a great relationship before we went to the hospital, and when we returned with our son, communication was really difficult . . . Our son was a real screamer, and if you have this screaming baby and you don't know where the diapers are, it's really frustrating . . . It sounds really lame, but knowing where the diapers were and how we were organizing the stuff was really important to making things run smoothly. So having a place for the diapers that we both agreed on was a really important decision.

Glenda, mom of two, stepmom of one

- *Accept help:* People will ask what they can do for you. Tell them. It might be picking up some milk or it might be watching the baby for thirty minutes while you take a walk around the block or nap. Let others be there to help you out; you don't have to do it all on your own. If it's in your budget, you may find it helpful to hire someone to help you out in those first weeks—a baby nurse, postpartum doula, or a mother's helper for a few hours every day or every couple of days.

Postpartum Doulas

✦ The first certified doula in Connecticut, Janet Hall has been a birth doula for nearly twenty years. She now runs Birth Partners, an agency that offers both birth and postpartum doula services.

Q: What's the difference between a postpartum doula and a baby nurse?

Janet Hall: A baby nurse's focus is on the baby. Since she's a nurse, she can do medical things, including administering medications and monitoring the baby's weight. A postpartum doula's focus is on the family—the mother especially—but really the whole family. The things we do vary from family to family: emotional support, watching for signs of postpartum depression, breastfeeding education, parenting education, helping with the bath, which is a really big deal—a lot of first-time parents are nervous about the bath—light housework, running errands, meal preparation, caring for other children. We do overnight care and daytime care. If you're breastfeeding and it's nighttime, we get up with the baby and bring him to you. If you're bottle feeding, we'll feed the baby. It's the whole gamut.

Q: What kind of parenting education do postpartum doulas provide?

JH: That part is about giving new parents the permission to parent their child in ways that they feel comfortable with—as long as it's safe. They might have their parents saying, "Don't pick up the baby! You'll spoil the baby!" And friends that say, "Oh no! Hold the baby all the time." It's nice to have that person there, the doula, who can just say, "What do you think? What is your gut telling you?" It's helping new parents to feel more comfortable in their new roles and helping them to feel good about the choices they make. Again, getting input from a professional and not a family member or a friend makes a really big difference. Everyone around you is telling you the right way to parent, and a doula isn't.

Q: How are postpartum doulas trained?

JH: Postpartum certification has just recently become available through DONA (Doulas of North America, *www.dona.org*). Before that, there really wasn't anything. The agency I run has been around for fourteen years, so over time we've gotten our own training together. It includes breastfeeding training, a parenting workshop, adult and infant CPR certification, and staying up-to-date on the latest books in postpartum care.

Q: What should someone look for when they're interviewing a postpartum doula?

JH: I think they have to trust their gut. Is this someone that you're comfortable having in your home? There are all those intangible qualities. Yes, a doula will be trained—but you can't teach everything there is to being a postpartum doula. If you're going through an agency, you want to make sure that the agency has been around awhile, and everyone should ask for references. But mostly ask yourself, "Does this person feel comfortable for our family?"

Q: Would you interview a postpartum doula before you give birth?

JH: Absolutely. You can meet in person or, if it's a referral from a friend, talk on the phone. But I think it's important to have as much as possible in place while you're still pregnant, and that includes a postpartum doula if you're planning to have one.

• *Build a network:* Once again, don't try to go it alone. Reach out to other women who have children, who've been where you are now and who can help you. They can be new acquaintances you meet in the park, or old friends who live across the country. Some women find that mothers' groups are enormously helpful; you might find a group to join through a community association, your caregiver, hospital or birthing center, on the bulletin board at a local market, or through a friend. The point is that a support network of other women can provide both a reality check and companionship at a time in life when it's easy to feel isolated and overextended.

REAL VOICES

I bought a headset for my phone about two weeks after my son was born. It was a lifesaver. I really needed to talk to my girlfriends, and with the headset, I could! I learned that hands-free isn't just for driving.

Beth, mom of one

When you're ready, join a mothers' group. If you feel particularly close to any mother or mothers, make playdates with them. When I was on maternity leave, I spent nearly every weekday with my mom friends, either at my place, their place, at a coffeehouse, or in the park. It broke up the monotony of each day, gave me support, helped me normalize my baby's behavior, and provided me with an outlet for adult conversation and thought.

Tina, mom of one

• *Breathe:* I don't typically recommend mind-body exercises to women during the postpartum period, because I know from personal experience that if you've got fifteen minutes of quiet to close your eyes, odds are you're going to fall asleep—and you should! But one thing you can do is simply breathe. If you find you're feeling overwhelmed, or if the baby is fussing and you're trying to get him to nurse, or if you think you won't be able to go five more minutes without sleep but the baby is wide awake and ready to go, take a step back and breathe deeply for a few seconds. Let the breath center and calm you. Physiologically, deep, slow breaths help your body slow down and relax, and even if you're at your wit's end, your breath is always there for you. When you're calm, you can help your baby be calm as well.

REAL VOICES

Being pregnant is just an exercise in how much you can surrender to get prepared for having a kid—you know?

Lisa, mom of one

• *Sleep:* Sleep is an enormous issue for new parents. Newborns typically don't sleep for more than two or three hours at a time, and they need to be fed throughout the day and night. The old advice to sleep when your baby sleeps can really help. If it's three o'clock in the afternoon, your baby's asleep, and you have a choice between folding the laundry and napping, choose napping. Try to develop a schedule with your partner that allows you both to get the rest you need.

When things have gotten really tough, many of the women I've worked with over the years have told me that one night away—at a friend's, a family member's, or even a hotel—during which they can get eight or ten hours of uninterrupted sleep, can be enormously helpful. Obviously, a night away isn't an option for everyone, especially if you're breastfeeding and not pumping. But if you feel like you've really "hit the wall" when it comes to sleep, a night away might be something to consider if it's an option for you. Alternatively, a weekend in a nice hotel with your partner and baby can also be really nice. After all, the hotel staff will make your bed and cook your food. (Watch for an off-season special at a local hotel.)

REAL VOICES

A friend told me that I should sleep when the baby's sleeping, even if that meant not showering or brushing my teeth. But on the days that I didn't shower, I just felt gross. It was much better for me to just put my daughter wide awake in the bouncy seat where I could see her from the shower and take the five minutes I needed to clean up and feel like myself again. *Then* I could sleep when she slept.

Johanna, mom of one

The First Six Weeks: The Baby Blues and Postpartum Depression

• *The baby blues:* The American College of Obstetricians and Gynecologists estimates that between 70 and 85 percent of women experience what's known as "the baby blues." A very mild form of depression that usually starts around three days after birth, "the baby blues" can last for around two weeks. In this phase, you might find yourself crying, and/or feeling anxious, upset, overextended, or irritable. Even if you're madly in love with your baby, you may find yourself wondering, "What have I done?" These feelings are absolutely normal. With new parenthood come new responsibilities, hormonal changes, breast engorgement, lack of sleep, changes in lifestyle, and changes in the dynamic with your partner, all of which can contribute to anxiety and uncertainty. There's no cure for the baby blues. Simply try to take care of yourself, sleep when you can, let others help you out, get outdoors (with or without the baby), and trust you'll soon feel better and adjust to life with baby.

• *Interventions for the baby blues:* If you feel like your mood isn't improving as much as you'd like, here are some basic interventions you can try. If you're *at all* concerned about your mood, or find you don't feel like yourself, please don't hesitate to talk to your care provider or a mental health professional.

– *Nutritional interventions:* Because protein provides amino acids, the building blocks for the brain chemicals that help stabilize mood, eating a high-protein diet when you're feeling low may help improve your mood. Try to consume about 100 grams of protein a day. (See page 229 for high-protein foods.) In addition to protein, supplement your daily diet with 2,000 mg of omega-3 essential fatty acids (at least 1,000 mg each of EPA and DHA). Both in preliminary studies and in my experience, omega-3 essential fatty acids help to stabilize mood in women suffering from both the baby blues and postpartum depression (PPD).

– *Sunlight:* It's helpful to spend time in the sun, particularly if you know you're susceptible to feeling down during the winter (seasonal affective disorder). If you know this is a problem for you and you're due in the winter, consider using a full-spectrum lamp for ten minutes a day.

– *Go outside:* Spend some time walking outside each day. Getting out of the house and breathing fresh air will help revive your spirits—no matter the weather.

• *Postpartum depression (PPD):* About 10 percent of new mothers develop postpartum depression at some point within the first year of giving birth.

— *Risk factors:* Factors that could influence the condition or increase your risk for it include a family or personal history of depression; if your pregnancy wasn't planned; if your spouse isn't supportive; and if you're experiencing chronic stress from financial problems, a move or job loss, or a divorce or separation. Your risk is also greater if you had a difficult pregnancy or if you have a history of abuse. Having a risk factor doesn't make PPD inevitable, but it might make it worth spending some time (before you give birth) thinking about your support network: Who can help you with your new baby? Whom can you call for help if you start to feel bad?

— *Symptoms:* Signs of PPD include feeling like you can't take care of the baby, you're not interested in the baby, or you want to hurt the baby. If you experience any of these, call your caregiver and find someone to help you care for the baby. Other symptoms of PPD are similar to symptoms of depression in general: insomnia, weepiness or persistent sadness, difficulty concentrating, irritability, panic attacks, and suicidal thoughts.

— *Treatment:* PPD needs to be treated by a mental health professional. Some women are helped by talk therapy, others by medication, still others by a combination of therapy and medication. What's important, though, is to let yourself be helped.

Note: Preliminary studies suggest that supplementing the diet with 2,000 mg of omega-3 essential fatty acids (1,000 each of EPA and DHA) daily can help stabilize mood in women suffering from both the baby blues and PPD.

The First Six Weeks: Nutrition and Medication, Exercise and Sex

Giving yourself time to rest and recover is the most important thing you can do for your body during the first six weeks postpartum. This is especially true if you're nursing, which is physically and emotionally demanding. While it may seem impossible to imagine, try to take things easy and nurture yourself in whatever way you can. By taking care of yourself, you really are taking care of your family.

Don't focus on socializing with friends or family members unless you want to. If people drop by unannounced, don't worry about being a good host. Ask people to call before they come over. If it's not a good time for you, ask them to come another time. And, needless to say, if your house isn't as neat as you'd like, don't worry about that, either. Soon enough, you'll develop a routine and rhythm for your daily life. Until then, don't push anything.

• *Nutrition:* Many women worry about losing weight after they give birth. During the first six weeks, though, a healthy diet is more important than a weight-loss diet. Continue to eat a balance of fruits, vegetables, whole grains, protein, calcium, and iron. Whether or not you're breastfeeding, your body is still recovering from the pregnancy and birth, and a nutritionally balanced diet will help you feel better faster.

Your care provider may recommend that you take a non-constipating iron supplement for the first six weeks postpartum, while your body recovers from the blood loss of birth.

If you're breastfeeding, it's especially important to eat a well-balanced diet, since you're still sharing all the calories you're consuming. Try to eat frequent small meals and a healthy mix of nutritious foods, including fruits, vegetables, whole grains, and proteins. (If you count calories, a breastfeeding woman should consume the same amount as she did before pregnancy to maintain her weight plus about 500 calories. For many, this means about 2,500 to 2,700 calories a day, which will support milk production and allow for moderate weight loss of half a pound per week.)

Continue to avoid fish that are high in methylmercury. (See page 231.) Other foods, such as sushi, raw milk products, and deli meats, are less risky now, but you should still take reasonable precautions to avoid food-borne illnesses. Precautions include cooking meat and poultry all the way through (see page 247 for guidelines), washing all cooking utensils thoroughly, washing all fruits and vegetables thoroughly, and only eating raw foods like sushi from a dependable source.

• *Weight loss:* If you're breastfeeding, a good bit of the pregnancy weight will come off fairly quickly. But this isn't a time to try to lose weight. Whether or not you're breastfeeding, your body won't recover as well or as quickly if you cut back drastically on your portions or calorie intake. If you ate a lot of sweets or treats during your pregnancy, you can start to cut back on those. But otherwise, there's no need to add the extra pressure of dieting to an already stressful period.

• *Medication—herbal and over-the-counter (OTC):* If you're breastfeeding, take the herbs and OTC medication that you would if you were pregnant. (See chapter 12.) The one exception is ibuprofen, which you can take when you're breastfeeding.

If you're not breastfeeding, there are no restrictions on which conventional or herbal medications you can take.

• *Exercise:* It's a good idea to start taking short, easy walks as soon as it feels comfortable for you. Most caregivers recommend waiting until the six-week postpartum checkup before starting more vigorous exercise, but that's a somewhat arbitrary time frame, based on the typical model of obstetric care. If you're no longer bleeding, if your stitches seem to have healed, and if you *want* to be more active, moderate exercise before the six-week postpartum visit shouldn't be a problem.

Listen to your body. Don't push yourself hard; start out slowly; and if you find you're tired or uncomfortable, take your activity level down a notch. There's no reason to rush the healing process; there will always be time for exercise.

• *Sex:* As with exercise, caregivers recommend waiting until the six-week postpartum checkup before having intercourse, to make sure you've healed properly. In my practice, some couples wait for the checkup and others don't. I believe that it's better to wait to be examined. But if *you* feel up to it—meaning you're no longer bleeding, any stitches seem to have healed, and sexual activity feels comfortable and enticing—it's not necessarily a problem to have sex before the six-week checkup. Remember to use birth control, even if you're nursing, because you could, theoretically, conceive again. The chances are slim, but they're not none. (See postpartum birth control, page 512.)

Q: My hair's falling out. A lot of it. Will it ever stop?

Dr. Evans: Yes. By the end of the first year postpartum any hair loss you're experiencing should stop. Hair loss happens for the same reason as hair growth during pregnancy—changing hormone levels. Usually, by three months postpartum, hair growth patterns return to normal.

The Six-week Postpartum Checkup

The six-week postpartum visit is a simple check-in with your caregiver. You'll be weighed, have your blood pressure taken, and you'll be asked about any problems going to the bathroom or with nursing (if you're breastfeeding). Your care provider will also try to get a sense of how you're doing emotionally and watch for warning signs of PPD. Finally, your care provider will examine your perineum, cervix, ovaries, and uterus, after which she'll probably give you the green light on both exercise and intercourse.

• *Postpartum birth control:* Your care provider will go over your birth control options with you. Most of them are similar to the options you had before your pregnancy: IUDs, diaphragms, condoms, and birth control pills. If you're nursing, even once a day, there's a progesterone-only birth control pill that's safe to use. If you're not nursing, then the progesterone-only pill isn't a good choice. It's less effective than the standard birth control pill, must be taken continuously and can be associated with more side effects.

If you're thinking of tracking your mucus/basal body temperature in order to avoid unprotected sex during the week of peak fertility (see page 40), keep in mind that it could take up to six months for your period to return to normal, and longer if you're nursing. While it's less likely for nursing mothers to conceive, it's certainly not unheard-of.

• *Postpartum sex:* Sex after pregnancy is different. Most women say that penetration is more painful and there's less natural lubrication. Breastfeeding can thin the vaginal tissue, further contributing to discomfort. These changes are usually temporary, though some women say there are subtle, more lasting changes in how sex feels physically and emotionally. The best advice for when you become sexually active again is to use plenty of lubricant, tell your partner what feels good and what doesn't, explore different positions and activities, and don't rush anything.

• *A postpartum body—the big picture:* After all the physiological changes of pregnancy—the increased blood volume, shifting of organs, etc.—within six weeks of giving birth, a woman's body will return almost to how it was before pregnancy. But pregnancy does bring some lasting changes, some we can see and others we can't.

 — *Breasts:* After pregnancy, and especially after breastfeeding, breasts mature; they no longer have the same internal support and elasticity that they had before pregnancy.
 — *Stretch marks:* Stretch marks can fade over time, and some can be treated with a laser but they rarely disappear entirely.
 — *Feet:* Some women find that their shoe size changes permanently; others find that their feet return to pre-pregnancy size after they lose the baby weight.
 — *The cervix:* Only an obstetric caregiver will notice this change. After a vaginal birth, the shape of the opening of the cervix (the external os) changes from circular to oval. Sometimes the caregiver can see tiny scars where the cervix has healed from the birth. These small, inconsequential tears will remain along the edges of the cervix permanently.

- *Vaginal tone:* Some women notice a dropped bladder/uterus and difficulty holding their urine when they cough or sneeze. This is totally normal in the first few months after pregnancy, and Kegel exercises done consistently will usually remedy it.

  Note: Every woman, whether she gave birth vaginally or by C-section, should do ten Kegels every time she goes to the bathroom during the first six weeks postpartum. After that, continue to do five sets of at least ten Kegels each day until you hit the three-month postpartum mark.

- *Rectal tone:* Because of pressure on pelvic nerves during childbirth, some women may lose the ability to control passing gas from their rectum or sometimes lose stool when they don't want to. If this happens, notify your care provider, who will check to see that there's no damage that would need a surgical repair. Usually surgery is unnecessary and the situation improves on its own over time as the nerves heal.

Note: Kimberli McEwen, MPH, reviewed the breastfeeding material. She has studied lactation for eight years and has worked with hundreds of breastfeeding mothers as a breastfeeding counselor. She provides breastfeeding education to both professionals and families.

Afterword: Personal Reflections

In writing this book I've realized my dream of sharing my approach to prenatal care with more women than I could reach in my practice. Over the years, it's become increasingly clear that my way of caring for prenatal patients is not at all common. What is unusual is that in addition to providing quality medical care, I work with my pregnant patients to find answers to questions they have that aren't in conventional obstetric texts and support them in trying out different treatments. For example, I have researched which herbs pregnant women can safely take; how they can change their diets before, during, and after pregnancy to achieve optimal health; if and when modalities like acupuncture, massage, and craniosacral therapy are safe and effective during pregnancy; and how women can best foster an emotional connection with their babies before birth.

When these questions first started coming up in my practice, I didn't have the answers. But in setting out to gather solid information for my patients, with safety as my number-one priority, I thoroughly investigated complementary and alternative (CAM) interventions before recommending them in my practice or in this book.

But my process of assessing CAM treatments didn't end with research; it continued in discussions with pregnant patients about what's most useful, helpful, and important to them. After all, a lack of scientific data proving efficacy isn't the same as scientific justification *not* to *try* a safe intervention to see if it works *for you.*

Working with my patients helped me develop an expanded and holistic philosophy of prenatal care. It's this combination of a holistic approach, CAM therapies, conventional medical care, and the nuances of my patients' real-life experiences that I originally set out to present in *The Whole Pregnancy Handbook*.

I wanted to motivate women to demand a new type of prenatal care—and I wanted to encourage all those who care for pregnant women (obstetricians, residents, medical students, midwives, nurses, and doulas) to bring a broader way of thinking to their prenatal care.

Why was this so important to me? From what I can see, the unfortunate fact is that prenatal care, and especially care in childbirth, all too often breaks down into "conventional" and "natural" camps, with little room for overlap or even constructive debate. As I've tried to show throughout this book, I believe there's a way to approach prenatal care that takes advantage of the best of the natural and conventional worlds and allows for a high level of mutual respect and communication between provider and patient.

Women should be able to choose from the full range of prenatal care and childbirth options without having to "choose sides." It is my sincere hope that *The Whole Pregnancy Handbook* will move both pregnant women and their caregivers to embrace a more comprehensive, open, and collaborative approach to prenatal care and childbirth.

Cultivating a holistic approach in my medical practice hasn't been a simple or straightforward process, but it has been enormously rewarding for me, and I hope for my patients as well. I believe a similar challenge faces all those who are involved with prenatal care—both parents and care providers. How is it that we can treat a developing baby holistically? How can we understand the whole life of a fetus in the womb? Can we build on what we know insures the basics of good health and incorporate a fetus's developing sensory experiences and emotional connection with the parents? If we can find a way to do so, I believe we as parents and caregivers can establish not only a strong bond with each other and our children, but also create a powerful source of physical, emotional, and spiritual wellness from which our children can grow.

I offer here both some of what I've learned from the latest research in prenatal psychology and my own thoughts about the spiritual and emotional worlds of pregnancy and birth. I hope this will spark your own thoughts about the life of a child in the womb, and about how you can deepen the already profound connection you share with your child and the world during this extraordinary moment in life. Research in prenatal psychology shows that:

- A baby begins active listening by the twenty-fourth week, and the sense of hearing is the most developed sense before birth.

- Starting in the second trimester, a baby gets excited at sudden noises and calms down when the mother talks quietly.
- A baby hears the mother's voice with little distortion, whereas other external voices are more muffled.
- After the sixth month, a baby moves in rhythm with the mother's speech. The fetal heart rate slows when the mother is speaking, suggesting not only that a baby hears his mother's voice, but finds it calming.
- A baby learns the sound patterns and frequencies of a language while still in the womb.
- Babies show a preference for stories, rhymes, and poems first heard in the womb.
- Newborns show a preference for a melody their mother sang during pregnancy over a new song heard after birth. Newborns are calmed by lullabies first heard in the womb.

In the future, I believe that further research in prenatal psychology will show how a baby "picks up" on many of the physical sensations from her environment and many of her parents' emotions. I believe it will become clear that there is a benefit from working with a provider who supports you and recognizes the importance of caring therapeutic encounters. I also believe that the loving care and intentions of parents during pregnancy and childbirth will spill over to foster a baby's emotional and physical development after birth.

As a prenatal care provider, I've thought long and hard about the emotional and spiritual aspects of pregnancy and birth. Here, I'd like to share my most personal and intimate thoughts on the spirituality of pregnancy. These words reflect *my beliefs,* not scientific fact. They inform how I've approached my work as a prenatal care provider, and it's my hope that they will encourage you to explore your own thoughts about the emotional and spiritual world of pregnancy.*

---

*I would like to thank Tullia Forlani Kidde, holistic psychotherapist, and Pat Rodegast, author of the Emmanuel books, for sharing their wisdom with me over the years as I developed my own understanding of the metaphysics of pregnancy. I also want to thank the Association for Pre- and Perinatal Psychology and Health, and acknowledge the work of Giselle Whitwell, RMT, and Fred J. Schwartz, MD, as resources that fostered my growing interest in the sensory development of the fetus. I encourage everyone interested in this topic to visit the Web site *www.birthpsychology.com.*

- There is no higher calling on earth than acting to create a new life with love.
- Throughout your pregnancy, try to allow all of your emotions to surface, whatever they may be.
- Treat yourself with compassion and great respect. There is great power and dignity in the journey through pregnancy and in the courage to accept the responsibility to offer to another soul the opportunity to live on earth with all the joys and sorrows that life brings.
- If you're pregnant for the first time, it's like embarking on a new journey with a road map that you see only at the end of the trip. Take comfort in the fact that so many women have completed this journey before and with you.
- During the months of pregnancy, you create a closeness and physical bond with your child that can never be duplicated.
- Pregnancy is a time of heightened awareness and creates an opportunity to nurture your intuition.
- Pregnancy and parenting create the opportunity to care, love, and cherish; to teach as well as to learn; to guide as well as to respect; and to simultaneously expand your understanding of the physical, emotional, spiritual, and intellectual needs of yourself and another human being who has chosen to join you on this earth.
- You and your partner truly are the co-creators of new life, a "becoming," which is an event that science can't fully understand. Science understands the language of hormones, chromosomes, cells, and blood supply, but science can't give breath, life, love, or spirit. You are the channel that makes life possible.
- You connect with your baby through your thoughts, touch, words, and songs. Try to keep this connection alive in whatever way comes naturally to you—whether it is putting your hands on your belly or thinking about, or actually talking and singing to, your baby. Through your voice, thoughts, and emotions your baby can connect with you and your love.
- Birth is an event of joy and continuity; it's life and breath. It's joining with everything in nature, from humans to animals to plants, that is part of the process of creation.
- Birth is a spiritual adventure with a physical outcome. In giving birth to a child, you're also giving birth to yourself.

By acknowledging your fears and honoring the spirit that connects you, your baby, and all of nature, you can help your baby come into this world feeling loved and safe. If you spend time thinking about and loving your baby with a quiet mind and an open heart, you will deepen your already powerful spiritual connection, which will lead to healthier, happier, more peaceful moms, babies, and families. I believe, deep in my soul, that this is the important next step in helping us achieve what we so desperately need: a world that honors and respects what unites, rather than divides, us all.

Namaste,
Joel M. Evans, MD
Stamford, Connecticut

Resources

BOOKS

Holistic and Functional Medicine

Clinical Nutrition: A Functional Approach, 2nd edition, the Institute for Functional Medicine, Healthcomm International, Inc., 2004. (Note: This book is written for health professionals.)

Encyclopedia of Natural Medicine, revised 2nd edition, by Michael Murray and Joseph Pizzorno, Prima Lifestyles, 1998.

Imagery in Healing: Shamanism and Modern Medicine, by Jeanne Achterberg, Shambhala, 2002.

Manifesto for a New Medicine: Your Guide to Healing Partnerships and the Wise Use of Alternative Therapies, by James S. Gordon, Perseus Books, 1996.

Mind-Body Unity: A New Vision for Mind-Body Science and Medicine, by Henry Dreher, Johns Hopkins University Press, 2004.

Power Healing: Use the New Integrated Medicine to Cure Yourself, by Leo Galland, Random House, 1998.

Total Renewal: 7 Steps to Resilience, Vitality and Long-Term Health, by Frank Lipton, MD, Jeremy P. Tarcher, 2003.

General

Risk: A Practical Guide for Deciding What's Really Safe and What's Really Dangerous in the World Around You, by David Ropeik and George Gray, Mariner Books, 2002.

Environmental Issues in Pregnancy

Having Faith: An Ecologist's Journey to Motherhood, by Sandra Steingraber, Berkley, 2003.

Fertility and Pregnancy

Healing Fibroids: A Doctor's Guide to a Natural Cure, by Alan Warshowsky, Fireside, 2002.
Preventing Miscarriage: The Good News, revised edition, by Jonathan Scher, Perennial, 2005.
Taking Charge of Your Fertility: The Definitive Guide to Natural Birth Control, Pregnancy Achievement, and Reproductive Health, revised edition, by Toni Weschler, Perennial Currents, 2001.

Birth

The Birth Book: Everything You Need To Know To Have a Safe and Satisfying Birth Experience, by Martha Sears and William Sears, Little, Brown, 1994.
Birthing from Within: An Extra-ordinary Guide to Childbirth Preparation, by Pam England and Rob Horowitz, Partera Press, 1998.
The Birth Partner: Everything You Need To Know To Help a Woman Through Childbirth, by Penny Simkin, National Book Network, 1989.
Ina May's Guide to Childbirth, by Ina May Gaskin, Bantam, 2003.
When Survivors Give Birth: Understanding and Healing the Effects of Early Sexual Abuse on Childbearing Women, by Penny Simkin and Phyllis Klaus, Classic Day Publishing, 1998.

Breastfeeding

The Womanly Art of Breastfeeding, La Leche League International, Plume, 2004.
That's What They're There For: Breastfeeding Basics, by Janet Tamaro, Adams Media Corporation, 1998.

OMEGA-3 ESSENTIAL FATTY ACIDS

Carlson Nutritional Supplements: *www.carlsonlabs.com*
Metagenics: *www.metagenics.com*
Nordic Naturals: *www.nordicnaturals.com*
Vital Nutrients: *www.vitalnutrients.net*

HERBS AND TINCTURES

Note: If you notice any adverse side effects after taking any botanical medication or herbal tea, stop taking the blend immediately. Botanical medicine is best taken under the supervision of a trained herbalist.

Avena Botanicals (teas, tinctures, etc.). Phone: (866) 282-8362. Web site: *www.avenaherbs.com.*

The Center for Women's Health (herbal fertility and labor tonics). Phone: (203) 656-6635. Web site: *www.centerforwomenshealth.com.*

Eclectic Institute, Inc. (tinctures, capsules, supplements). Phone: (800) 332-4372. Web site: *www.eclecticherb.com.*

Herbalist & Alchemist (mostly tinctures, also salves, ointments, some Chinese teas and bulk herbs). Phone: (800) 611-8235. Web site: *www.herbalist-alchemist.com.*

HerbPharm (mostly tinctures). Phone: (800) 348-4372. Web site: *www.herb-pharm.com.*

Pacific Botanicals (bulk herbs for teas). Phone: (541) 479-7777. Web site: *www.pacificbotanicals.com.*

Rainbow Light (herb and vitamin supplements). Phone: (800) 635-1233. Web site: *www.rainbowlight.com.*

Turtle Moon Health (herbal tea blends, including pregnancy tea, lactation tea, lactation/colic tea, and postpartum uplift). Phone: contact Kimberly Dubois, (203) 629-1166. Web site: *www.turtlemoonhealth.com.*

MUSIC

For Relaxation and Meditation*

Music progresses by steps, rhythm is smooth and flowing, dynamics are soft to moderate, texture is simple, emotional content is minimal.

Alpha Relaxation System, Jeffrey D. Thompson, Relaxation, 1999.
Angel Love, Aeoliah, Oreade Music, 1992.

---

*Thanks to Lora Matz at the Center for Mind-Body Medicine for her help with music recommendations.

Eagle Canyon, William Gutierrez, original release, 1995.

Earth Spirit, R. Carlos Nakai, Canyon Records, 1987.

The Heard of Reiki, Merlin's Magic, Inner Worlds Records, 2000.

In the Key of Healing, Steven Halpern, Relaxation, 1996.

Motets, J. S. Bach (multiple recordings).

Oriental Sunrise: New Music for Zen Meditation, Riley Lee, Narada, 1996.

Quiet Heart/Spirit Wind, Richard Warner, Narada. 1996.

Silk Road (1), Kitaro, New World Music, 2002.

Ritual

For more focused meditations and visualization exercises.

Center her Mind-Body Medicine, Training for Health Professionals 5225 Connecticut Avenue, NW, Washington, DC, 20015. (202) 966-7338. *www.cmbm.org*

El Hadra, Klaus Wiese, Aquarius International, 1996.

Hymns from the Vedas and Upanishads, Vedic Chants, Jetendra Abisheki, Delos Records, 1996.

Institute for Functional Medicine, 4411 Point Fosdick Drive, NW, P.O. Box 1697, Gig Harbor, Washington, 98335. (800) 228-0622. *www.functionalmedicine.org*

A Portrait of Anonymous Four, Anonymous Four, Harmonia Mundi, 1997.

Sacred Sounds, Jorge Alfano, Relaxation, 1996.

Singing Bowls, Xumantra, Xonic Records, 1999.

A Glossary of CAM (Complementary and Alternative Medicine) Terms*

- *Acupressure:* Acupressure is an element of traditional Chinese medicine (TCM), but instead of using needles as in acupuncture, it involves applying firm pressure (primarily with fingers but sometimes with thumbs, palms, and elbows) to specific acupuncture points in order to release built-up energy and restore balance to the body.

- *Acupuncture:* A mode of treatment in traditional Chinese medicine (TCM) that's over five thousand years old, acupuncture is based on the principle that good health is the result of a proper balance in the body's energy, or qi (pronounced *chee*), and that illness and injuries can be treated by correcting imbalances and restoring the flow of qi. This is accomplished by placing very thin needles in specific points on the body's fourteen energy pathways, or meridians. Acupuncture is now one of the most accepted and widely used modalities of complementary medicine in the U.S.

- *Aromatherapy:* Fragrant, natural essential oils are extracted from plants, leaves, bark, roots, seeds, resins, and flowers and inhaled or absorbed into the skin (often in a massage) to take advantage of their meditative, restorative, and medicinal properties.

- *Ayurvedic medicine:* Ayurveda is a comprehensive medical system that developed in ancient India. It's built on the basic premise that by creating a healthy, balanced lifestyle, you can prevent illness, promote immunity, treat physical and mental illnesses, and support spiritual growth. Yoga practice is an element of ayurvedic philosophy and medicine.

- *Chiropractic:* Chiropractic doctors manipulate the spine and sometimes other joints in

---

*Note: Complementary and alternative medicine (CAM) is comprised of a huge range of modalities and practices. Those I've included here are used throughout the book or related to modalities described within the book.

order to allow nerve impulses to move freely, which encourages the body's natural ability to heal. The practice is best known for helping relieve skeletal and joint pain, particularly back and neck pain, as well as headaches. Many chiropractors combine classic chiropractic manipulation with other healing modalities.

• *Craniosacral therapy (CST):* The craniosacral system is comprised of the bones of the skull, the brain, the spinal column, the sacrum, the cerebrospinal fluid (the fluid that bathes the brain and spinal cord), and the protective membranes that surround the brain and spinal cord. The cerebrospinal fluid (CSF) moves in a distinct rhythmic pattern through the craniosacral system. The proper flow of CSF is an important component of health and wellness. CST involves applying gentle pressure (of about the weight of a nickel) to different points on the body and the craniosacral system in order to restore the balance and rhythm of the craniosacral system and improve overall health.

• *Dietary supplements:* Dietary supplements like vitamins, minerals, omega-3 essential fatty acids, etc., are taken to provide nutrients that may not be consumed in large enough quantities through food to be beneficial in maintaining overall health and preventing disease. According to Congress, in the Dietary Supplement Health and Education Act of 1994, a dietary supplement contains one or more ingredients such as vitamins, minerals, botanicals, amino acids, and other substances or their constituents; is intended to be taken by mouth as a pill, capsule, tablet, or liquid; and is labeled on the front panel as being a dietary supplement. Dietary supplements are regulated by the FDA, but not the way food and drugs are; the FDA doesn't regulate supplements for safety. However, it has established manufacturing guidelines. The National Nutritional Foods Association (NNFA) issues certificates of good manufacturing practices (GMP) based on FDA guidelines. Look for supplements that have GMP certification.

• *Herbal medicine (aka botanical or phytomedicine):* Herbal medicines are made from botanicals, which are plants or parts of plants that are used for their medicinal or therapeutic properties. There are different schools of herbal medicine around the world, including ayurveda, traditional Chinese medicine (TCM), and Western herbal medicine. Western herbal medicine doesn't have an overriding philosophy of health or disease, unlike ayurveda or TCM. In the United States, herbs aren't regulated by the Food and Drug Administration (FDA), but supplements are. (See "Dietary Supplements.") Herbs, which typically act gently and slowly on the body, can be taken in several forms. These include:

— *Tea (aka infusion):* Made by adding boiling water to fresh or dried botanicals and steeping them—drink either hot or cold.

— *Decoction:* Roots, bark, and berries that are simmered in boiling water for longer periods than a tea or infusion. A decoction can be drunk hot or cold.

— *Tincture:* A botanical is soaked in a solution of alcohol and water to concentrate and preserve it. Tinctures are made in different strengths.

— *Extract:* Made by soaking the botanical in a liquid to remove specific types of chemicals. The liquid is either used as is or evaporated to make a dry extract for use in capsules or tablets.

• *Homeopathy:* Homeopathy mixes plants, herbs, animal products, minerals, and chemicals to create remedies that in larger amounts would stimulate a mimicking of the symptoms of a disease, and in very small amounts will tap into the body's ability to cure itself of the disease or condition. (The very small dose of active agent in a homeopathic cure is one of homeopathy's claims to safety, particularly for pregnant and breastfeeding women.) This approach is known as the "principle of similars" or the belief that "like cures like." In classic homeopathy, homeopaths tailor remedies to an individual and her symptoms, but general homeopathic remedies are available in health food stores and natural markets.

• *Hypnotherapy:* In hypnotherapy, a person turns her attention inward to establish a deeply relaxed state in which she is both concentrating and responsive to suggestion. In a hypnotized state, blood pressure drops, heart rate slows, and certain brain waves (alpha and theta) are more active. Hypnotherapy is often used to help with psychological issues and physical ailments, to lower anxiety levels, to reduce the need for medication (for example if you're managing a chronic illness), and to make medical procedures more comfortable. It's also used to reduce discomfort during labor. Not everyone can be hypnotized.

• *Imagery and visualization:* Imagery involves utilizing thoughts and/or sensory experiences—including sight, smell, taste, and sound—to affect the physical body. Visualization is a variant of imagery that focuses more on sight, but the distinction between the two isn't important. Both are used extensively in mind-body medicine, for example in autogenics and progressive muscle relaxation (see page 399). Also, meditation techniques that involve sound (like a mantra) or an object (like a candle) can be said to use imagery.

Imagery and visualization are used to prepare for medical procedures by relieving anxiety or fears associated with a procedure. They're also used to help clinicians and patients alike work with physical symptoms of disease and to help identify major emotions associated with specific events (such as birth, see page 389).

• *Massage:* In therapeutic massage, the body's soft tissue (skin, muscle, body fat) is systematically touched and manipulated to release tension, relieve pain, and improve circulation and overall health. The best-known massage movements involve stroking and gliding (effleurage), kneading (petrissage), and percussion (tapotement). There are many different schools of massage and techniques that are widely used and available.

• *Mind-body medicine:* Mind-body medicine is an approach to medical care that recognizes the basic connection between the mind, body, and spirit. It embraces the idea that a person's attitudes, beliefs, personality, and outlook can play major roles in her physical experience of health and illness, in maintaining a sense of well-being, and in limiting the effects of stress. Techniques such as meditation, breathing exercises, movement, imagery and visualization, and psychotherapy are all part of mind-body medicine.

• *Naturopathic medicine:* Emphasizing prevention and the body's ability to heal itself, naturopathy utilizes a variety of complementary and alternative modalities, including acupuncture/TCM, exercise, massage, physical manipulation techniques, herbal medicine, nutritional medicine, ayurveda, and psychotherapy, to prevent and treat illness and promote the body's natural ability to heal itself. Naturopathic doctors (NDs) may function as primary care physicians and, in some states, can write prescriptions. NDs encourage patients to be active participants in their own care and to make lifestyle changes that promote good health.

• *Osteopathic medicine:* Osteopathy combines conventional medical diagnosis and treatment with an emphasis on musculoskeletal health and its relationship to the whole body. Doctors of osteopathy (DOs) have the same range of practice as conventional MDs, including prescribing, diagnosing, performing surgery, and providing emergency medical treatment. In addition, they incorporate manipulations of the spine and joints, postural alignment, and physical therapy into their treatments.

• *Qi gong:* Pronounced "chee gong," qi gong is a modality of traditional Chinese medicine that uses breathing exercises, physical movement, and meditation to develop an awareness of qi (the body's vital energy) and its flow through the body. There are two basic types of qi gong, internal and external. In external qi gong, a qi gong master uses his awareness to heal others. Internal qi gong is much more widely used in the U.S. and consists of a person using qi gong techniques and exercises *himself* to tap into and balance his qi.

• *Reflexology:* A form of acupressure, reflexology manipulates pressure points in the feet, hands, and sometimes outer ears to stimulate certain organs and glands, relieve pain and stress, and promote an optimal flow of energy throughout the body.

• *Reiki:* Reiki uses very light touch on specific points of the body to channel "universal healing energy" to the recipient, who's fully clothed during the treatment. With training, Reiki can also be done on one's own body.

• *Shiatsu:* A Japanese form of acupressure, in shiatsu a practitioner will use thumbs, fingers, and palms to apply pressure to specific points along pathways (meridians) on the body, to improve the flow of energy (qi), relieve pain, and heal injury.

• *Traditional Chinese medicine (TCM):* Traditional Chinese medicine is a comprehensive system of health and healing. It prevents and cures disease and injury by promoting a balanced lifestyle (including diet, exercise, and work) and encouraging and maintaining a steady flow of vital energy (qi) through the body's fourteen meridians, or energy channels. TCM utilizes a variety of modalities, including acupuncture, Chinese herbs, qi gong, tui na (a Chinese form of physical manipulations similar to osteopathy), diet, and exercise. TCM practitioners choose a method of healing (e.g., acupuncture, herbs, qi gong, diet, or some combination thereof) based on physical signs like pulse, look of the tongue, tone of voice, and body temperature.

• *Yoga:* Yoga is part of a six-limbed Indian philosophical system. It combines physical postures (*asanas*) with breathing exercises (*pranayamas*) and meditation (*dhyana*), to help an individual integrate her body, mind, and spirit. *Yoga* is derived from the Sanskrit word *yukti*, which can be translated as "union." The principles of yoga were written in the Yoga Sutras of Patanjali in the second century B.C.E. There are many different types of yoga practiced in the United States, including:

- *Astanga:* An intense, athletic practice, *astanga* yoga involves coordinating the breath with a predetermined series of postures (the series was established by Sri K. Pattabhi Jois). It's sometimes (incorrectly) called "power yoga."
- *Hatha: Hatha* can be taken as an umbrella term that describes the physical dimension of yoga (i.e., the postures and breathing exercises). The word breaks down into *ha* ("sun") and *tha* ("moon"), which reflects the goal of harmonizing opposites when practicing yoga postures.
- *Iyengar:* Developed by B. K. S. Iyengar, *Iyengar* yoga emphasizes precision and alignment in each posture. The sequence of postures is also extremely important; postures should build one on the next to achieve the most beneficial effect on the body. Props such as blocks, straps, and blankets are used to help a student find and experience proper alignment in every pose.
- *Vinyasa: Vinyasa* yoga refers to a "flowing" style of yoga. Practitioners move from one pose to the next using the breath as a guide. Unlike *astanga* yoga, sequences in vinyasa yoga are not predetermined before a class or practice.

Prenatal Yoga—
Additional Sequences

In this appendix you'll find*:

- General Information: Yoga Poses for Pregnancy
- First Trimester
- Second and Third Trimesters

GENERAL INFORMATION: *YOGA POSES FOR PREGNANCY*

The following poses are especially beneficial during pregnancy. You can use them in the sequences here or in chapter 14, or create your own sequences. Some brief descriptions are given here. Where noted, complete instructions and illustrations are in chapter 14. If you're not sure of a pose and there isn't a description, or if a pose is entirely new to you, don't do it on your own the first time; instead, do it in a class where a certified prenatal yoga instructor can help you. Please review general instructions and restrictions in chapter 14 before practicing yoga on your own.

- *Seated poses:* These poses open up the pelvis and improve circulation. They can be practiced throughout pregnancy as long as you don't experience any complications.

---

*Joan White, certified advanced Iyengar yoga teacher, contributed all the prenatal yoga material here and in chapter 14 in collaboration with Geeta Iyengar. Joan would like to thank Geeta for her help with this, and B. K. S. Iyengar for his pioneering work in the field.

- *Parvatasana:* Sit on shins (on bent legs) with arms overhead, fingers interlaced, and palms facing the ceiling.
- *Supta virasana (reclined hero's pose):* Sit with legs bent to either side of the buttocks and recline back over bolster or folded blankets. If your neck feels strained, use a small pillow. (See illustration and description on page 264.)
- *Upavista konasana (seated wide-angle pose):* Sit upright with legs wide apart in a V-shape—you should be able to hold onto both big toes with your fingers and extend your spine upward. If you can't, your legs are too wide. For a gentle twist, place a belt around right foot and turn, holding onto the belt. Switch sides. (See illustration and description on page 276.)
- *Baddha konasana (seated bound angle pose):* Sit upright with knees bent out to the sides and soles of feet together. If your knees stick up in the air and are uncomfortable, place rolled blankets, towels, pillows, or books under them for support. (See illustration and description on page 276.)

• *Supta sukhasana (aka Supta swastikasana) (reclined crossed leg pose):* Sit with your legs crossed, and lie back over a bolster or folded blankets. (See illustration and description on page 262.)
• *Supta baddha konasana (reclined bound angle pose):* Sit with knees bent out to the sides and soles pressed together, and lie back over a bolster or folded blankets. Knees may be supported on rolled blankets, towels, pillows, or books. Put a small pillow under your head if your neck is uncomfortable. (See illustration and description on page 263.)
• *Supta padangusthasana II:* Lie on your back with right leg straight and left leg out to the left side. Switch sides.
• *Shoulder poses:* These poses open the shoulders and chest. They can be practiced throughout pregnancy, and you can either stand or sit to do them.

- *Urdhva hastasana:* Stand up straight, raise your arms overhead, turn your palms to face forward.
- *Gomukhasana arms:* Take the right arm up over your head, bend at the elbow, and let your right hand drop behind your head. At the same time, take your left arm behind your back. Reach up to clasp hands. Switch sides. (See illustration and description on page 271.)
- *Paschima namaskarasana:* Stretch your arms out to the sides and turn them from the shoulders so your palms face the back wall. Bend your arms at the elbows and bring your palms together behind you into "prayer hands." If this isn't possible, hold onto either elbow with hands behind the back.

• *Standing poses:* These poses strengthen the spine and legs. If you feel tired or nauseous, don't do them. After the first trimester, do standing poses with your back against a wall and the back of a couch or a kitchen counter for extra support. Try to keep your spine extended in each pose.

- *Utthita trikonasana (triangle pose):* After 20 weeks or so, do against a wall.
- *Utthita parsvakonasana (extended side angle pose)*

– *Virabhadrasana II (warrior 2):* After 20 weeks or so, you can use a chair for support under your pelvis and bent leg if that's more comfortable.

– *Ardha chandrasana (half moon pose):* After the first trimester, do against a wall.

– *Parsvottanasana (standing forward bend):* Bend halfway down, place hands on blocks or a chair, and form a concave spine to open chest and extend spine itself.

– *Prasarita padottanasana (forward bend with wide legs):* Legs should be at least five feet apart, with hands on the floor or blocks and back extended in concave spine.

– *Utthita hasta padangusthasana II*

– *Adho mukha svanasana (downward dog pose):* Head and hands supported on block. (See illustration and description on pages 272–273.)

• *Inversions and simple back bends:* These poses open chest and relieve both fatigue and depression.

– *Cross bolsters (variation one of setu bandha sarvangasana):* Use two yoga bolsters or rolled-up blankets tied to form a bolster. Place one horizontally and the other vertically over the center of the first bolster. Lie down so that the pelvis is supported with shoulders on the ground. Legs can be supported on blocks or even the chair if you feel back pain. (See illustrations and description on pages 261–262.)

– *Supported setu bandha sarvangasana, second variation (supported bridge pose):* Lie over bolsters or blanket bolsters with shoulders resting on the floor. (See illustration and description on page 268.)

– *Sirsasana (headstand):* If you've practiced yoga and this pose for a year before becoming pregnant, continue for as long as you're comfortable.

– *Salamba sarvangasana (shoulderstand):* If you know the pose, continue for as long as you're comfortable doing it.

– *Ardha halasana (half plow pose):* In the first trimester, legs may be on the floor. After that, place legs on a chair. Continue for as long as you're comfortable in the pose.

– *Viparita karani (legs up the wall):* Place buttocks on folded blankets or bolster set close to wall. Place legs up the wall. Have someone help you into this pose so you don't strain your abdomen.

• *Forward bends:* These are usually done after inversions. Even in the first trimester, don't bend forward but work on extending the spine to form a concave back.

– *Janu sirsasana (head to knee pose):* (See illustration and description on page 273.)

– *Paschimottanasana (seated forward bend):* (See illustration and description on page 274.)

• *Relaxation*

– *Savasana (corpse pose):* Lie on your back for as long as it's comfortable (usually until 20 to 24 weeks). After that, lie on your left side. (See illustration and description on page 293.)

FIRST TRIMESTER

An extended sequence for when you're feeling strong. This sequence is best for students with some yoga experience.

- *Cross bolsters* (See illustration and description on pages 261–262.)
- *Utthita trikonasana (triangle pose)*
- *Virabhadrasana II (warrior II)*
- *Parsvakonasana (extended side angle)*
- *Parsvottanasana* (use blocks and keep spine concave)
- *Prasarita padottanasana* (use blocks)
- *Utthita hasta Padangustasana II supported*
- *Sirsasana (headstand):* For those practicing it, headstand should be done with feet resting on the wall and legs apart (you can ask someone to put a roll of paper towels between the tops of your thighs in order to maintain the proper width) or in bound angle pose. Stay up for as long as you're used to, or one to five minutes.
- *Salamba sarvangasana (shoulderstand)*
- *Halasana (plow pose)*
- *Janu sirsasana (head to knee pose):* Keep spine concave. (See illustration and description on page 273.)
- *Baddha konasana (bound angle pose):* (See illustration and description on page 276.)
- *Upavista konasana (Seated wide-angle pose, add gentle twist);* (See illustrations and description on 276.)
- *Supta virasana (reclined hero's pose):* (See illustration and description on page 264.)
- *Parvatasana in virasana (hero's pose with arms extended over head, hands clasped and inverted)*
- *Savasana (corpse pose):* (See illustrations and description on page 269.)

SECOND AND THIRD TRIMESTERS

An extended sequence for when you're feeling strong. This sequence is best for students with some yoga experience.

Advanced students: If you're comfortable in headstand, you can start this sequence with a half forward bend (*uttanasana*) done with hands on blocks, books, or the back of a chair and a concave spine. Move on to downward facing dog (*adho mukha svanasana*), and then a headstand (*sirsasana*). Headstand should be done with feet resting on the wall and legs apart (you can ask someone to put a roll of paper towels between the tops of your thighs in order to maintain the proper width) or in bound angle pose. Stay up for as long as you're used to, one to five minutes, then continue with the rest of the sequence, starting with *supta virasana*.

- *Cross bolster*
- *Supta virasana (reclined hero's pose):* (See illustrations and description on page 264.)
- *Supta baddha konasana (reclined bound angle pose):* (See illustrations and description on page 263.)
- *Utthita trikonasana (triangle pose):* Stand against a wall or counter. Use a block or book under your lower arm for support. Support should get higher as pregnancy progresses. (See illustrations and description on page 271.)
- *Parsvakonasana (extended side angle):* Use a block or book under lower hand for support.
- *Ardha uttanasana (half standing forward bend):* Legs apart and hands resting on the back of a chair or the kitchen counter.
- *Ardha chandrasana (half moon pose):* Stand against a wall or counter. Use a block or book under lower hand to create more space in hip.
- *Virabhadrasana III (warrior 3):* Place hands on back of chair and back foot resting on stool.
- *Adho mukha svanasana (downward dog):* Use blocks under head and hands. (See illustrations and description on page 272.)
- *Bharadvajasana (gentle seated twist):* Do not do this pose after 28 weeks. Sit on a chair with knees apart. Focus more on lifting trunk and extending spine than twisting. (See illustrations and description on page 275.)
- *Sarvangasana (shoulder stand):* Use a chair for support if you know how, *or Viparita karani (legs up the wall):* Ask for help getting into this pose. (See description on 278.)
- *Supta konasana (plow pose with legs apart):* Legs can be on one or two chairs.
- *Supta padangusthasana II:* With leg supported on wall.
- *Janu sirsasana (head to knee pose):* Sit on blankets for height; use a belt. (See illustrations and description on page 265.)
- *Upavistha konasana (seated wide-angle pose):* You can sit against a wall, using a small pillow for low back support. (See illustrations and description on page 276.)
- *Baddha konasana (bound angle pose):* You can do this seated against wall, using a small pillow for low back support. (See illustrations and description on page 276.)
- *Setu bandha (supported bridge pose):* Bend your knees and rest your legs on a chair if that's more comfortable. If your legs are straight, keep them apart. (See illustrations and description on page 268.)
- *Savasana (corpse pose):* (See illustration and description on page 269.)

For more information on how to do the poses, refer to these books:

Yoga: A Gem for Women, Geeta S. Iyengar, Allied Publishers, 1998.
Light on Yoga, B. K. S. Iyengar, Schocken, 1995.
Yoga and Pregnancy, Sophy Hoare, Unwin Paperbacks, London, 1985.
See also: *Light on Pranayama*, B. K. S. Iyengar, Crossroads, 1995.

APPENDIX 4

BMI Table and
Pregnancy Food Journal

Please see table on following page.

BODY MASS INDEX TABLE

Body Weight (pounds)

	Normal						Overweight					Obese										Extreme Obesity														
BMI → / **Height (in)** ↓	19	20	21	22	23	24	25	26	27	28	29	30	31	32	33	34	35	36	37	38	39	40	41	42	43	44	45	46	47	48	49	50	51	52	53	54
58	91	96	100	105	110	115	119	124	129	134	138	143	148	153	158	162	167	172	177	181	186	191	196	201	205	210	215	220	224	229	234	239	244	248	253	258
59	94	99	104	109	114	119	124	128	133	138	143	148	153	158	163	168	173	178	183	188	193	198	203	208	212	217	222	227	232	237	242	247	252	257	262	267
60	97	102	107	112	118	123	128	133	138	143	148	153	158	163	168	174	179	184	189	194	199	204	209	215	220	225	230	235	240	245	250	255	261	266	271	276
61	100	106	111	116	122	127	132	137	143	148	153	158	164	169	174	180	185	190	195	201	206	211	217	222	227	232	238	243	248	254	259	264	269	275	280	285
62	104	109	115	120	126	131	136	142	147	153	158	164	169	175	180	186	191	196	202	207	213	218	224	229	235	240	246	251	256	262	267	273	278	284	289	295
63	107	113	118	124	130	135	141	146	152	158	163	169	175	180	186	191	197	203	208	214	220	225	231	237	242	248	254	259	265	270	278	282	287	293	299	304
64	110	116	122	128	134	140	145	151	157	163	169	174	180	186	192	197	204	209	215	221	227	232	238	244	250	256	262	267	273	279	285	291	296	302	308	314
65	114	120	126	132	138	144	150	156	162	168	174	180	186	192	198	204	210	216	222	228	234	240	246	252	258	264	270	276	282	288	294	300	306	312	318	324
66	118	124	130	136	142	148	155	161	167	173	179	186	192	198	204	210	216	223	229	235	241	247	253	260	266	272	278	284	291	297	303	309	315	322	328	334
67	121	127	134	140	146	153	159	166	172	178	185	191	198	204	211	217	223	230	236	242	249	255	261	268	274	280	287	293	299	306	312	319	325	331	338	344
68	125	131	138	144	151	158	164	171	177	184	190	197	203	210	216	223	230	236	243	249	256	262	269	276	282	289	295	302	308	315	322	328	335	341	348	354
69	128	135	142	149	155	162	169	176	182	189	196	203	209	216	223	230	236	243	250	257	263	270	277	284	291	297	304	311	318	324	331	338	345	351	358	365
70	132	139	146	153	160	167	174	181	188	195	202	209	216	222	229	236	243	250	257	264	271	278	285	292	299	306	313	320	327	334	341	348	355	362	369	376
71	136	143	150	157	165	172	179	186	193	200	208	215	222	229	236	243	250	257	265	272	279	286	293	301	308	315	322	329	338	343	351	358	365	372	379	386
72	140	147	154	162	169	177	184	191	199	206	213	221	228	235	242	250	258	265	272	279	287	294	302	309	316	324	331	338	346	353	361	368	375	383	390	397
73	144	151	159	166	174	182	189	197	204	212	219	227	235	242	250	257	265	272	280	288	295	302	310	318	325	333	340	348	355	363	371	378	386	393	401	408
74	148	155	163	171	179	186	194	202	210	218	225	233	241	249	256	264	272	280	287	295	303	311	319	326	334	342	350	358	365	373	381	389	396	404	412	420
75	152	160	168	176	184	192	200	208	216	224	232	240	248	256	264	272	279	287	295	303	311	319	327	335	343	351	359	367	375	383	391	399	407	415	423	431
76	156	164	172	180	189	197	205	213	221	230	238	246	254	263	271	279	287	295	304	312	320	328	336	344	353	361	369	377	385	394	402	410	418	426	435	443

Source: Adapted from *Clinical Guidelines on the Identification, Evaluation, and Treatment of Overweight and Obesity in Adults: The Evidence Report.*

Food, Beverage, Physical Activity, and Symptom Journal for Pregnancy

Height _____   Weight _____

Read instructions first.

1. Record all foods and beverages ingested for six (6) consecutive days.
2. Record quantity of foods and beverages, physical activity, and any physical symptoms felt.

Describe Foods and Beverages	Quantity	Describe Physical Activity	How Long	Describe Symptoms	When Felt
DAY ONE					
		Afternoon (12:00 Noon to 5:00 P.M.)			
		Evening (5:00 P.M. to Bedtime)			

Describe Foods and Beverages	Quantity	Describe Physical Activity	How Long	Describe Symptoms	When Felt
DAY TWO					
Afternoon (12:00 Noon to 5:00 P.M.)					
Evening (5:00 P.M. to Bedtime)					

Describe Foods and Beverages	Quantity	Describe Physical Activity	How Long	Describe Symptoms	When Felt
DAY THREE					
Afternoon (12:00 Noon to 5:00 P.M.)					
Evening (5:00 P.M. to Bedtime)					

DAY FOUR

Describe Foods and Beverages	Quantity	Describe Physical Activity	How Long	Describe Symptoms	When Felt
Afternoon (12:00 Noon to 5:00 P.M.)					
Evening (5:00 P.M. to Bedtime)					

Describe Foods and Beverages	Quantity	Describe Physical Activity	How Long	Describe Symptoms	When Felt
DAY FIVE					
		Afternoon (12:00 Noon to 5:00 P.M.)			
		Evening (5:00 P.M. to Bedtime)			

Describe Foods and Beverages	Quantity	Describe Physical Activity	How Long	Describe Symptoms	When Felt
DAY SIX					
		Afternoon (12:00 Noon to 5:00 P.M.)			
		Evening (5:00 P.M. to Bedtime)			

Acknowledgments

Many people have helped make *The Whole Pregnancy Handbook* a reality. The attention and insight that our editor, Erin Bush Moore, brought to this project helped us every step of the way. Thanks to the whole Gotham team for their energy and enthusiasm. This book would not have reached completion without the unflagging support and clear-eyed guidance of our agent, Janis Donnaud. Many thanks to the CAM practitioners, doulas, doctors, and midwives who gave of their expertise and time; their input has been invaluable. Finally, we can't thank enough the women who generously shared their time and experiences for the "Real Voices" of conception, pregnancy, childbirth, and life postpartum.

From Dr. Evans:

I would never have developed into the authentic holistic physician and author I dreamed I could be without the teaching, guidance, and support of many extraordinary people. It is with heartfelt gratitude that I acknowledge all those who have supported and encouraged me.

When I was an undergraduate, Pyser Edelsack of the City College of New York helped me understand, on a human level, the tremendous impact socioeconomic factors can have on health and wellness. I am indebted to Irwin Merkatz, MD, for both recognizing my potential when I was a medical student and teaching me the necessary skills to become a highly qualified and respected ob/gyn.

Thanks to Tullia Forlani Kidde, dear friend, colleague, and teacher, for being a source of unconditional love over the past eight years. Jim Gordon, MD, the founder and director of the Center for Mind-Body Medicine, enabled me to have the "aha" moment that helped me see it was time to bring mind-body-spirit medicine into my personal and professional life. In fact, Jim taught me most of the mind-body techniques I write about and utilize; he has served as a mentor, friend, role model, and brother to me since 1997. I want to thank Dr. Michael Culp for introducing me to the wonder of the world of functional medicine, and Dr.

Jeff Bland for both taking me under his wing to help me become an authority on nutrition, supplements, and women's health, and offering me his friendship. Speaking of friendship, special thanks go to Peter Poser for his continuous and heartfelt support. My dear friends Jeffery Perry, Mark Sandler, and Andy Kuritzkes always had words of encouragement and humor to successfully ground me in times of stress.

I am indebted to Robin Evans, my wife, who through her tireless devotion and commitment to our family, lovingly gave me the freedom to spend inordinate amounts of family time on this project. Her parents, Rose and Howard Gunty, have always been there to love and support me, as well as to cheerfully lend a helping hand at home. I thank my sister, Eve Evans, for her ever-present ear and wise words of support. I thank my children, Jarad and Spencer Evans, for being constant reminders of the joy that parenthood brings and the importance of this work.

I am grateful to my parents, Leo and Shirley Evans, for always giving me the message that I could do anything, which helped make me believe I really could write this book. But, in reality, I couldn't have written this book without the assistance of Robin Aronson, whose research and wordsmithing skills are second to none. It is no small coincidence that the birth of her twins coincided with the completion of the manuscript, and I am truly blessed that Robin magically came into my life.

Finally, Monique Class, my original office nurse, who has become a gifted nurse practitioner, first introduced me to holistic medicine by whispering suggestions of interventions to try with my patients. She deserves to be recognized for modeling holistic pregnancy care before I even knew what that meant. By listening to my patients and making them feel comfortable and safe, she has helped the Center for Women's Health evolve into the leading holistic integrative women's center it is today.

From Robin Aronson:

I first want to thank Joel Evans, who, with his humor and big spirit, went from being a colleague to being a friend. A special thank you to John Firestone for his generous and wise counsel. Dr. Jonathan Scher was a collaborator, teacher, supporter, and friend from long before this book was a twinkle in anyone's eye. Thanks to Mindy Brown for brainstorming with me at key moments. I'm extremely grateful to Ana Deboo, who was a perfect copy editor and friend when I needed her most. I'm extremely lucky to have a group of friends who are always ready to share their time, knowledge, and opinions. Special thanks to: Ami Aronson, Suzanne Biemiller, Melissa Clark, Natalie Dohrmann, Sarah Hill, Dorothy Novick Kenney, Nicole Marwell, Amy Ross, Elsie Stern, and Mary Recine Struthers.

As always, my parents, Myrna and Edward Aronson, have been unflagging cheerleaders. For this project, they've opened up an entirely new niche market for a pregnancy book: empty nesters in New England. David Stone, my husband, makes everything that much sweeter, and I can't thank him enough for his steady encouragement.

Finally, I must thank our kids. As of this writing, they're still known as Baby A and Baby B, and since they made their miraculous presence known, they've taught me something new every day about the joys, fears, and extraordinary blessings of pregnancy.

Index

About the Authors

JOEL M. EVANS, MD, is a board certified OB/GYN and the founder and director of the Center for Women's Health, an integrative holistic health center located in Darien, Connecticut. He is a member of the teaching faculty of both the Albert Einstein College of Medicine and the College of Physicians and Surgeons of Columbia University. As a member of the senior faculty at the acclaimed Center for Mind-Body Medicine in Washington, D.C., Dr. Evans teaches health professionals from around the world advanced skills in mind/body medicine and nutrition. He is a recognized leader in the holistic medicine movement, a founding diplomate of the American Board of Holistic Medicine, and lectures extensively across the country as well as internationally. In addition to the Center for Women's Health in Darien, Connecticut, he maintains an office in New York City. Dr. Evans lives in Stamford, Connecticut, with his wife, Robin, and their two sons. For information about Dr. Evans' clinical and consulting practice, or lecture and workshop schedule, log onto *www.wholepregnancy.com.*

ROBIN ARONSON is the former editor in chief of *Parents.com,* the Web site for *Parents* magazine. She lives with her family in Philadelphia, Pennsylvania.